Clinical Nursing Education:
CURRENT REFLECTIONS

Nell Ard, PhD, RN, CNE, ANEF
Theresa M. Valiga, EdD, RN, FAAN, ANEF
Editors

National League
for **Nursing**

National League for Nursing
61 Broadway
New York, NY 10006
212-363-5555 or 800-669-1656
www.nln.org

ISBN   978-1-934758-07-6

This is to acknowledge that the following are included in this book with the permission of the copyright owners:

OCNE Models and OCNE Exercise — *Oregon Consortium*

QSEN Exercise — *Leli Pedro, University of Colorado at Denver School of Nursing*

QSEN Tables — *Elsevier*

The Simulation Framework, Annotative Literature Review of Clinical Nursing Education, Final Report of the NLN Task Group on Clinical Nursing Education, Abbreviated Final Report of the NLN Think Tank on Transforming Clinical Nursing Education, and NLN Blue Ribbon Model of Clinical Education — *National League for Nursing*

Cover Design and Art Direction by Mara Jerman

Printed in the United States of America

Clinical Nursing Education:
CURRENT REFLECTIONS

CLINICAL NURSING EDUCATION

TABLE OF CONTENTS

LIST OF TABLES

LIST OF FIGURES AND BOXES

Many years ago, I opened my doctoral dissertation with a quote from Mary Dineen, who noted: "clinical laboratory experiences stand at the very heart of nursing education" (Dineen, 1959). That observation is integral to the historical development and rich traditions of nursing education, and it remains as true in the hearts and minds of nurse educators today as it was 50 years ago. But the 21st century has brought a new set of challenges and issues to what was already a complicated context for teaching and learning. The extraordinary expansion of knowledge used by nurses today has produced extensive changes in nursing practice, and underscored the critical role of the nurse in early detection of untoward responses. Such changes make clinical learning even more important than has been the case in the past. Yet, in the present environment, especially acute care patient settings, nursing students are often marginalized. Ironically, it seems that the high acuity level, in and of itself, presents restrictions on the ability of the learner to be a full participant in providing care. It seems that, while the technical requirements for safe and efficient nursing care have increased, our ability to provide students with ample opportunities to practice those very skills are being diluted.

Furthermore, we do not have a strong history of significant educational change. Despite consistent and tireless efforts, we seem to be constantly "tinkering with parts" of our clinical education processes, but generating limited significant change. In the early 1990s, there were many of us who made the leap to community-based education and tried to incorporate principles of health promotion and disease prevention into the traditional hospital "core." While sporadic but genuine success came from these measures, the force of history and a frame of reference generated from the apprenticeship model of old has maintained the notion of the new graduate who can "hit the ground running" as part of our mythology.

Embedded in this history and faced with these issues, how do nurse educators prepare professionals for a world of practice? The gurus of education would refer to the landmark studies from the Carnegie Foundation for the Advancement of Teaching, and reflect on the "habits of mind, habits of hand and habits of heart" that characterize education for the professions (Shulman, 2004, 2005). These "habits" are developed through the rigorous application of specific pedagogies, one of which is the pedagogy of practice.

Nursing has built its approach and strategies about education on a model of clinical education that differs markedly from that of other health professions and other practice professions. Most of those groups — pharmacists, physical therapists, physicians, lawyers, and so on — rely on the experts in practice to oversee the development of neophytes. Nursing, as the one exception, has required, and in fact legally mandates, in most state nurse practice acts, that the faculty of the school of nursing provide that direct instruction. I wonder what that says about us?

Given the centrality of this approach and the extent to which it appears to be valued in nursing education, one would expect that nurse educators would be consummate masters at teaching the art of clinical practice. Yet discussion, analysis, critiques and angst about clinical teaching, and clinical learning, abound.

Recognizing all of these issues, the National League for Nursing has taken the lead in creating groups and forums in which dialogue and discovery about clinical education can occur. One such group was the Task Group on Clinical Nursing Education, which worked diligently from 2006 to 2008 in collaboration with the editors of this book. Dr. Nell Ard served as Chair of the Task Group, while Dr. Terry Valiga (in her role as Chief Program Officer at the NLN) provided staff support to the group. This book has been created in direct response to the realization of the nurse educators involved in the Task Group that the nursing education community needs more resources to facilitate their work.

Ard and Valiga have endeavored within this work to pull together emerging ideas and innovative approaches to clinical education. This book challenges nurse educators to reconceptualize and DREAM about the possibilities as we prepare the next generations of nurses to practice their craft at the highest level. You will want to read it from cover to cover!

Eileen P. Zungolo, EdD, RN, CNE, FAAN, ANEF
Dean, Duquesne University School of Nursing
Pittsburgh, PA

References

Dineen, M. (1959). *The allocation of college credit for the clinical laboratory experience in the pre-service baccalaureate nursing program.* Unpublished doctoral dissertation, Columbia University, New York, NY.

Shulman, L. (2004). *The wisdom of practice: Essays on teaching, learning, and learning to teach.* San Francisco: Jossey-Bass.

Shulman, L. (2005). Pedagogies of uncertainty. *Liberal Education, Spring.* Retrieved from http://www.aacu.org/liberaleducation/le-sp05/le-sp05feature2.cfm

Nursing education has seen significant changes throughout its history. With the evolving and expanding roles for which nurses must be prepared and the current shortage of faculty, nurse educators are being challenged to rethink all components of nursing education and consider innovative ways to design and implement each. One of the most challenging areas in nursing education today — and one that requires significant reenvisioning — is that of providing effective clinical learning experiences for students throughout their programs of study.

Currently, faculty in all types of programs — from prelicensure to advanced practice — are challenged to find clinical learning experiences for students that are adequate in number, effectively involve clinicians in the experience, and provide the opportunities that will help students achieve learning goals. In response to these challenges, schools of nursing are exploring many options, including partnerships with clinical agencies to employ staff as clinical instructors, creation of dedicated education units (DEUs), increased use of high quality simulation in place of experiences in the actual clinical setting, immersion-like clinical experiences, and curriculum revisions that provide for more integrated thinking and learning.

These innovations are exciting, and faculty are encouraged to continue their exploration. But such exploration must be accompanied by a concern for maintaining high standards of education, attending to quality and safety in the provision of patient care, continuing accreditation and regulation standards, and making appropriate use of faculty and staff. This book provides readers with the opportunity to explore these and many more issues in clinical nursing education and, as such, offers a unique resource for educators.

While the literature provides educators with rich resources for the whole of nursing education (Billings & Halstead, 2009; Caputi & Englemann, 2005; DeYoung, 2009; Herrman, 2008) or the evaluation of learning in nursing education (Oermann, 2006), those that focus exclusively on clinical education in nursing (Emerson, 2007; O'Connor, 2006) are too few. Thus, there is a need for a scholarly book about the challenges and opportunities of clinical nursing education. Clinical Nursing Education: Current Reflections has been created as such a resource.

The need for a book such as this grew out of the editors' work with the National League for Nursing's (NLN) Task Group on Clinical Nursing Education, Blue Ribbon Panel on Research in Nursing Education, and Think Tank on Transforming Clinical Nursing Education. Each of these august groups, in which leaders in the field participated, pointed to the need to (a) reexamine the design and nature of clinical education in nursing; (b) systematically explore the impact of new models of clinical education on student learning, staff nurse recruitment and retention, faculty satisfaction, economic efficiency, and quality patient care; and (c) reflect seriously on the evidence base that underlies our teaching practices in clinical education. Indeed, there is much work to be done to ensure that graduates of today's (and tomorrow's) nursing programs are prepared to practice effectively in the complex, uncertain, ambiguous health care arena.

This book provides nurse educators and students enrolled in graduate-level teacher preparation programs with a variety of reflections on clinical education, simulation, performance evaluation, student experiences, and faculty responsibilities related to these critical aspects of a nurse's education. Through such reflections, the reader is provided with an extensive review of the current literature on clinical education and has the amazing opportunity to learn from today's leaders in nursing education, accreditation and regulation.

We are honored to have colleagues like Dr. Marsha Adams, Dr. Patricia Benner, Dr. Judith Halstead, Dr. Pamela Ironside, Dr. Pamela Jeffries, Dr. Gwen Sherwood, Dr. Nancy Spector, Dr. Elaine Tagliareni, Dr. Sharon Tanner and Dr. Eileen Zungolo, among so many others, contribute components of this book that will stimulate the reader's thinking and open their eyes and minds to new possibilities. Our hope is that this book will challenge graduate students, new faculty and seasoned faculty to reflect on the complexities of clinical education in nursing, propose strategies that can transform that component of nursing education to ensure its effectiveness, and pursue scholarly activities that will help the nursing education community develop evidence-based practices for clinical education.

As noted, our hope is that Clinical Nursing Education: Current Reflections will serve as a scholarly resource for what many believe to be the most crucial component of nursing education, namely clinical learning. We welcome you on this journey to explore how rethinking clinical education in nursing can serve to transform our educational programs in ways that best prepare nurse clinicians, scholars and leaders who can create a preferred future for our profession.

Nell Ard, PhD, RN, ANEF, CNE
Collin County Community College District
Director & Professor of Nursing

Theresa M. "Terry" Valiga, EdD, RN, ANEF, FAAN
Duke University School of Nursing
Director, Institute for Educational Excellence
& Clinical Professor

References

Billings, D., & Halstead, J. (2009). *Teaching in nursing: A guide for faculty* (3rd ed.). Philadelphia: Saunders.

Caputi, L., & Engelmann, L. (2005). *Teaching nursing: The art and science* (Volumes 1-4). Glen Ellyn, IL: College of DuPage.

DeYoung, S. (2009). *Teaching strategies for nurse educators* (2nd ed.). Upper Saddle River, NJ: Prentice Hall.

Emerson, R. J. (2007). *Nursing education in the clinical setting.* St. Louis, MO: Mosby.

Herrman, J. W. (2008). *Creative teaching strategies for the nurse educator.* Philadelphia: F.A. Davis.

O'Connor, A. B. (2006). *Clinical instruction and evaluation: A teaching resource* (2nd ed.). Sudbury, MA: Jones and Bartlett.

Oermann, M. H. (2006). *Evaluation and testing in nursing education* (2nd ed.). New York: Springer Publishing.

ACKNOWLEGMENTS

The editors wish to extend sincere thanks to all those who contributed chapters to this book. We were most fortunate to have so many of nursing education's leaders involved in this project, and acknowledge that the book is richer because of them. Their expertise, innovation, scholarliness, and collegiality are things for which we will always be grateful.

A very special thanks goes to all the members of the NLN's Task Group on Clinical Nursing Education. This group of talented nurse educators worked diligently and collaboratively to bring new perspectives to clinical education practices, share those perspectives with the nursing education community for validation of their merit, and keep important questions about the nature and meaning of clinical education "front and center" so they could be addressed thoughtfully. We all worked hard, but we also had fun. All those in the group learned from one another and with one another, and each of us learned something about ourselves throughout the process. We are enriched because of the work we did together, and we thank you.

Our thanks go to the National League for Nursing for its commitment to advancing excellence in nursing education and supporting the lifelong development of nurse educators. Through the work of task groups like the ones on which we served, the publication of books such as this, conferences, research grants, the Academy of Nursing Education, certification for nurse educators and many other initiatives, attention is given to heroes in our profession who often go unsung, namely, nurse faculty and nursing education scholars. We are grateful that the NLN maintains its focus on education, faculty development, and advancing the science of nursing education.

DEDICATIONS

This book is dedicated to the four players in clinical education. To the student whose purpose is to be actively involved in the process of learning how to be a nurse. To the faculty whose role is to formulate and guide the process. To the patient who allows students to learn from their illnesses, losses, and emotions. To the clinical staff who allow "extra" people on the unit and assist in educating the students by their words and examples. The future of nursing education and the nursing profession will be better because of these players.

This book is also dedicated to my family. To my parents, especially my late father, who always believed in me and encouraged me to aspire for higher goals. To my husband, Wayne, who has been my rock to lean on and my daily source of encouragement and support. God has truly blessed me and I'm grateful.

Nell Ard

This book is dedicated to all those in nursing education who work diligently to craft exquisite clinical learning experiences for students. Clinical education is complex and challenging, and it calls upon faculty, students, and clinical partners to give tirelessly of themselves. Yet clinical teachers and staff colleagues often go unrecognized for the significant roles they play in the formation of tomorrow's nurses. It is hoped that this book serves to publicly acknowledge the vital role of clinical teachers and clinical education in creating a preferred future for our profession, and to thank them for their contributions.

The book also is dedicated to all those patients, families, and community members who invite nursing students into their lives as a way to help them learn what it means to be a nurse and how to practice that role with compassion and intellect. Without them, there would be no such thing as clinical education.

Finally, I would like to dedicate this book to my parents who, though no longer alive, provided me with values that keep me in constant pursuit of excellence…my sister and fellow nurse, Diane, whose passion for humanistic patient care always keeps me grounded in the reality of the clinical practice world…and my husband, Bob, whose tireless support and encouragement continues to amaze me. I will be forever grateful.

Terry Valiga

Chapter 1

REVIEW OF LITERATURE

Kristen Rogers, MSN, RN, CNE
Sharon Vinten, MSN, RNC, WHNP, CNE

Traditionally, clinical education is an arena that fosters the learner's transformation from novice to beginning nurse. In 2006, the National League for Nursing (NLN) convened a task group to explore clinical nursing education. The group conducted an extensive review of the recent literature on clinical education in nursing as well as other disciplines and compiled an annotated bibliography of many of these rich resources (see Appendix B). Through this exploration, the task group identified five components of clinical education — the WHAT (i.e., what defines clinical education?), the WHY (i.e., what are the reasons clinical education is so integral to the preparation of a nurse?), the WHERE (i.e., in what kinds of settings can clinical learning take place?), the WHEN (i.e., when in their total educational program should nursing students be engaged in clinical practice activities?), and the WHO (i.e., who are the "players" that need to be involved if an experience is to be called "clinical"?). This chapter provides an overview of the literature related to each of these components.

WHAT Is Clinical Education?

According to the NLN Clinical Nursing Education Task Group, clinical nursing education is a holistic experience attending to the intellectual, physical, and passion components of learning what it means to be a nurse and developing one's identity as a nurse (Ard, Rogers, & Vinten, 2008). The concept of holism is a very important aspect of clinical education, as it allows one to focus on one aspect of the patient's care but appreciate how that aspect impacts the entire individual, or to focus on a larger community or system (Slater, 2005). Holism also attends to the mind-body-spirit connection in patients and nurses alike, and, as such, is critical in clinical education.

The barriers and strategies to integrating concepts of holism into undergraduate nursing education have been reviewed (King & Gates, 2006) as has the impact of having an undergraduate theory course in holistic nursing (Downy, 2007). Spiritual care and spirituality have also been seen as components of holism, yet few references (Hoffert, Henshaw, Mvududu, 2007; Meyer, 2003) were found that addressed it. Regardless of one's particular perspective on the concept of holism, few would argue that a significant aspect of clinical education is helping students learn about its meaning in patient care and for one's own practice. As noted, the concept of holism in clinical education refers to the integration of the intellectual, physical and passion of learning, each of which will be addressed.

Intellectual

Intellectual components of clinical nursing education are the cognitive skills of knowledge acquisition, critical thinking, decision making, priority setting and knowledge transfer (NLN Task Group on Clinical Nursing Education, 2006). These components are often tied to overall cognitive learning (Thompson, 2009), with critical thinking being the concept most frequently discussed in the literature.

The American Association of Colleges of Nursing (AACN) describes critical thinking as: "All or part of the process of questioning, analysis, synthesis, interpretation, inference, inductive and deductive reasoning, intuition, application, and creativity. Critical thinking underlies independent and interdependent decision making" (AACN, 2008, p. 36). Critical thinking is a program outcome for many schools of nursing and is a core competency identified in the *AACN Essentials of Baccalaureate Education for Professional Nursing Practice* (AACN, 2008).

During the 1980s and 1990s, much of the clinical education literature addressed intellectual skills necessary for decision making in nursing (Brooks & Thomas, 1997; Jenkins, 1985; Pardue, 1987; Shin, 1998; Tschikota, 1993). More recent literature specifically addresses the decision making skills using an intrinsic case study approach (Baxter & Rideout, 2006) as well as the process used by students and those with whom they collaborate to make decisions (Baxter & Boblin, 2008).

Critical thinking is also associated with skill acquisition and improvement. The literature addresses multiple strategies employed by faculty to teach/learn, stimulate, and evaluate thinking (Ard, 2009). Some examples in the literature include the use of critical thinking scales and reflective writing (Kennison, 2006), writing assignments (Niedringhaus, 2001), role playing and simulation (Comer, 2005b), and transformative approaches that facilitate acquisition of critical thinking (McAllister, Tower, & Walker, 2007). Several articles also exist that deal with the basic concept of decision making in the clinical setting (Botti & Reeve, 2002; Cholowski & Chan, 2004; Comer, 2005a; Conger & Mezza, 1996; Durak, Caliskan, Bor, & Van Der Vlueten, 2007; Fitzpatrick, 2006).

Physical

Clinical education should also include the active involvement of the learner, patient, faculty, and staff, which constitutes the "physical" aspect. In the spirit of innovation, adaptation of theory-based learning to the clinical setting can be accomplished either individually (Baumberger-Henry, 2005; Bowles, 2006; Lottes, 2008) or using a team-based approach (Clark, Nguyen, Bray, & Levine, 2008). Several articles discuss specific strategies such as gaming (Royse & Newton, 2007), MUDD mapping (Barrington & Campbell, 2008), concept maps (Hill, 2006), and using an online environment (Buckley, Beyna, Dudley-Brown, 2005) to assist the student in actively engaging in the overall learning process in the clinical setting.

In the clinical setting, active participation by students is a given. Although observational, experiences such as observing the legislative process or hospital ethics committee meetings can actively support student learning. In addition, a code blue situation, with minimal student participation or the student in an observational role, can offer valuable insight into clinical skills of cardiopulmonary rescuitation, medication administration, collaboration, critical thinking and a host of physical, cognitive and psychosocial skills.

The physical aspect of clinical education also incorporates the concept of psychomotor learning (Jeffries, Kost, & Sweitzer, 2009) and the acquisition of skills. The clinical environment is an optimal opportunity to transfer knowledge of skills previously acquired in the lab setting into the student's care of the patient (Bjork & Kirkevold, 1999; Clarke, Davies, & McNee, 2002; Davies & Clarke, 2004; Mayne et al., 2004).

Passion

The passion of clinical education is the final component of learning necessary in the clinical setting. This includes professional involvement, values, and the psychosocial aspects of caring for patients. Caring as a value is most frequently seen in nursing literature and is also an NLN core value (2009). There is a paucity of recent literature on the concept of caring (Beck, 1999, Beck, 2001; Charon, 2001; Lee-Hsieh, Kuo, & Tseng, 2005). This is also the aspect of clinical education where affective learning (Shultz, 2009) occurs.

WHY Do We Do Clinical Education?

Clinical learning experiences have been a component of nursing education programs from the beginning of our history. In the early years of nursing education, students went to homes and hospitals to care for patients, and they often were expected to provide service to the hospital as a requirement of their education. This service consisted of caring for patients and was the primary focus of the education program; theory/classroom learning was a secondary focus (Donahue, 1985).

Through the evolution of nursing education, clinical education continues to be an integral component. In 2005, the National Council of State Boards of Nursing (NCSBN) issued a position paper, *Clinical Instruction in Prelicensure Nursing Programs*, which states that experiences with actual patients were necessary in all prelicensure programs. NCSBN further stated that these experiences with actual patients needed to be of sufficient quality to allow students to meet outcomes (NCSBN, 2005). (See Chapter 12 — Clinical Education and Regulation).

Several books have discussed the "why" of clinical education. According to O'Connor (2006), clinical education provides students with an environment to apply the concepts learned in the classroom setting. Through application in this environment, students develop critical thinking and communication skills, refine technical skills, and implement therapeutic nursing interventions. Reilly and Oermann (1992) state that clinical education is a fertile environment for student learning that engages students through "hands-on" activities. Students are active participants in this environment and, as active participants, experience challenges that build confidence and foster growth into the role of nurse. According to Oermann and Gaberson (2006), clinical education fosters growth through exposing students to ambiguous environments that challenge them to think and implement action. Also in this environment, students observe the nurses and other professionals carrying out their roles, which facilitates the students' learning and socialization to the profession.

Evaluating the competence of the student in direct patient care is also one of the aspects of the "why" (Arcand & Neumann, 2005; Bradshaw, 1998; Bradshaw & Woodring, 1999; Casey, 2000; Urquhart & Comeau, 2002; Utley-Smith, 2004). Students learn a variety of concepts in the classroom and lab setting that must be effectively used in the clinical setting. Competence can be evaluated through a variety of methods, each of which presents some issues and challenges (see Chapter 6 — Evaluation of Clinical Performance).

WHERE Does Clinical Education Take Place?

The NLN Task Group on Clinical Nursing Education has indicated the locations of clinical education should be in settings where students can collaborate with the patient, clinical staff, faculty and other health professionals in the design and delivery of patient care. Placements also should be in settings where students are challenged to integrate the intellectual, physical and passion components of what it means to be a nurse (Ard et al., 2008). The learning outcomes/goals of the student should also assist in determining the environment in which clinical experiences occur (NLN Task Group on Clinical Nursing Education, 2006), and settings should be selected based upon the overall clinical objectives/outcomes and the site's ability to facilitate the achievement of them.

Technology Impact on Clinical Sites

Technological advances have been a catalyst for changes in the health care system. It is now a thread rather than an innovation and transcends theory and clinical. The Institute of Medicine (Greiner & Knebel, 2003) recommendation to integrate technology into health care has been followed by initiatives from other organizations. Both the Technology Informatics Guiding Educational Reform (TIGER) Initiative (2006) and the Alliance for Nursing Informatics (2009) encourage collaboration among nursing organizations. The NLN (2008) has published an informatics position paper with goals to prepare practitioners for electronic health records of 2014. The NLN Task Group on Informatics Competencies of the Educational Technology and Information Management Advisory Council (ETIMAC, 2007) survey of nursing faculty and administrators concluded that it remains unclear what composes nursing informatics and what knowledge base is required for nursing practice.

A framework supporting information literacy is evolving. Equipping future nurses with the information literacy skills and knowledge essential for practice through their educational programs is discussed by Barnard, Nash, and O'Brien (2005). Collaborative efforts between library systems and nursing can also educate students about information literacy and technologies (Innes, 2008).

Concepts associated with online learning are being utilized clinically. The instructional best practices developed by Chickering and Gamson (1987) provide a framework for development of online courses and have implications for clinical education. Nurse educators should consider learning styles, feelings of connection, and building a community of collaboration among participants when determining the use of online learning related to clinicals (Billings, Skiba, & Connors, 2005).

There are variety of examples of the use of technology in clinicals, such as Blackboard (Green et al., 2006; Raines, 2007), discussion boards where students reflect on clinical practice and share experiences, observations and insights with peers (Buckley, Beyna, and Dudley-Brown, 2005; Moran, 2005), WebQuest (Lahaie, 2007), and webcasting (Jeffries, 2005; Salyers, 2007). Frequently, students may be assigned some type of computer program as a component of clinicals. Bloomfield, While and Roberts (2008) reviewed computer assisted learning (CAL) research published between 1997 and 2006 and discussed its limitations. They concluded that there are published positive effects of CAL and encouraged more rigorous studies to develop an evidence base. Evaluation of the quality of courses continues to be an area where further research is needed (Billings & Connors, 2001).

Computer-based clinical conferencing has been shown to have several positive effects on students, such as a positive impact on student self-efficacy, support group connections, and increased self-confidence (Babenko-Mould, Andrusyszyn, & Goldenberg, 2004); increasing flexibility and promoting equal student participation (Cooper, Taft & Thelen, 2004); and support of clinical students' refinement of reasoning skills and receipt of timely feedback from faculty and peers (DeBourgh, 2001). A less traditional application of technology is the development and maintenance of an Internet database for student clinical placement in a capstone course (Stone & Rowles, 2007).

The most rapidly developing technology area is the use of simulation. Bitzer (1966) described laboratory simulation in nursing education. Simulations are being expanded to be very course and task specific. Use of simulation is seen in critical care (Henneman & Cunningham, 2005), obstetrics (Bantz, Dancer, Hodson-Carlton, & Van Hove, 2007), mock codes (Spunt, Foster & Adams, 2004), medication administration (Bearnson & Wiker, 2005), and cardiac surgery (Rauen, 2004). Particular populations can also be targeted, such as novice students (Bremner, Aduddell, Bennett & VanGeest, 2006).

Simulation provides faculty with the ability to facilitate learning without jeopardizing human life or safety, bridge theory and clinical, and stimulate critical thinking (Bremner et al., 2006; Jeffries, 2006). Simulation provides insight into student assessment and prioritization skills, critical thinking, team building and problem-solving ability. Well-developed, realistic simulations provide for active learning and an opportunity for debriefing and immediate feedback (Eaves & Flagg, 2001; Larew, Lessans, Spunt, Foster, & Covington, 2006; McCausland, Curran, & Cataldi, 2004; Medley & Horne, 2005; NLN, 2006). With limited clinical sites and skill availability, simulation has expanded the potential for clinical learning (Jarzemsky & McGrath, 2008) and provides an opportunity for remediation for marginal students (Haskvitz, & Koop, 2004). Standardized patients are less commonly used in undergraduate nursing education and more frequently seen in advanced practice nursing (Becker, Rose, Berg, Park, & Shatzer, 2006; Bosek, Li, & Hicks, 2007; Errichetti, Gimpel, & Boulet, 2002; Festa, Baliko, Mangiafico, & Jarosinski, 2000; Gibbons et al., 2002). (See Chapter 10 — Simulation: Integral to Clinical Education).

Academic and Service Partnerships in Clinical Education

The need for acute care clinical sites exceeds availability and challenges service and education (Palmer, Cox, Callister, Johnsen, & Matsumura, 2005; Rice, 2003). Academic-service partnerships are developing to improve this situation, with both groups benefiting from collaborative efforts (Becker, 2004; Campbell & Dudley, 2005; Campbell, Prater, Schwartz, & Ridenour, 2001; Henderson, Heel, & Twentyman, 2007; Hewlett & Eichelberger, 1999; Kirkpatrick, Byrne, Martin, & Roth, 1991; Murray, 2007; Porter & Baker, 2005; Stevens & Roper, 2004). Service organizations stand to gain employees at the conclusion of the educational process and benefit when there is time to understand and develop a relationship with the future nurse (Hill & Walker, 2004).

Partners in Action, a public health program for BSN students in Delaware, described a public health/academic partnership creating programs, outreach, and public policy activities benefiting underserved populations. Approximately 75 percent of those students became nurses in the community/public health field upon graduation, validating the benefit of the service connection while a student (Hall-Long, 2004).

Sowan, Moffatt, and Canales (2004) discuss a partnership between a university and health department for clinical experiences. Bartz and Dean-Barr (2003) describe a community-based/academic partnership providing a consumer-provider interdependent care setting. This setting met "the expectations of the baccalaureate nursing student population for lifelong learning, career building and sophisticated and effective delivery systems" (Bartz & Dean-Barr, p. 221).

Alternative Locations for Clinical Experiences

Alternative locations for clinical experiences are becoming more available and reported. Kirkham, Harwood, and Van Hofwegen (2005) studied the implications of using clinical sites other than the public health setting. International, rural, and correctional sites support transformative learning experiences with students' reports of increased awareness of social justice, knowledge of disparity, and economics. Schmidt (2007) discusses a camp nurse clinical elective course where students take ownership of their learning, and participate in syllabi and program development while actively engaged in camp life. Other nursing programs have used the concept of Service Learning to expand clinical experiences (Bentley & Ellison, 2005; Kemsley & Riegle, 2004; Ligeikis-Clayton & Denman, 2005). Additional alternative sites include elementary schools (Charron & Parns, 2004), working with those in poverty (DeLashmutt & Rankin, 2005), private practice (Doubt, Paterson, & O'Riordan, 2004), larger communities (Eide, Hahn, Bayne, Allen, & Swain, 2006), and the nursing home (McCallum, 2004).

Faculties and students have found value and positive outcomes in combining concepts and clinical experiences. Faculty have described using hospice as mental health clinicals with students emerging with improved communication skills and understanding of death and dying (Hayes, 2005). Lasater, Luce, Yolpin, Terwilliger and Wold (2007) combined community and mental health courses. They suggested that, as health trends continue and care becomes more community based, providing community-based experiences earlier and threaded through the curriculum may be beneficial for students and the health care of the community. Brancato (2006) modified clinical rotations to include evidence-based practice components of the overall clinical rotation versus direct patient care. Ehrenberg & Haggblom (2007) combined clinical learning with problem-based learning to assist students in bridging the gap between theory and practice.

Interdisciplinary Approaches to Clinical Education

Clinical education can occur in a silo or it can incorporate a variety of health care disciplines. There are several examples of interdisciplinary approaches in the literature. (See Chapter 11 — Interdisciplinary Clinical Education). Some examples of this type learning can be found in dedicated education units and in "partnerships" with other health-related disciplines. Moscato, Miller, Logsdon and Weinberg (2007) describe the Dedicated Education Unit (DEU) as a university and clinical partnership focusing on development and recognition of clinical instructors, communication, student critical thinking, and including a mix of students on the unit. Ranse and Grealish (2007) discuss student perception of learning in this type of unit. (See Chapter 4 —Innovative Approach to Clinical Education: Dedicated Education Units).

The literature also has examples of partnering nursing students with other health care providers to facilitate learning. Coyle-Rogers and Putman (2006) partnered nursing students with Certified Nursing Assistants (CNAs) to learn the basic aspects of the nursing role as well as orientation to the unit. Halse and Hage (2006) partnered novice nursing students with peers who were further in the program. This facilitated the growth of the novice nurses while assisting the peers to learn essential delegation skills.

WHEN Should Clinical Education Occur?

When clinical education occurs can vary dependent upon the program, location, size, and overall emphasis/outcomes. The NLN Task Group on Clinical Nursing Education survey identified three areas of consensus among faculty regarding the "when" of clinical education:

- Clinical education should occur throughout the nursing program;
- Students should have a "capstone" or "immersion" experience just before graduation that provides them with a synthesis opportunity; and
- Clinical education should begin shortly after entry into the nursing program as a way to assist students who may be uncertain about this career choice and engage those who definitely want to be nurses (Ard et al., 2008).

Having a clinical component throughout the nursing curriculum allows students to grow clinically as they gain additional knowledge in the theory setting. Students are able to apply the information they are learning as they learn it. Clinical also provides students with opportunities to gain additional confidence in their abilities in providing patient care.

The traditional capstone experience is a student-chosen, precepted clinical experience in a particular area or discipline, with supervision by a preceptor as well as faculty. Ideally, this experience is "characterized by intensive interaction among faculty, students, and/or community members and focuses on real-world problems from a multidisciplinary perspective" (Schroetter & Wendler, 2008, p. 77). The literature describes two types of capstone experiences that vary from the traditional. The first involves experiences in agencies that offer the student a stipend for working with the institution (Brockopp, Hardin-Pierce, & Welsh, 2006) and the second involves students who complete an evidence-based project for the clinical agency (Brancato, 2006).

Early introduction to the clinical environment is key to assisting students in determining whether the profession is a good "fit" for themselves. Many students in today's world are coming into the nursing profession because of job availability and may not realize what nurses actually do. Some students are not able to make the transition to providing care to patients as well as the stress of making decisions that could mean life or death. Early exposure to the clinical environment is vital.

Nursing associations call for innovation in nursing education (ANA, 2002; Ard et al., 2008; NLN, 2003). Several different clinical models have been seen in the literature that support an innovative approach to the "when" of clinical education. As a response, a clinical immersion residency model has been developed by the University of Delaware and addresses socialization, student accountability, and a refined transition to the practice of nursing. This undergraduate clinical education model exposes the student to simulation, field experiences, and a work requirement during the first three years and clinical immersion during the fourth year (Diefenbeck, Plowfield, & Herrman, 2006). Catholic University developed a Bridge to Practice model where students complete all med/surg experiences in a student-chosen setting. A university faculty, housed in the hospital setting, oversees students and serves as a clinical resource to hospital staff, who are preceptors (Paterson & Grandjean, 2008). The Oregon Consortium for Nursing Education (OCNE) has developed a clinical education curriculum utilizing planned clinical learning experiences scaffolded to the curriculum, the course outcomes and the level of the students (Gubrud-Howe & Schoessler, 2008). (See Chapter 3 — OCNE Clinical Education Model.)

The literature has several other "models" of clinical education that are not considered a traditional approach. Cox (2002) describes a model that has students in didactic for two weeks and then clinical for two weeks. This model enables two groups of students to utilize the same clinical units. Cooperative learning and education are also seen as examples in the literature as a clinical approach (Hoffart, Diani, Connors, & Moynihan, 2006; Ladyshewsky, 2000; Mallette, Loury, Engelke, & Andrews, 2005; Secomb, 2008). These demonstrate how multiple patients can be assigned the same student because each student has a different objective for the care. The concept of assigning mentors can also be used in clinical education (Aston & Molassiotis, 2002; Leyshon, 2005; Sowan et al., 2004). Tobar, Wall, and Parsh (2007) describe how 12-hour shifts improve student learning and allow additional students access to the clinical units. Finally, Memshick and Shepard (1996) describe a model used in physical therapy with two students to one instructor.

WHO Needs to Be Involved in Clinical Education?

The players involved in clinical education include the student, teacher, patient and clinical staff (Ard et al., 2008). The involvement of these players is addressed in the position statement on Innovation in Nursing Education, which calls for teachers, students, and clinical staff to collaborate in developing programs that support the delivery of health care to consumers in the current environment and future environment (NLN, 2003).

Student

The student is the primary player in clinical education. Reilly and Oermann (1992) state that students must be active participants in clinical education and need to accept responsibility for their role in the clinical environment. This role incorporates a sense of freedom to explore and challenge the knowledge gleaned from the classroom setting, to gather information, apply it to the situation, and evaluate possible solutions.

Oermann and Gaberson (2006) discuss the need for students to consider the clinical environment as a place for learning to learn. In this environment, students' active participation through observation and utilization of interpersonal and assessment skills allow them to handle challenging situations. In these challenging situations, students need to question care decisions and outcomes to foster their growth and change.

Tanner (2002) believes that students need to be immersed in clinical environments that stimulate them to learn. These types of environments will challenge students to be active participants in their learning, to learn to think like nurses, and to develop decision making skills. This can occur when nurses dialogue with students about their thinking in various patient care situations.

There are a variety of student attributes that need to be considered in developing effective learning environments (Ard, 2009). Nurse educators need to consider the students' learning priorities (Ballard & Trowbridge, 2004), autonomy and motivation (Chan & Wai-Tong, 2000), stress (Firth, 1986), and teacher characteristics (Ard, 2009; Kelly, 2006).

(See Chapter 7 — Student Perspectives on Clinical Learning.)

Teacher

The second player in clinical education is the teacher/educator. Porter-O'Grady (2001) describes the teacher role as a facilitator of learning who ensures that students have the tools for learning available and provides guidance to students in utilization of these tools. In this role, the teacher is less responsible for delivering content and more responsible for guiding students through self-directed learning situations.

Novotny and Griffin (2006) emphasized that the teacher is important in providing supervision during clinical experiences. The teacher's role is to assist students so they glean everything they can during clinical experiences. They also serve as role models for students. It is essential to student learning in the clinical setting that teachers create a comfortable environment that decreases anxiety for students and facilitates their learning. Also a comfortable environment allows teachers to observe students, facilitate their thinking and evaluate their growth.

O'Connor (2006) indicated that the teacher is key in moving the student from assuming a dependent role to an independent role. The teacher creates a relationship of trust with students. Through this trusting relationship, teachers mentor students' learning in various situations. In the beginning, the situations are driven by teachers. As students grow, teachers should decrease their control of the learning situation so the transition to a collegial relationship can occur.

Oermann and Gaberson (2006) state that teachers serve as guides to students on their path to beginning nurses. Teachers direct students to resources that facilitate their learning in the clinical environment. They provide support to students as they experience challenges in caring for patients. Through this support, they help students complete a self-assessment to determine gaps in their learning.

According to Emerson (2007), teachers have the responsibility to ensure that students have experiences that facilitate learning. These experiences can be supervised directly or indirectly by teachers, but the teacher assumes ultimate responsibility in providing situations that allow students to achieve outcomes. So when teachers delegate supervision of students in clinical situations to others, they must guarantee that these individuals have the skills necessary to guide student learning. (See Chapter 8 — Educator Perspectives on Transitioning Clinicians to the Academic Faculty Role With Emphasis on Clinical Teaching, and Chapter 9 — Demonstrating Expertise in Clinical Education: Essential Faculty Compentencies.)

Patient

An underlying purpose in clinical education is to care for the client/patient, who is the third player. In today's current education environment, controversy exists regarding the concept of the client/patient and who/what this may be. According to Reilly and Oermann (1992), it is essential that students provide care to real patients, because nursing is a practice discipline. In interacting with real patients, students utilize critical thinking plus affective and humanistic skills to individualize the care provided. With real patients, students learn to think on the spot, because the environment is unpredictable.

Curran, Elfrink, and Mays (2009) developed a computer-generated environment where students provide care to virtual patients within a community. In this environment, students are challenged to identify risk factors for health, environmental factors that impact health, and recognize clinical manifestations. The purpose of this virtual community is to assist students in developing critical thinking skills. In this program, students care for a patient with multiple traumas, and a patient with uncontrolled diabetes or a group of patients exposed to an environmental disaster.

Medley and Horne (2005) utilize high fidelity simulators as patients. These simulated clinical experiences promote critical thinking development by exposing students to complex situations that require independent thinking and interventions. In the simulated environment, students experience the consequences of their actions. After completion of the simulation, students explore their actions with peers and teachers in a debriefing session.

The effectiveness of using standardized patients in clinical experiences is also discussed in the literature (Becker et al., 2006; Yoo & Yoo, 2003). Standardized patients are people that have been trained to act like patients. These patients engage students in an interactive scenario within a safe, nonthreatening environment. (See Chapter 10 for additional information on the use of simulators and standardized patients in clinical education.)

Clinical Staff

According to the Clinical Education Task Group, the final player necessary in clinical education is the clinical staff. The staff could be serving in the capacity of preceptors or "buddy nurses" to students, with clinical faculty readily available. Minimally, staff nurses will serve as role models to the students on their units.

O'Connor (2006) defines clinical staff expectations when participating with students during clinical experiences. Clinical staff expect that the teacher will collaborate with them regarding the objectives for the clinical experience and students' skill/assessment abilities. They want the teacher to involve them in the selection of patient assignments, not necessarily in the final decision regarding patient assignments. In addition, staff believe that communication with students is essential in providing quality care to patients. Oermann and Gaberson (2006) state that health care professionals serve as valuable role models to students during clinical experiences. Through observing and collaborating with health care professionals, students learn about effective interactions. In addition, students learn how to handle patient issues/problems.

According to Freiburger (2001), clinical staff nurses play an essential role in students' growth during preceptor experiences. In these experiences, clinical staff nurses supervise students when caring for patients. Nurses have identified that this type of experience has a positive impact by providing students with an environment for skill refinement and development of self-confidence. Students have identified that these experiences improve their communication and organizational skills and confidence in decision making.

Blum (2009) describes a preceptor-guided nursing practice education model for clinical education. In this design, students and clinical staff develop a collaborative relationship, since students remain on the same unit for a year. Through this design, clinical staff develops ongoing relationships with students and are able to provide consistent guidance to them. This consistency in placement creates a less stressful environment for students, which enhances their learning and development of self-confidence. The literature has many additional articles dealing with the concept of preceptors in graduate education (Amelia, Brown, Resnick, & McArthur, 2001), preparation necessary for success (Baltimore, 2004), a literature review (Barn, 1996), preceptor job satisfaction and its effect on clinical performance of the student (Barrett & Myrick, 1998), the preceptor experience (Berry, 2005; Charleston & Happell, 2004; Charleston & Happell, 2005a, 2005b; Happell & Charleston, 2004; Lusk, Winne, & DeLeskey, 2007; Mamchur & Myrick, 2003; Matsumura, Callister, Palmer, Cox, & Larsen, 2004; Usher, Nolan, Reser, Owens, & Tellefson, 1999), and the recruitment and retention of preceptors (Ryan-Nicholls, 2004).

Conclusion

While a great deal has been written about clinical education, there is a paucity of research-based literature that can provide for evidence-based practices in this area. Rigorous research studies need to be conducted and their findings published so that educators can make decisions about the components of clinical education (i.e., the when, where, etc.) based on evidence, not merely tradition. Such evidence will help nursing education scholars design new models of clinical education that are transforming.

What will those new models and clinical education of the future look like? Perhaps the answers to questions such as the ones that follow will guide us as we create that preferred future.

- Is there a difference in a student's ability to transfer knowledge to the clinical setting when information is learned in the didactic versus laboratory versus simulation setting?

- What framework or guidelines will help faculty effectively use simulation as part of clinical education?

- What outcomes emerge when students do not all have the same clinical rotations?

- What would be gained or lost if clinical experiences in specific medical specialty areas (e.g., pediatrics, obstetrics, mental health, medical/surgical) were not required for all students?

- Would clinical learning be more effective if it were guided more by outcomes to be achieved than by hours to be "put in"?

- How beneficial is a preceptor experience in a capstone course?

- How does the role of the teacher change when clinical partners are more actively involved in designing clinical learning experiences and collaborating with students in providing patient care?

References

Amelia, E. J., Brown, L., Resnick, B., & McArthur, D. B. (2001). Partners in NP education: The 1999 AANP preceptor and faculty survey. *Journal of the American Academy of Nurse Practitioners, 13*(11), 517-523.

American Association of Colleges of Nursing. (2008). *Essentials of baccalaureate education for professional nursing practice.* Retrieved January 22, 2009, from http://www.aacn.nche.edu/Education/pdf/BaccEssentials08.pdf

American Nurses Association. (2002). Nursing's agenda for the future. Retrieved February 1, 2009, from https://www.ncsbn.org/Plan.pdf

Arcand, L. L., & Neuman, J. (2005). Nursing competency assessment across the continuum of care. *Journal of Continuing Education in Nursing, 36*(6), 247-254.

Ard, N. (2009). Essentials of learning. In C. Shultz (Ed.), *Building a science of nursing education: Foundation for evidence-based teaching and learning* (pp. 25-131). New York: National League for Nursing.

Ard N., Rogers K., & Vinten, S. (2008). [Headlines from the NLN]. Summary of the survey on clinical education in nursing. *Nursing Education Perspectives, 29*(4), 238-245.

Aston, L., & Molassiotis, A. (2002). Supervising and supporting student nurses in clinical placements: The peer support initiative. *Nurse Education Today, 23*(3), 202-210.

Babenko-Mould Y., Andrusyszyn, M. A., & Goldenberg, D. (2004). Effects of computer-based clinical conferencing on nursing students' self-efficacy. *Journal of Nursing Education, 43*(4), 149-155.

Ballard, P., & Trowbridge, C. (2004). Critical care experience for novice students: Reinforcing basic nursing skills. *Nurse Educator, 29*(3), 103-106.

Baltimore, J. (2004). The hospital clinical preceptor: Essential preparation for success. *Journal of Continuing Education in Nursing, 35*(3), 133-140.

Bantz, D., Dancer, M. M., Hodson-Carlton, K., & Van Hove, S. (2007). A daylong clinical laboratory: From gaming to high-fidelity simulators. *Nurse Educator, 32*, 274-277.

Barn, L. (1996). Preceptorship: A review of the literature. *Journal of Advanced Nursing, 24*, 104-107.

Barnard, A., Nash, R., & O'Brien, M. (2005). Information literacy: Developing lifelong skills through nursing education. *Journal of Nursing Education, 22*(11), 505-510.

Barrett, C., & Myrick, F. (1998). Job satisfaction in preceptorship and its effect on the clinical performance of the preceptee. *Journal of Advanced Nursing, 27*, 364-371.

Barrington, K., & Campbell, B. (2008). MUDD mapping: An interactive teaching-learning strategy. *Nurse Educator, 33*(4), 159-163.

Bartz, C., & Dean-Baar, S. (2003). Reshaping clinical nursing education: An academic-service partnership. *Journal of Professional Nursing, 19*, 216-223.

Baumberger-Henry, M. (2005). Cooperative learning and case study: Does the combination improve students' perception of problem-solving and decision making skills? *Nurse Education Today, 25*, 238-246.

Baxter P. E., & Boblin S. (2008). Decision making by baccalaureate nursing students in the clinical setting. *Journal of Nursing Education, 47*, 345-350.

Baxter P., & Rideout, E. (2006). Second-year baccalaureate nursing students' decision making in the clinical setting. *Journal of Nursing Education, 45*(4), 121-127.

Bearnson, C., & Wiker, K. (2005). Human patient simulators: A new face in baccalaureate nursing education at Brigham Young University. *Journal of Nursing Education, 44*(9), 421-425.

Beck, C. (1999). Quantitative measurement of caring. *Journal of Advanced Nursing, 30*(10), 24-32.

Beck, C. (2001). Caring within nursing education: A metasynthesis. *Journal of Nursing Education, 40*(3), 101-109.

Becker, C. (2004). Taking initiative on training: providers push expansion of nursing education. *Modern Healthcare, 34*(24), 26,34.

Becker, K. L, Rose, L. E., Berg, J. B., Park, H., & Shatzer, J. H. (2006). The effectiveness of standardized patients. *Journal of Nursing Education, 45*(4), 103-111.

Bentley, R., & Ellison, K. J. (2005). Impact of a service-learning project on nursing students. *Nursing Education Perspectives, 26*(5), 287-290

Berry, J. (2005). A student and RN partnered clinical experience. *Nurse Educator, 30*(6), 240-241.

Billings, D., & Connors, H. (2001). *Best practices in online learning.* Retrieved January 15, 2009, from http://www.electronicvision.com/nln/chapter02/index.htm

Billings, D. M., Skiba, D. J., & Connors, H. R. (2005). Best practices in web-based courses: Generational differences across undergraduate and graduate nursing students. *Journal of Professional Nursing, 21*, 126-133.

Bitzer, M. (1966). Clinical nursing instruction via the PLATO simulated laboratory. *Nursing Research, 15*(2), 144-150.

Bjork, I. T., & Kirkevold, M. (1999). Issues in nurses' practical skill development in the clinical setting. *Journal of Nursing Care Quality, 14*(1), 72-84.

Bloomfield, J., While, A., & Roberts, J. (2008). Using computer assisted learning for clinical skills education in nursing: Integrative review. *Journal of Advanced Nursing, 63*(3), 222-235.

Blum, C. A. (2009). Development of a clinical preceptor model. *Nurse Educator, 34*(1), 29-33.

Bosek, M .S., Li, S., & Hicks, F. D. (2007). Working with standardized patients: A primer. *International Journal of Nursing Education Scholarship, 4*(1), 1-12, Article 16.

Botti, M., & Reeve, R. (2002). Role of knowledge and ability in student nurses' clinical decision-making. *Nursing & Health Sciences, 5*, 39-49.

Bowles, D. J. (2006). Active learning strategies…not for the birds! *International Journal of Nursing Education Scholarship ,3*(1), 1-11, Article 22.

Bradshaw, A. (1998). Defining "competency" in nursing (part II): An analytical review. *Journal of Clinical Nursing, 7*, 103-111.

Bradshaw, M. J., & Woodring, B. (1999). Clinical pathways: A tool to evaluate clinical learning. *Journal of the Society of Pediatric Nurses, 4*(1), 37-40.

Brancato, V. (2006). An innovative clinical practicum to teach evidence-based practice. *Nurse Educator, 31*(5), 195-199.

Bremner, M. N., Aduddell, K., Bennett, D. N., & VanGeest, J. B. (2006). The use of human patient simulators: Best practices with novice nursing students. *Nurse Educator, 31*(4), 170-174.

Brockopp, D., Hardin-Pierce, M., & Welsh, J. (2006). An agency-financed capstone experience for graduating seniors. *Journal of Nursing Education, 45*(4), 137-140.

Brooks, E. M., & Thomas, S. (1997). The perception and judgment of senior baccalaureate student nurses in clinical decision making. *Advances in Nursing Science, 19*(3), 50-69.

Buckley, K. M., Beyna, B., & Dudley-Brown, S. (2005). Promoting active learning through on-line discussion boards. *Nurse Educator, 30*(1), 32-36.

Campbell, S. E., & Dudley, K. (2005). Clinical partner model: Benefits for education and service. *Nurse Educator, 30*(6), 271-274.

Campbell, S. L., Prater, M., Schwartz, C., & Ridenour, N. (2001). Building an empowering academic and practice partnership model. *Nursing Administration Quarterly, 26*(1), 35-44.

Casey, A. (2000). Nursing competencies for 2010. *Paediatric Nursing, 12*(5), 3.

Chan, S., & Wai-Tong, C. (2000). Implementing contract learning in a clinical context: Report on a study. *Journal of Advanced Nursing, 31*(2), 298-305.

Charleston, R., & Happell, B. (2004). Evaluating the impact of a preceptorship course on mental health nursing practice. *International Journal of Mental Health Nursing, 13*, 191-197.

Charleston, R., & Happell, B. (2005a). Attempting to accomplish connectedness within the preceptorship experience: The perceptions of mental health nurses. *International Journal of Mental Health Nursing, 14*, 54-61.

Charleston, R., & Happell, B. (2005b). Coping with uncertainty within the preceptorship experience: The perceptions of nursing students. *Journal of Psychiatric and Mental Health Nursing, 12*, 303-309.

Charon, R. (2001). Narrative medicine: A model for empathy, reflection, profession, and trust. *Journal of the American Medical Association, 286*, 1897-1902.

Charron, S. A., & Parns, M. (2004). Promoting emotional wellness: Undergraduate clinical experiences in elementary schools. *Nurse Educator, 29*(5), 208-211.

Chickering A. W., & Gamson, Z. F. (1987). Seven principles for good practice in undergraduate education. *American Association for Higher Education Bulletin, 39*(7), 3-7.

Cholowski, K. M., & Chan, L. K. S. (2004). Cognitive factors in student nurses' clinical problem solving. *Journal of Evaluation in Clinical Practice, 10*, 85-95.

Clark M. C., Nguyen H. T., Bray C., & Levine R. E. (2008). Team-based learning in an undergraduate nursing course. *Journal of Nursing Education, 47*(3), 111-117.

Clarke, D., Davies, J., & McNee, P. (2002). The case of children's skills laboratory. *Paediatric Nursing, 14*(7), 36-39.

Comer, S. K. (2005a). Clinical reasoning: Turning your students into clinical detectives. *Nurse Educator, 30*(6), 235-237.

Comer, S. K. (2005b). Patient care simulations: Role playing to enhance clinical understanding. *Nursing Education Perspectives, 26*(6), 357-361.

Conger, M. M., & Mezza, I. (1996). Fostering critical thinking in nursing students in the clinical setting. *Nurse Educator, 21*, 11-15.

Cooper, C., Taft, L., & Thelen, M. (2004). Examining the role of technology in learning: An evaluation of online clinical conferencing. *Journal of Professional Nursing, 20*(3), 160-166.

Cox, L. S. (2002). Focused Learning: 2 weeks of class — 2 weeks of clinical. *Nurse Educator, 27*(1), 15.

Coyle-Rogers, P., & Putman, C. (2006). Using experiential learning: Facilitating hands-on basic patient skills. *Journal of Nursing Education, 45*(4), 142-143.

Curran, C. R., Elfrink, V., & Mays, B. (2009). Building a virtual community for nursing education: The town of Mirror Lake. *Journal of Nursing Education, 48*(1), 30-35.

Davies, J., & Clarke, D. (2004). Clinical skills acquisition in children's nursing: An international perspective. *Paediatric Nursing, 16*(2), 23-26.

DeLashmutt M. B., & Rankin, E. A. (2005). A different kind of clinical experience: Poverty up close and personal. *Nurse Educator, 30*(4), 143-149.

DeBourgh, G. (2001). Using web technology in a clinical nursing course. *Nurse Educator, 25*(5), 227-233.

Diefenbeck, C., Plowfield, L., & Herrman, J. (2006). Clinical immersion: A residence model for nursing education. *Nursing Education Perspectives, 27*(2), 72-79.

Donahue, M. P. (1985). *Nursing, the finest art: An illustrated history*. St. Louis, MO: Mosby.

Doubt, L., Paterson, M., & O'Riordan, A. (2004). Clinical education in private practice: An interdisciplinary project. *Journal of Allied Health, 33*(1), 47-50.

Downey, M. (2007). Effects of holistic nursing course. *Journal of Holistic Nursing, 25*(2), 119-125.

Durak, H. I., Caliskan, S. A., Bor, S., & Van Der Vleuten, C. (2007). Use of case-based exams as an instructional teaching tool to teach clinical reasoning. *Medical Teacher, 29*, 170-174.

Eaves, R. H., & Flagg, A. J. (2001) The U.S. Air Force pilot simulated medical unit: A teaching strategy with multiple applications. *Journal of Nursing Education, 40*, 110-115.

Educational Technology and Information Management Advisory Council (2007). *Survey results.* Retrieved January 29, 2009, from http://www.himss.org/content/files/CBO/Meeting9/Nursing_Informatics_Survey.pdf

Ehrenberg, A. C., & Haggblom, M. (2007). Problem-based learning in clinical nursing education: Integrating theory and practice. *Nurse Education in Practice, 7*(2), 67-74.

Eide, P. J., Hahn, L., Bayne, T., Allen, C. B., & Swain, D. (2006). The population-focused analysis project for teaching community health. *Nursing Education Perspectives, 27*(1), 22-27.

Emerson, R. J. (2007). *Nursing education in the clinical setting.* St. Louis, MO: Mosby.

Errichetti, A., Gimpel, J., & Boulet, J. (2002). State of the art in standardized patient programs: A survey of osteopathic medical schools. *Journal of the American Osteopathic Association, 102*(11), 627-631.

Festa L. M., Baliko B., Mangiafico T., & Jarosinski J. (2000). Maximizing learning outcomes by videotaping nursing students' interactions with a standardized patient. *Journal of Psychosocial Nursing & Mental Health Services, 38*(5), 37-44.

Firth, J. (1986). Levels and sources of stress in medical students. *British Medical Journal, 92*, 1177-1180.

Fitzpatrick, J. J. (2006). [Editorial]. Blinking: The art of clinical judgment? *Nursing Education Perspectives, 27*(1), 5.

Freiburger, O. A. (2001). A tribute to clinical preceptors: Developing a preceptor program for nursing students. *Journal for Nurses in Staff Development, 17*(6), 320-327.

Gibbons, S. W., Adamo, G., Padden, D., Ricciardi, R., Graziano, M., Levine, E., et al. (2002). Clinical evaluation in advanced practice nursing education: Using standardized patients in health assessment. *Journal of Nursing Education, 41*(5), 215-222.

Green, S. M., Weaver, M., Voegeli, D., Fitzsimmons, D., Knowles, J., Harrison, M., et al. (2006). The development and evaluation of the use of a virtual learning environment (Blackboard 5) to support the learning of pre-qualifying nursing students undertaking a human anatomy and physiology module. *Nurse Education Today, 26*(5), 388-395.

Greiner, A., & Knebel. E. (Eds.). (2003). *Health professions education: A bridge to quality.* Washington, DC: National Academies Press.

Gubrud-Howe, P., & Schoessler, M. (2008). From random access opportunity to a clinical education curriculum. *Journal of Nursing Education, 47*(1), 3-4.

Hall-Long, B. (2004). Partners in Action: A public health program for baccalaureate nursing students. *Community and Community Health Nursing, 27*(4), 338-345.

Halse, K., & Hage, A. M. (2006). An acute hospital ward, densely populated with students during a 12-week clinical study period. *Journal of Nursing Education, 45*(4), 133-136.

Happell, B., & Charleston, R. (2004). Good preceptorship: The way forward. *Australian Nursing Journal, 12*(3), 39.

Haskvitz, L., & Koop, E. (2004). Students struggling in clinical? A new role for the patient simulator. *Journal of Nursing Education, 43*(4), 181-184.

Hayes, A. (2005). A mental health nursing clinical experience with hospice patients. *Nurse Educator, 30*(2), 85-88.

Healthcare Information and Management Systems Society (2009). Alliance for nursing informatics. Retrieved June 19, 2009, from http://www.himss.org/ASP/topics_FocusDynamic.asp?faid=119

Henderson, A., Heel, A., & Twentyman, M. (2007). Enabling student placement through strategic partnerships between a health-care organization and tertiary institutions. *Journal of Nursing Management, 15*(1), 91-96.

Henneman, E. A., & Cunningham, H. (2005). Using clinical simulation to teach patient safety in an acute/critical care nursing course. *Nurse Educator, 30*, 172-178.

Hewlett, P. O., & Eichelberger, L. W. (1999). Creating academic/service partnerships through nursing competency models. *Journal of Nursing Education, 38*(7), 295-298.

Hill, C. (2006). Integrating clinical experiences into the concept mapping process. *Nurse Educator, 31*(1), 36-39.

Hill, K. S., & Walker, L. (2004). Partnerships pack recruitment power. *Nursing Management, 35*(12), 14.

Hoffart, N., Diani, J. A., Connors, M., & Moynihan, P. (2006). Outcomes of cooperative education in a baccalaureate program in nursing. *Nursing Education Perspectives, 27*(3), 136-143.

Hoffert, D., Henshaw, C., & Mvududu, N. (2007). Enhancing the ability of nursing students to perform a spiritual assessment. *Nurse Educator, 32*(2), 66-72.

Innes, G. (2008). Faculty-librarian collaboration: An online information literacy tutorial for students. *Nurse Educator, 33*(4), 145-146.

Jarzemsky, P., & McGrath, J. (2008). Look before you leap: Lessons learned when introducing clinical simulation. *Nurse Educator, 33*(2), 90-95.

Jeffries, P. (2005). Technology trends in nursing education: Next steps. *Journal of Nursing Education, 44*(1), 3-4.

Jeffries, P. (2006). A framework for designing, implementing, and evaluating simulations used as teaching strategies in nursing. *Nursing Education Perspectives, 26*(2), 96-103.

Jeffries, P., Kost, G., & Sweitzer, V. (2009). Teaching-learning in the psychomotor domain. In C. Shultz (Ed.), *Building a science of nursing education: Foundation for evidence-based teaching and learning* (pp. 177-215). New York: National League for Nursing.

Jenkins, H. M. (1985). Improving clinical decision making in nursing. *Journal of Nursing Education, 24*, 242-243.

Kelly, R. E. (2006). Engaging baccalaureate clinical faculty. *International Journal of Nursing Education Scholarship, 3*(1), 1-16, Article 14.

Kemsley, M., & Riegle, E. (2004). A community-campus partnership: Influenza prevention campaign. *Nurse Educator, 29*(3), 126-129.

Kennison, M. (2006). The evaluation of students' reflective writing for evidence of critical thinking. *Nursing Education Perspectives, 27*(5), 269-273.

King, M., & Gates, M. (2006). Perceived barriers to holistic nursing in undergraduate nursing programs. *Journal of Science and Healing, 2*(4), 334-338.

Kirkham, S., Harwood, C., & Hofwegen, L. (2005). Capturing a vision for nursing: Undergraduate nursing students in alternative clinical settings. *Nurse Educator, 30*(6), 263-270.

Kirkpatrick, H., Byrne, C., Martin, M. L., & Roth, M. L. (1991). A collaborative model for the clinical education of baccalaureate nursing students. *Journal of Advanced Nursing, 16*, 101-107.

Ladyshewsky, R. K. (2000). Peer-assisted learning in clinical education: A review of terms and learning principles. *Journal of Physical Therapy Education, 14*(2), 15-22.

Lahaie, U. (2007). WebQuests: A new instructional strategy for nursing education. *CIN: Computers, Informatics, Nursing, 25*(3), 148-156.

Larew, C., Lessans, S., Spunt, D., Foster, D., & Covington, B. (2006). Innovations in clinical simulation application of Benner's theory in an interactive patient care simulation. *Nursing Education Perspectives, 27*(1), 16-21.

Lasater, K., Luce, L., Yolpin, M., Terwilliger, A., & Wold, J. (2007). When it works: Learning community health nursing concepts from clinical experience. *Nursing Education Perspectives, 28*, 88-92.

Lee-Hsieh, J., Kuo, C., & Tseng, H. (2005). Application and evaluation of a caring code in clinical nursing education. *Journal of Nursing Education, 44*(4), 177-184.

Leyshon, S. (2005). Making the most of teams in the mentorship of students. *British Journal of Community Nursing, 10*(1), 21-23.

Ligeikis-Clayton, C., & Denman, J. (2005). Service learning across the curriculum. *Nurse Educator, 30*, 191-192 .

Lottes, N. (2008). Fire up: Tips for engaging student learning. *Journal of Nursing Education, 47*(7), 331.

Lusk, J., Winne, M., & DeLeskey, K. (2007). Nurses' perceptions of working with students in the clinical setting. *Nurse Educator, 32*(3), 102-103.

Mallette, S., Loury, S., Engelke, M., Anderews, A., (2005). Ihe integrative clinical preceptor model: Anew method for teaching undergraduate community health nursing. *Nurse Educator.* 30(1), 21-26.

Mamchur, C., & Myrick, F. (2003). Preceptorship and interpersonal conflict: A multidisciplinary study. *Journal of Advanced Nursing, 43*(2), 188-196.

Matsumura, G., Callister, L. C., Palmer, S., Cox, A. H., & Larsen, L. I. (2004). Staff nurse perceptions of the contributions of students to clinical agencies. *Nursing Education Perspectives, 25*, 297-303.

Mayne, W., Jootun, D., Young, B., Marland, G., Harris, M., & Lyttle, P. (2004). Enabling students to develop confidence in basic clinical skills. *Nursing Times, 100*(24), 36-39.

McAllister, M., Tower, M., & Walker, R. (2007). Gentle interruptions: Transformative approaches to clinical teaching. *Journal of Nursing Education, 46*,(7) 304-312.

McCallum, C. (2004). Clinical education in a nursing home setting: A structured framework for student learning. *International Journal of Therapy and Rehabilitation, 11*(8), 374-380.

McCausland, L., Curran, C., & Cataldi, P. (2004). Use of a human patient simulator for undergraduate nurse education. *International Journal of Nursing Education Scholarship, 1*(1), Article 23.

Medley, C. F., & Horne, C. (2005). Using simulation technology for undergraduate nursing education. *Journal of Nursing Education, 44*(1), 31-34.

Memshick, M. T., & Shepard, K. F. (1996). Physical therapy clinical education in a 2:1 student-instructor education model. *Physical Therapy, 76*(9), 968-981.

Meyer, C. (2003). How effectively are nurse educators preparing students to provide spiritual care? *Nurse Educator, 28*(4), 185-190.

Moran, R. (2005). Enriching clinical learning experiences in community health nursing through the use of discussion boards. *International Journal of Nursing Education Scholarship, 2*(1), Article 23.

Moscato, R., Miller, J., Logsdon, K., & Weinberg, S. (2007). Dedicated education unit: An innovative clinical partner education model. *Nursing Outlook, 55*, 31-37.

Murray, T. A. (2007). Expanding educational capacity through an innovative practice education partnership. *Journal of Nursing Education, 46*, 330-334.

National Council of State Boards of Nursing. (2005). *Position paper: Clinical instruction in prelicensure nursing programs.* Retrieved February 2, 2009, from https://www.ncsbn.org/Final_Clinical_Instr_Pre_Nsg_programs.pdf

National League for Nursing. (2003). *Position statement: Innovation in nursing education — A call to reform.* Retrieved February 2, 2009, from http://www.nln.org/aboutnln/PositionStatements/innovation082203.pdf

National League for Nursing. (2006). *Designing and implementing models for the innovative use of simulation to teach nursing care of ill adults and children: A national, multi-site, multi-method study.* Retrieved January 19, 2009, from https://www.nln.org/research/LaerdalReport.pdf

National League for Nursing. (2008). *Position Statement: Preparing the next generation of nurses to practice in a technology-rich environment: An informatics agenda.* Retrieved February 16, 2009, from http://www.nln.org/aboutnln/PositionStatements/index.htm

National League for Nursing. (2009). *Core Values.* Retrieved January 30, 2009, from https://www.nln.org/aboutnln/corevalues.htm

Niedringhaus, L. (2001). Using student writing assignments to assess critical thinking skills: A holistic approach. *Holistic Nursing Practice, 15*(3), 9-17.

NLN Task Group on Clinical Nursing Education. (N. Ard, Chair). (2006). Meeting minutes, July 6-7, 2006. New York: Author.

Novotny, J. M., & Griffin, M. T .Q. (2006). Supervising a clinical group. In *A nuts and bolts approach to teaching nursing.* (3rd ed., pp. 11-31). New York: Springer Publishing.

O'Connor, A. B. (2006). *Clinical instruction and evaluation: A teaching resource.* Sudbury, MA: Jones and Barlett.

Oermann, M. H., & Gaberson, K. B. (2006). Clinical evaluation. In *Evaluation and testing in nursing education* (2nd ed., pp. 199-211). New York: Springer Publishing.

Palmer, S., Cox, A., Callister, L. C., Johnsen, V., & Matsumura, G. (2005). Nursing education and service collaboration: Making a difference in the clinical learning environment. *Journal of Continuing Education in Nursing, 36*(6), 271-276.

Pardue, S. F. (1987). Decision-making skills and critical thinking ability among associate degree, diploma, baccalaureate, and master's-prepared nurses. *Journal of Nursing Education, 26*, 354-361.

Paterson, M., & Grandjean, C. (2008). The bridge to practice model: A collaborative program designed for clinical experiences in baccalaureate nursing. *Nursing Economic$, 26*(5), 302-306, 309.

Porter, J., & Baker, E. L. (2005). The management moment: Partnering essentials. *Journal of Public Health Management Practice, 11*(2), 174-177.

Porter-O'Grady, T. (2001). Profound change: 21st century nursing. *Nursing Outlook, 49*(4), 182-186.

Raines, D. A. (2007). Using the Blackboard platform — More than a course site. *Journal of Nursing Education, 46*, 243-244.

Ranse, K., & Grealish, L. (2007). Nursing students' perceptions of learning in the clinical setting of the dedicated education unit. *Journal of Advanced Nursing, 58*(2), 171-179.

Rauen, C. (2004). Simulation as a teaching strategy for nursing education and orientation in cardiac surgery. *Critical Care Nurse, 24*, 46-51.

Reilly, D. E. & Oermann, M. H. (1992). *Clinical teaching in nursing education* (2nd ed.). New York: National League for Nursing.

Rice, R. B. (2003). Collaboration as a tool for resolving the nursing shortage. *Journal of Nursing Education, 42*(4), 147-148.

Royse M., & Newton, S. (2007). How gaming is used as an innovative strategy for nursing education. *Nursing Education Perspectives, 28*(5), 263-267.

Ryan-Nicholls, K. D. (2004). Preceptor recruitment and retention. *Canadian Nurse, 100*(6), 18-22.

Salyers, V. L. (2007). Teaching psychomotor skills to beginning nursing students using a web-enhanced approach: A quasi-experimental study. *International Journal of Nursing Education Scholarship, 4*(1), Article 11.

Schmidt, L. (2007). Camp nursing: Innovative opportunities for nursing students to work with children. *Nurse Educator, 32*(6), 246-250.

Schroetter, S., & Wendler, C. (2008). Capstone experience: Analysis of an educational concept for nursing. *Journal of Professional Nursing, 24*(2), 71-79.

Secomb, J. (2008). A systematic review of peer teaching and learning in clinical education. *Journal of Clinical Nursing, 17*, 703-716.

Shin, K. R. (1998). Critical thinking ability and clinical decision-making skills among senior nursing students in associate and baccalaureate programmes in Korea. *Journal of Advanced Nursing, 27*, 414-418.

Shultz, C. (2009). Teaching-learning in the affective domain. In C. Shultz (Ed.), *Building a science of nursing education: Foundation for evidence-based teaching and learning* (pp. 217-300). New York: National League for Nursing.

Slater, V. (2005). Holistic nursing practice. *Journal of Holistic Nursing, 23*, 261.

Sowan, N. A., Moffatt, S. G., & Canales, M. K. (2004). Creating a mentoring partnership model: A university-department of health experience. *Family & Community Health, 27*, 326-337.

Spunt, D., Foster, D., & Adams, K. (2004). Mock code: A clinical simulation module. *Nurse Educator, 29*(5), 192-194.

Stevens, R. H., & Roper, W. L. (2004). The North Carolina experiment: Academia-practice partnerships. *Journal of Public Health Management Practice, 10*(4), 316-326.

Stone, C., & Rowles, C. (2007). Clinical site selection by students through use of an Internet database. *CIN: Computers, Informatics, Nursing, 25*(4), 236-240.

Technology Informatics Guiding Educational Reform Initiative. (2006) TIGER – Enabling full participation by nurses in the informatics revolution!. Retrieved January 16, 2009, from http://www.umbc.edu/tiger/index.html

Tanner, C. A. (2002). Clinical education, circa 2010. *Journal of Nursing Education, 41*, 51-52.

Thompson, C. (2009). Teaching-learning in the cognitive domain. In C. Shultz (Ed.), *Building a science of nursing education: Foundation for evidence-based teaching and learning* (pp. 133-176). New York: National League for Nursing.

Tobar, K., Wall, D., & Parsh, B. (2007). Use of 12 hour clinical shifts in nursing education: Faculty, staff and student response. *Nurse Educator, 32*, 190-191.

Tschikota, S. (1993). The clinical decision-making processes of student nurses. *Journal of Nursing Education, 32*, 389-398.

Urquhart, G., & Comeau, A. (2002). Maintaining specialized clinical competencies: Continous learning to renew clinical competencies can be difficult to achieve for nurses in acute care and frustrating for the educator. *Canadian Nurse, 98*(8), 25-28.

Usher, K., Nolan, C., Reser, P., Owens, J., & Tellefson, J. (1999). An exploration of the preceptor role: Preceptors' perceptions of benefits, rewards, supports, and commitment to the preceptor role. *Journal of Advanced Nursing, 29*(2), 506-514.

Utley-Smith, Q. (2004). Five competencies needed by new baccalaureate graduates. *Nursing Education Perspectives, 25*(4), 166-170.

Yoo, M. S., & Yoo, Y. (2003). The effectiveness of standardized patients as a teaching method for nursing fundamentals. *Journal of Nursing Education, 42*(10), 444-448.

NATIONAL SURVEY ON CLINICAL EDUCATION IN PRELICENSURE NURSING EDUCATION PROGRAMS

Angela McNelis, PhD, RN
Pamela Ironside, PhD, RN, FAAN, ANEF

Introduction

Clinical experiences are a critical part of prelicensure nursing education. The National Council of State Boards of Nursing (NCSBN) has reinforced the need for all prelicensure students to have clinical experiences with patients across the lifespan and to be supervised by qualified faculty (NCSBN, 2005). While many alternative experiences now supplement clinical learning, there is widespread agreement that students need "hands on" experiences with actual patients to learn the practice of nursing (Ard, Rogers & Vinten, 2008; NCSBN, 2005). A study of 2,218 faculty funded by the National League for Nursing (NLN) found general agreement among faculty that clinical education is an active and holistic experience where students apply theoretical knowledge to patient care involving faculty, students, staff, and clients (Ard, Rogers, & Vinten, 2008).

Despite widespread agreement in the discipline on the importance of clinical experiences to the preparation of new nurses for practice, very little research has been conducted to guide the design and implementation of these experiences and little is known about the strategies

Table 2 –1
Members of the National League for Nursing
Blue Ribbon Panel on The Future of Nursing Education Research

Patricia Benner, PhD, RN, FAAN University of California at San Francisco San Francisco, CA Carnegie Foundation for the Advancement of Teaching Stanford, CA
Judith Halstead, DSN, RN, ANEF Indiana University Indianapolis, IN
Pamela Ironside, PhD, RN, FAAN, ANEF Indiana University Indianapolis, IN
Marilyn Oermann, PhD, RN, FAAN, ANEF Wayne State University Detroit, MI (at the time the Blue Ribbon Panel was convened) University of North Carolina at Chapel Hill Chapel Hill, NC (current appointment)
Chris Tanner, PhD, RN, FAAN Oregon Health Sciences University Portland, Oregon
Theresa "Terry" Valiga, EdD, RN, FAAN National League for Nursing New York, NY (at the time the Blue Ribbon Panel was convened) Duke University Durham, NC (current appointment)
Lin Jacobson, EdD, RN, CPHQ NLN Staff Liaison

that foster desired student outcomes. The study described here, also funded by the NLN, was undertaken to examine the barriers and challenges faculty face in optimizing students' clinical learning, the strategies they use to address these barriers and challenges, the effectiveness of these strategies, and the teaching practices they employ in clinical settings.

Blue Ribbon Panel and Clinical Education Think Tank

In 2006, the NLN convened a Blue Ribbon Panel of leaders in nursing education (see Table 2–1) to identify and articulate the priorities for future nursing education research. Among these leaders, there was strong agreement that developing and testing new models for clinical education was critically important to assuring that new nurses were prepared for practice in contemporary health care systems. There was also recognition that new models of clinical education would require transformation of classroom teaching and the systems that support nursing teachers and students. Thus, the Panel identified three major areas of focus for future research in nursing education:

1. New models of clinical education that foster partnerships between schools and clinical agencies that align clinical learning with contemporary practice and health care needs

2. Patient-centered teaching that integrates classroom and clinical education

3. Educational system redesign that supports excellence in patient-centered, integrative teaching, and ongoing innovation in nursing education

Beginning with the first focal area, the NLN held an invitational think tank on transforming clinical nursing education in 2008. The purpose of this think tank was to gather nursing leaders from education, practice, and regulation as well as interdisciplinary scholars to explore current and emerging approaches to clinical education and the assessment of clinical performance. There was consensus among think tank members on the need to transform clinical nursing education, particularly in prelicensure programs. Members recognized that many innovative approaches and practices in clinical education were occurring at a local level, but those innovations were not widely disseminated or known.

Study Purposes

In an effort to document current practice in clinical education, the NLN commissioned this national survey to address barriers and challenges to clinical education. Specifically, this study was designed to (a) describe faculty members' perceived barriers to optimizing clinical learning experiences for students enrolled in prelicensure nursing programs, (b) identify strategies faculty members commonly employ to address barriers to optimizing clinical learning experiences for students enrolled in prelicensure nursing programs, (c) document the perceived effectiveness of strategies employed to address barriers to optimizing clinical learning experiences for students enrolled in prelicensure nursing programs, (d) describe faculty members' perceived challenges to optimizing clinical learning experiences for students enrolled in prelicensure nursing programs, (e) identify strategies faculty members commonly employ to address the challenges to optimizing clinical learning experiences for students enrolled in prelicensure nursing programs, and (f) document the perceived effectiveness of strategies faculty employ to address the challenges to optimizing clinical learning experiences for students enrolled in prelicensure nursing programs.

Methodology

The survey instrument was developed by the investigators. Survey items reflected insights obtained from the work of the NLN Task Group on Clinical Nursing Education, a review of the literature on clinical education in nursing, documents generated during the Blue Ribbon Panel and Think Tank on Clinical Nursing Education meetings, conversations with faculty currently engaged in clinical teaching, and the investigators' personal experience.

Survey Instrument

Survey items were organized into four sections, including both multiple choice and open-ended items. In section 1, respondents provided demographic information about their school, role, and experience in providing clinical education. In section 2, respondents were provided with a list of 17 barriers and asked to select and rank order the five most important barriers they faced that hindered their efforts to optimize students' clinical learning experiences during the previous two years. For each barrier selected, respondents were asked to identify the strategies they used or are presently using to address each and rate their perception of the effectiveness of each strategy. For this survey, barriers were defined as "those institutional, state, or federal guidelines/policies, as well as structural, programmatic, administrative, or procedural aspects of your program/school that influence students' clinical learning and over which you personally may have little or no control."

Section 3 focused on respondents' teaching practices in clinical settings. Respondents were provided with a list of 13 common clinical teaching activities and asked to identify the three activities that typically took up most of their time during a clinical day, and to estimate the percent of each clinical day they engaged in each of the identified activities. In this section, respondents also described their use of pre- and postclinical conferences, noting if these conferences occurred and identifying the activities that commonly occurred during them.

The fourth section focused specifically on the challenges respondents faced when teaching in clinical settings. Respondents were provided with a list of 29 common challenges, asked to select the five most significant challenges they faced during the previous two years and rank order them from the most to the least challenging. Respondents were then asked to select one of their ranked challenges, describe the single, most important strategy they used to address it, and rate how effective they perceived this strategy was in addressing the challenge. For this study, *challenges* were defined as "those course, context, professional, or personal aspects over which you, as a faculty member, exert some degree of control or influence or those aspects of your teaching practice that are influenced by the particular course, context or setting in which you teach and over which you, as a faculty member, exert some degree of control or influence."

The survey concluded with an opportunity for respondents to add any comments about clinical teaching or evaluation that would help other nurse educators better understand the barriers and challenges to optimizing clinical learning experiences for students enrolled in prelicensure nursing programs, strategies faculty members commonly employ to address those barriers, and the effectiveness of those strategies.

This chapter presents an overview of the demographic characteristics of faculty responding to the survey, their identified barriers and strategies for addressing their five most important barriers, activities that take the most time and energy during a clinical day, and the most significant challenges faced in teaching in a clinical setting. A more comprehensive, detailed report of the findings, to be published by the NLN, is forthcoming.

Pilot Testing

Prior to release, the survey underwent rigorous pilot testing. First, members of the NLN Blue Ribbon Panel and faculty known to the investigators who had clinical teaching responsibilities across types of programs and specialty courses reviewed an electronic copy of the survey for content, clarity, and comprehensiveness. The investigators used this feedback to refine the survey, which was then loaded onto the NLN website, but not released to the public. Members of the NLN Task Group on Clinical Nursing Education participated in a second pilot testing by completing the web-based version of the survey; providing feedback on the format, clarity and comprehensiveness; and reporting completion time for the survey in this format. The second testing also allowed investigators to test the ease of use and skip patterns, and to identify technical problems.

Procedures

Because the population of clinical nursing faculty is unknown, a convenience sample was used for this survey. Prior to launch, the membership of NLN was alerted to the upcoming survey via an announcement at the 2008 NLN Education Summit, in the October NLN Member Update, and in Fall 2008 NLN Faculty Development Bulletins. These announcements described the intent of the study and the date the survey would be available for online completion. An email blast to all NLN members accompanied the launch of the survey and provided the URL to access the survey. This message was also posted on three list-servs covering nursing education. In each message, respondents were asked to circulate the survey URL to other faculty they knew to be teaching in clinical settings. The NLN sent three reminder emails, occurring two weeks after launch, one month after launch, and several days before closure of the survey. The URL for the survey remained open for a total of nine weeks. Response to the survey served as consent.

Analysis of Survey Data

Survey data were compiled by the NLN and converted into SPSS data files for transfer to Indiana University School of Nursing for analysis. After receiving approval from the Institutional Review Board at Indiana University, all numerical data were analyzed using descriptive statistics.

Summary of Findings

Demographics

Respondents were 2,386 faculty members, representing all 50 states. The states with the highest faculty response rates were Pennsylvania (n = 172), New York (n = 155), Ohio (n = 148), Texas (n = 145) and Indiana (n = 89). In all states, faculty came from various types of institutions, with no one type predominating. The majority of respondents taught at a community college or a public college or university, and were predominantly full-time faculty members teaching both clinical and didactic courses. On average, respondents had been actively involved in prelicensure education for 12.3 years. Table 2-2 provides more detailed demographic characteristics.

Barriers to Students' Clinical Learning

Following the demographic section, respondents were asked about barriers faced in their efforts to optimize students' clinical learning. Thinking of the course in which they had the most extensive clinical teaching responsibilities, faculty respondents rank ordered the five most important barriers faced during the previous two years, where "1" was the most important barrier faced, "2" was the second most important barrier faced, and so on. A list of 17 barriers was provided from which respondents selected and rank ordered the barriers they perceived to be most important (see Table 2-3). Results shown are the total number of respondents who ranked the barrier as one of their top five, thus, the total responses to this question (11,279) exceeds the total number of respondents (2,386).

For each of the barriers respondents ranked as one of their top five, they were provided a list of possible strategies to address this barrier. They selected up to three strategies used most often to address each identified barrier and rated the effectiveness of each strategy on a 4-point scale from "very effective" to "not at all effective."

More than 50 percent of respondents indicated that the lack of quality clinical sites was an important barrier to optimizing students' clinical learning. The top strategies they used to address this barrier were 1) providing clinical rotations on evenings, nights, weekends, and/ or holidays, 2) substituting simulation activities for clinical hours (high-fidelity simulators, mannequins, role play, videos, case studies to assist students to learn and apply clinical concepts in the context of simulated clinical scenarios), and 3) providing more observational experiences for students during clinical time. Faculty perceived these strategies to be only somewhat effective in addressing the barrier.

Nearly 46 percent of respondents indicated that the lack of qualified faculty was a barrier to students' clinical learning. To address this barrier they most frequently reported 1) hiring faculty with little or no preparation in teaching, 2) hiring more part-time faculty, and 3) having faculty teach overload courses. Faculty perceived that hiring faculty with little or no preparation in teaching was only minimally effective, and hiring more part-time faculty and teaching overload courses were perceived to be somewhat effective.

The size of clinical groups was identified by almost 45 percent of respondents as one of the top five barriers to optimizing students' clinical learning. To address this barrier, respondents most commonly identified 1) providing more observational experiences for students during clinical time, 2) pairing students for clinical assignments, and 3) creating other kinds of learning experiences on the clinical unit to replace total patient care. Faculty indicated that all of these strategies were only somewhat effective in addressing the barrier.

Restrictions on numbers of students or limitations to students' experiences imposed by clinical agencies was identified as one of the top five barriers to students' clinical learning by more

Table 2 – 2
Demographic Characteristics of Respondents

Variable	N (%)
Type of institution	
• Vocation/technical	112 (4.7)
• Community college	839 (35.2)
• Hospital or medical center based college or university	332 (13.9)
• Liberal arts college or university	138 (5.8)
• Private not-for-profit college or university	232 (9.7)
• Private for-profit college or university	118 (4.9)
• Public college or university	558 (23.4)
• Other	50 (2.1)
Type of prelicensure program offered	
• Associate	1360
• Diploma	24
• Baccalaureate	1016
Role in the school of nursing	
• Director/Dean	180 (7.5)
• Department Chair	110 (4.6)
• Program Director	102 (4.3)
• Curriculum Director	29 (1.2)
• Level coordinator	67 (2.8)
• Course coordinator	232 (9.7)
• Member of curriculum committee	15 (.6)
• Faculty member full time	1321 (55.4)
• Faculty member part time, temporary or adjunct	212 (8.9)
• Other	111 (4.7)
Program of primary teaching responsibility	
• Associate	1242 (52.1)
• Diploma	190 (8.0)
• Baccalaureate	882 (37.0)
Highest degree held	
• MS in nursing	1056 (44.3)
• MS in nursing with specialization in nursing education	773 (32.4)
• MS in other field	122 (5.1)
• CNE certified	217 (9.1)
• PhD or other doctoral degree	503 (21.1)
• Expertise in teaching via CE	199 (8.3)

Table 2 – 3
Barriers to Optimizing Clinical Learning Experiences

Variable	N (%)
Lack of quality clinical sites that can accommodate the number of students in my group and/or provide experiences for the learning objectives of my course	1218 (51)
Lack of qualified faculty	1091 (45.7)
Size of clinical groups (ratio of faculty to students)	1061 (44.5)
Restrictions on numbers of students or limitations to students' experiences imposed by clinical agencies	971 (40.7)
Time-consuming nature of students learning multiple clinical agency systems (e.g., documentation systems are all different, hospital policies and procedures differ)	933 (39.1)
Clinical rotations now take too much time for orientation to the technology (e.g., electronic medical records, clinical information systems)	869 (36.4)
Students' inability to chart on new systems unless they are trained and certified	720 (30.2)
Rapid turnover of patients in the clinical setting	710 (29.8)
Lack of qualified clinicians to serve as preceptors	549 (23)
Unwillingness of qualified clinicians to serve as preceptors for students	519 (21.8)
Providing students with experience caring for patients with a variety of clinical conditions	518 (21.7)
Too few clinical hours in the curriculum	466 (19.5)
Lack of opportunities for effective, positive interprofessional teamwork	464 (19.4)
Acuity of patients in the clinical setting	430 (18)
Providing students with experience with culturally diverse client populations	343 (14.4)
Increased number of PRN staff in clinical settings	277 (11.6)
HIPAA restrictions limiting students' access to patient information	140 (5.9)

than 40 percent of respondents. To address this barrier, the most frequent strategies used were 1) substituting simulation activities for clinical hours (high-fidelity simulators, mannequins, role play, videos, case studies to assist students to learn and apply clinical concepts in the context of simulated clinical scenarios), 2) creating other kinds of learning experiences on the clinical unit to replace total patient care, and 3) increasing the number of rotations to observation areas. Again, respondents reported that these strategies were only somewhat effective in addressing the barrier.

Finally, nearly 40 percent of respondents identified how time-consuming it is for students to learn multiple clinical agency systems as a barrier to optimizing students' clinical learning. To address this barrier, respondents reported 1) mandating preclinical orientation sessions to prepare students for the different clinical information systems and other technologies, 2) not allowing students to enter electronic data during their rotation, and 3) decreasing the number of different units/settings to which students rotate to reduce the various clinical information systems and technology students must learn. Respondents reported that mandating pre-clinical orientation and decreasing the number of units to which students rotate to be somewhat effective, while not allowing students to enter electronic data was perceived as minimally effective.

Clinical Teaching Practices

The third part of the survey was designed to learn about respondents' clinical teaching practices. Respondents were asked to think of the course in which they had the most extensive clinical teaching responsibilities during the previous two years, and select the top three activities that typically took most of their time and energy during a clinical day. Table 2-4 lists the 13 activities from which respondents chose. Results shown are the total number of respondents who ranked the activity as one of their top three (6,765) which, again, of necessity exceeds the total number of respondents (2,386).

In addition, respondents were asked whether they designated time for pre- and postclinical conferences and what activities they used to promote students' clinical learning during these times. Only about 33 percent of respondents reported setting aside time to meet with students *individually* prior to the clinical experience. When this preclinical time was used, respondents

Table 2 – 4
Teaching in Clinical Settings

Variable	N (%)
Supervising students' skill performance (e.g., medication administration, IV therapy, wound care)	1636 (68.6)
Assisting students to synthesize clinical information and assessment findings	1164 (48.8)
Questioning students to assess their grasp of their assigned patients' clinical-status	874 (36.6)
Providing feedback to students on clinical paperwork/reports/recording	710 (29.8)
Assuring safety of assigned patients	449 (18.8)
Evaluating students' overall performance	387 (16.2)
Providing feedback to students on their clinical performance	348 (14.6)
Determining students' level of preparation to provide care	314 (13.2)
Rounding on patients assigned to students in clinical group	292 (12.2)
Interacting with clinical agency staff and other health professionals	218 (9.1)
Accessing the clinical information and electronic medical records for students	178 (7.5)
Intervening when conflicts or problems arise among students, staff, and other health professionals	102 (4.3)
Charting by proxy for students in electronic systems they do not have access to	93 (3.9)

indicated they used it to determine the student's level of preparation to provide care, review the status of patients to whom the student would provide care, and review the student's organization and priorities for the experience. When asked if they met with students *as a group* before clinical, nearly 77 percent of respondents indicated that they did. When these meetings occurred, the time was used to review students' organization and priorities for the experience, determine students' level of preparation to provide care, and review the status of patients to whom students would provide care.

Respondents were also queried about meetings with individual students that occurred after the clinical experience. There was a nearly even split between those who did and those who did not conduct postconferences with individual students. Faculty who did have postconferences used the time to discuss the kind of nursing practices the student observed (i.e., decisions nurses made, how nurses interacted with other health care professionals, tasks nurses completed), to conduct reflective activities where the student considered that day's experience in relation to their previous experiences, and to review the skills and procedures the student had completed during the clinical.

Finally, when asked about group postconference, approximately 89 percent of respondents acknowledged having this activity. Faculty used postclinical conferences to discuss the kind of nursing practices students observed (i.e., decisions nurses made, how nurses interacted with other health care professionals, and tasks nurses completed), to have students lead a discussion about the patients for whom they provided care that day, and to have students reflect on their experiences, considering their experience in relation to their previous experiences and that of their peers.

Challenges

In the final section of the survey, respondents were asked to identify the challenges they have faced when teaching in clinical settings during the previous two years. Listed in Table 2-5 are the 29 items from which respondents selected and ranked their five most significant challenges. Results shown are the total number of respondents who ranked the challenge as one of their five most significant (10,916); again, the total number of individual respondents was 2,386.

In the top five challenges faculty respondents faced in teaching in the clinical setting, approximately 50 percent identified providing appropriate guidance and supervision to each student, as well as teaching students to "think on their feet" and make clinical judgments. This challenge far exceeded all others as no other challenge identified was ranked in the top five by more than 30 percent of respondents, and 12 of the listed challenges were identified in the top five by fewer than 10 percent of respondents. In this section, respondents were also asked to select one of the top five challenges they identified and to comment on the single most important strategy they have used to address it.

Strategies for addressing the two most frequently cited challenges included a wide range of approaches. Many faculty described ways they remained accessible to students as a way to deal with the challenge of providing appropriate guidance and supervision to students.

Table 2 – 5
Challenges to Teaching in Clinical Settings

Variable	N (%)
Providing appropriate guidance and supervision to each student	1173 (50.2)
Teaching students to "think on their feet" and make clinical judgments	1147 (49.1)
Providing meaningful feedback to each student	667 (28.6)
Managing clinical teaching responsibilities with other expectations of faculty role	573 (24.5)
Supervising students' skill performance	570 (24.4)
Evaluating students' clinical performance	560 (24)
Students' focus on task completion and skill demonstration	549 (23.5)
Fostering a spirit of inquiry among students while in the clinical setting	542 (23.2)
Matching clinical experiences with classroom content	541 (23.2)
Pressure to have students "ready to hit the ground running"	492 (21.1)
Integrating learning across classroom, clinical, and lab settings	469 (20.1)
Finding ways to avoid too much student "down time"	428 (18.3)
Documenting students' learning via meaningful paperwork or assignments	400 (17.1)
Integrating new technology, such as clinical information systems and electronic health records, into the clinical experience when the school's resource centers do not have this type of system	347 (14.9)
Staying current clinically/Maintaining clinical competence and skills	304 (13)
Monitoring students in multiple agencies or on multiple units at the same time	273 (11.7)
Attending to students' attitudes toward the clinical experience	239 (10.2)
Finding ways to support overburdened staff in the clinical setting	207 (8.9)
Resistance to changing the way clinical experiences are structured	191 (8.2)
Helping students learn strategies for using resources during clinical	189 (8.1)
Fostering integrity in practice	172 (7.4)
Developing and using new models for clinical education	170 (7.3)
Helping students appreciate/understand health care systems issues	150 (6.4)
Helping students appreciate a patient's trajectory across clinical settings (e.g., acute care to home care)	94 (3.9)
Students negatively affecting the productivity of staff in the clinical agency	58 (2.5)
Attending to students' attitudes toward the clinical faculty	50 (2.1)

"I stay very busy, always accessible, stay on the unit at all times, do not take lunch break. Very organized, have lots of 'check-off lists,' ask students lots of questions, major multitasking."

"I have not really found a way to address this [providing appropriate guidance and supervision to students]. I think 10 students in a clinical group are too many, but it isn't the students' fault that I am so busy. I run constantly during the clinical day and do the best I can to teach them."

Similarly, many faculty described ways they addressed the challenge of teaching students to "think on their feet" and make clinical judgments.

"We created clinical forms in which students have to prioritize care and address these priorities. We use different activities in postconference such as concept maps. We have students present interesting cases/experiences during postconferences."

"My students know that they must be able to answer 'why' to everything they do. Some are reluctant to do this at first because they fear they will be wrong. When they realize there is no penalty for thinking, they are more likely to try to figure out the response to my frequent question, 'WHY?' This strategy has helped them develop the ability to think on their feet."

"Make rounds with students, have them do their assessments and then develop their plan for the day."

While an exhaustive analysis of respondents' descriptions of the most important strategies they have used to address the challenges faced in optimizing students' clinical learning is beyond the scope of this chapter, faculty have clearly devised many creative ways to address these challenges. Overall, faculty rated the strategies they described as somewhat to very effective in addressing the challenges of optimizing students' clinical learning.

Discussion and Conclusions

The findings from this study highlight the barriers and challenges faculty face when teaching in prelicensure RN programs. The lack of quality clinical sites and lack of qualified faculty were the most frequent barriers identified by respondents. These findings are noteworthy in light of the persistent demand for schools to admit more students to ease the shortage of nurses nationally. Although faculty reported employing a wide range of strategies to address the barriers they face, most of these strategies were perceived to be only somewhat or minimally effective. These findings support Tanner's contention that the traditional model of clinical education is no longer effective (Tanner, 2006). That is, many of the barriers faced by faculty may not be fixable by merely adopting new strategies, no matter how creative. Substantively new models for clinical education are needed if these barriers and challenges are to be overcome without further straining limited scarce resources (both clinical sites and faculty).

Initiatives that create new partnerships among academia and service and among faculty and staff nurses to better leverage the expertise of each and create learning opportunities that improve clinical education are promising (Connolly & Wilson, 2008; Edgecombe, Gonda, Wotton, & Mason, 1999; McNelis, Jeffries, Hensel, & Anderson, in press; Messina, Steckel, & Voelpel, 2008; Preheim, Casey & Krugman, 2006). Such innovative clinical models may also address the barriers faculty face from restrictions on what students can do in the clinical setting and the challenge of providing appropriate supervision, because students are working directly with staff nurses to provide patient care. In addition, such models may further alleviate other barriers and challenges such as supervising students' skill performance, assuring safety of patients, and learning new documentation systems and technology for multiple agencies. Further development and testing of such models is crucial to the identification of best practices in teaching and learning in clinical settings.

Faculty respondents frequently identified the challenge of supervising students' skill performance and this was the most time-consuming aspect of teaching in clinical settings. Ideally, new clinical models comprised of innovative partnerships among faculty and staff could decrease this burden for faculty, and give them time to focus time and attention on the higher-level cognitive skills that they also ranked as a time-consuming aspect of teaching in clinical settings. Similarly, these new models can assure that the burden of clinical education does not merely shift from faculty to staff nurses, but rather that the expertise of staff and faculty is accessed by students in ways that best support learning without adversely affecting patient care.

More research is needed to identify the critical aspects of students' experiences in clinical settings and the strategies that most effectively support their achievement. In addition, research that assists faculty to differentiate the skills that must be learned in a clinical setting from those that can just as effectively be learned in a simulation lab, virtual clinical experience or classroom is imperative if faculty are to maximize the use of limited clinical sites and their limited time with students.

Finally, despite the numerous barriers and challenges they face, the majority of faculty respondents create opportunities to meet with students as a group before and after each clinical experience to assess students' preparation and to assist them to learn from their experiences through reflection and discussion with peers. They identified many innovative strategies for addressing the challenges they face, including (but not limited to) providing appropriate guidance, teaching students to "think on their feet," and providing students with meaningful feedback. Yet, few of these strategies have been tested and disseminated in the nursing literature. The need to advance the science of nursing education for clinical experiences is imperative to assure future pedagogical decisions are evidence-based and that our educational practices keep pace with the rapidly changing field in which students learn.

References

Ard, N., Rogers, K., & Vinten, S. (2008). Summary of the survey on clinical education in nursing [Headlines from the NLN]. Nursing Education Perspectives, 29, 238-245.

Connolly, M. A., & Wilson, C. J. (2008). Revitalizing academic-service partnerships to resolve nursing faculty shortages. AACN Advanced Critical Care, 19(1), 85-97.

Edgecombe, K., Gonda, J., Wotton, K., & Mason, P. (1999). Dedicated education units: A new concept for clinical teaching and learning. Contemporary Nurse, 8, 166-171.

McNelis, A. M., Jeffries, P. R., Hensel, D. E., & Anderson, M. (in press). Simulation: Integral to clinical education. In N. Ard & T. M. Valiga (Eds.). Clinical nursing education: Current reflections. New York: National League for Nursing.

Messina, B. A. M., Steckel, A., & Voelpel, P. E. (2008). A pilot program for maximizing faculty productivity in the clinical setting. Nursing Education Perspectives, 29, 198-199.

NCSBN (National Council of State Boards of Nursing). (2005). Clinical instruction in prelicensure nursing programs. [Position Paper]. Retrieved from http://www.ncsbn.org/Final_Clinical_Instr_Pre_Nsg_program.pdf

Preheim, G., Casey, K., & Krugman, M. (2006). Clinical scholar model: Providing excellence in clinical supervision of nursing students. Journal for Nurses in Staff Development, 22(1), 15-20.

Tanner, C. A. (2006). The next transformation: Clinical education. [Editorial]. Journal of Nursing Education, 45, 99-100.

3 Chapter

OCNE CLINICAL EDUCATION MODEL

Paula Gubrud, EdD, RN
Mary Schoessler, EdD, RN-BC

There is little doubt that health care has changed dramatically in the last 20 years, yet the teaching practices utilized by nursing education in clinical settings have not been reformed. Challenges to creating optimum learning experiences that emphasize the development of competencies that address today's clinical environment were presented in the landmark Institute of Medicine (IOM) Health Professions Education report (Greiner & Knebel, 2003). In response to changes in practice and to the call for reform in health care education practices, the Oregon Consortium for Nursing Education (OCNE) created a new model of clinical education that completes the competency-based curriculum that is designed to prepare graduate nurses for today's health care environment (Tanner, Gubrud-Howe, & Shores, 2008).

The Oregon Consortium for Nursing Education (OCNE) is a collaboration that includes eight community colleges and the five campuses of the Oregon Health & Science School of Nursing (OHSU). The consortium was created in response to the nursing shortage as a strategy to increase capacity in Oregon's nursing programs (Gubrud-Howe et al., 2003). The shared competency-based curriculum was designed through a multiyear collaborative process in response to the need for a new kind of nurse to care for Oregon's aging and increasingly diverse population (Tanner et al., 2008). Through OCNE, students can complete course work for the Bachelor of Science degree in nursing from OHSU without leaving their home community. After completing a full year of prerequisite courses, when students have completed the first two years of the shared, competency-based curriculum at a partner community college, they may earn an associate degree in nursing and are eligible to sit for the RN licensure examination. Course work and clinical experiences for the full four-year program are available through any campus of the consortium using distance delivery from baccalaureate programs, and by utilizing joint faculty appointments to offer upper division course work.

The shared curriculum is based on a set of core competencies consortium members and practice partners deemed essential to prepare nurses to provide care to individuals, families and communities in health promotion, acute or chronic illness, and at the end of life. Graduates from an OCNE program are skilled in clinical judgment, culturally appropriate and relationship-centered care, systems thinking, leadership, and evidence-based practice. A full description of the OCNE curriculum design process and explanation of courses and infrastructure that supports the consortium can be found in Tanner et al., 2008.

The OCNE curriculum development has included a multiphase project aimed at redesigning clinical education. The OCNE clinical education redesign project seeks to ensure that clinical learning experiences reflect deliberate integration of core OCNE concepts and provides ample opportunity for students to develop in all ten competencies. The purpose of this chapter is to explain the development and implementation of the OCNE Model of Clinical Education, which complements the overall curriculum design.

Background

New approaches to teaching for clinical practice are essential, both for effective education and to strengthen partnerships between faculty and clinical staff. Students need experience that leads to deep understanding of the knowledge, skills and attitudes used when caring for patients across the lifespan. Clinical learning activities should expose students to ill-structured problems and provide ample opportunity to manage clinical problems for patients experiencing prevalent illnesses and diseases (Gaberson & Oermann, 2007; Tanner, 2006). In addition, clinical learning experiences that assure students understand the trajectory of chronic illness and management of end-of-life care are essential. Consequently, the Clinical Education Model Project[1] for the Oregon Consortium for Nursing Education was launched in February 2006. A comprehensive, statewide assessment process confirmed that the predominant current model of clinical education is taxing for faculty, facilities, students, and clinical staff[2] and is increasingly driven by availability of clinical placements, not by experience that correlates with course outcomes or competency development.

As a result of these findings, a Clinical Education Redesign Group (CERG) was formed to develop a comprehensive Clinical Education Model that would span the OCNE curriculum. This 25-member group was equally composed of representatives from academic and service organizations and included faculty from OCNE community colleges and OHSU; staff nurses from acute, long-term care and community settings; and nurse executives. The group met for six all-day sessions and, through facilitated dialogue, developed the OCNE Clinical Education Model, which was then disseminated among faculty on each OCNE campus. The Model was also disseminated among nursing staff, staff developers and nursing executive groups in the clinical agencies represented in CERG for feedback and revision. The revised Model that evolved from this feedback is currently being integrated on all OCNE campuses. Grant funds have been secured[3] to provide for full implementation and evaluation of all elements of the Model on four OCNE campuses. The Model will continue to be refined as collected data is analyzed and the effects of implementation become evident. The Model will also continue to be refined based on findings from the comprehensive evaluation.

The Process — A Comprehensive Strategy

The first two meetings of the Clinical Education Redesign Group (CERG) involved identifying agreed-upon assumptions that would frame the new Model. Assumptions were clarified and validated through an on-line Delphi technique. The Model assumptions appear in Table 3.1. (insert table here)

Using the nominal group process, the group participants spent several sessions studying the literature, discussing traditional and recent innovative clinical activities and brainstorming new possibilities that reflected the assumptions identified. Once the Model was established, each CERG member vetted the Model with her/his colleagues and partners. A statewide summit was then held, and constituents from both academia and health systems were invited. At the Summit, the Model was presented, including exemplars of each Model element. Small group discussions provided feedback on the Model. Based on this feedback, a few refinements were made to provide clarity and enhance the understanding of each element. The OCNE

1 Funded by Northwest Health Foundation and Kaiser Community Fund.
2 Paula Gubrud-Howe, Bonnie Driggers, Christine A. Tanner, Louise Shores, Mary Schoessler, [2007]. [White paper]. OCNE clinical education redesign. Unpublished manuscript.
3 Funded by the Fund for Improvement of Postsecondary Education (FIPSE), U.S. Department of Education.

Table 3 – 1
Assumptions of the OCNE Clinical Education Model

Curriculum Assumptions

The OCNE competencies are integral to the model.

The OCNE curriculum emphasizes highly prevalent conditions across populations and settings, seeking deep understanding of situations most likely to be encountered.

There is variety in the types of clinical learning activities and clinical settings.

Every learning activity has a deliberate intention related to learning and development of competencies. Reflection is a deliberate part of every learning activity.

Pedagogical Assumptions

Learning activities are as close to actual nursing as feasible in order to help students think, feel, and behave like a nurse throughout the curriculum.

Optimal learning is contextual (situated in real nursing practice) and conceptual (includes knowledge, know-how, and ethical comportment of nursing practice) whether in the classroom, lab or clinical setting. The line between classroom and clinical is intentionally blurred to support the blending of contextual with the conceptual learning.

The model moves away from total patient care in an acute care setting as a primary instructional approach to one that uses a variety of learning activities in a variety of settings and includes experiences for advancing clinical judgment and ethical reasoning and comportment.

Learning is enhanced by an environment with support that is appropriate to the level of the student.

Clinical learning experiences are scaffolded. For example, faculty provide support and difficulty regulated to the developmental level of the student so that the level of challenge is optimal.

Partnership Assumptions

A collaborative partnership between the clinical agency and the nursing education program supports learning using shared language and values to enhance communication and relationships.

Optimal learning requires a learning environment with a relationship between staff, faculty, and students in which all are learning together.

Efficient use of student, faculty and staff time and resources is considered in the design of learning activities.

The new model is designed to reduce the workload for faculty and staff of the clinical agencies that are used for student experience.

faculty from each partner school then affirmed the Model. OCNE schools were encouraged to begin integrating the Model as a framework to guide planned and deliberate clinical activities that complement the OCNE curriculum. All OCNE schools have begun to adjust aspects of their clinical education program to correspond to the Model.

Overview of the Model

The OCNE Clinical Education Model challenges traditional thinking about how clinical education is situated in curricula and how it is enacted in the practice setting. The Model moves away from "total patient care" in an acute care setting as the predominate instructional approach to a curriculum that uses a variety of learning activities in multiple settings to focus on advancing clinical judgment and ethical reasoning skills. In the OCNE Model, optimal learning, whether in the classroom, laboratory or clinical setting, is designed to be (a) contextual (i.e., situated in real nursing practice) and (b) conceptual (i.e., focused on knowledge, know-how, and ethical comportment). Within the OCNE curriculum, there is purposeful blurring of lines between the traditional classroom and clinical education in order to most effectively synthesize contextual and conceptual learning. Learning activities that closely mimic actual clinical situations are created in order to help students think, feel, and behave like a nurse throughout the curriculum.

The Model requires thoughtful linking of clinical activities to theoretical course work by creating opportunity for students to fill out and extend their understanding of essential concepts by engaging in a variety of clinical learning activities. The Model is defined by five discrete elements and clinical activity scaffolding is purposively incorporated into the planned clinical experiences over time. Scaffolding involves deliberate consideration of the level of student clinical proficiency in comparison with the complexity and uncertainty of the clinical learning environment. As students demonstrate increasing proficiency in the OCNE competencies, the context of the learning activities are designed to become more complex and patient problems and clinical situations are planned to be increasingly ambiguous and uncertain. Clinical nursing faculty support students' learning at this increased level of difficulty by providing scaffolds. These scaffolds often take the form of coaching, cuing, prompting and expert modeling. As students demonstrate increased confidence and proficiency with increased complex and ambiguous situations the scaffolds are progressively withdrawn through a process called fading (Cope, Cuthbertson, & Stoddard, 2000). The cycle of increasing the complexity and uncertainty of the clinical learning situation, providing scaffolds and then fading, continues until the student has demonstrated abilities required to engage in learning and to respond to situations in the actual patient care environments in a safe and effective manner. All elements of the Model are integrated to assist the students' progression in competency development.

Elements of the Model

The OCNE Clinical Education Model plans and stages learning activities to accomplish course outcomes and takes into account the learning needs and developmental level of the student, as well as the complexity and opportunities available in the learning environment (Gubrud-

Howe & Schoessler, 2008). The following five types of learning experiences are elements of the proposed OCNE Clinical Education Model:

1. **Concept-Based Experiences** are designed to support student learning of pattern recognition. Through multiple encounters with clients experiencing the same problem, students learn to recognize patterns associated with a specific concept, illness, disease or health problem. The patterns related to recognition and treatment of illness/disease and health problems are intentionally uncovered and addressed. The defining characteristic of this element of the Model is that students study the concept or issue at hand through involvement with several clients in an authentic clinical learning environment. Students compare and contrast findings among several individual clients as they collect, organize and analyze assessment data collected in actual clinical situations. Similarities and differences between patients experiencing the same or closely related patient care problems are emphasized through collaborative learning activity such as nursing rounds (Gaberson & Oermann, 2007) and reflective group discussion. The activities are designed to help students understand the normal trajectory of a particular problem and standard treatments with intent to help them notice when the normal trajectory is disrupted. Students function as active participants in collecting and analyzing data, and, although they do not deliver client care, they remain accountable for meeting standards for client safety and for communicating significant observations and findings to the appropriate clinical staff.

2. **Case-Based Experiences** present students with authentic clinical problems they will likely encounter in practice, and they provide for practicing clinical judgment and nursing performance through client case exemplars. Such experiences encompasses seminar discussion of faculty-designed or computer-based cases, as well as a variety of simulations, including use of high-, mid- and low-fidelity environments using human patient simulators, standardized patients, expert modeling and role-playing. Case-based experiences promote the development of clinical reasoning as situations unfold and as students learn to notice both obvious and subtle clinical changes as they interpret findings; consider appropriate responses; communicate with physicians and other providers about their observations and interpretations; and reflect on practice. Clinical, case-based learning activities are often presented using simulation experiences. Simulations include cases involving prevalent and low volume/high stakes clinical problems and also provide opportunities for developing team communication skills, as well as working collaboratively with physicians, pharmacists and other health professionals.

3. **Intervention-Skill-Based Experiences** build proficiency in the "know-how" and "know-why" of nursing practice. Skill-based experiences are usually introduced in the nursing laboratory and often include repetitive practice. Students are provided ample opportunity to rehearse skill performance, because repetition facilitates skill mastery and the development of embodied know-how (Benner, 2004; Ericsson, 2004; Gaberson & Oermann, 2007). These experiences include psychomotor skills, as well as communication, teaching, advocacy, motivational interviewing and health coaching.

Interpersonal skills required for appropriate leadership activity such as delegating and supervising unlicensed assistive personal are included as an intervention-skill experience as students practice these nursing care activities in the laboratory setting.

4. **Direct-Focused Client Care Experiences** enable students to gain experience in providing nursing care and building relationships with patients. "Focused" patient care is different from traditional "total patient care," in that students engage only in activities that will help them achieve course outcomes, which include a developing sense of self as a therapeutic agent. Students learn to notice the salient features of patient care situations through coming to know the client's individual and unique responses to disease, illness and treatment. Students also learn practical knowledge of how care is delivered in the organizational context and how care is structured throughout the client's stay. During focused, direct client care experiences, students may or may not be responsible for all aspects of the client's care, but they are accountable for those aspects pertinent to the learning experience and for clearly communicating relevant information to the client's nurse and other providers. Students are also accountable for communicating with their faculty members regarding their learning about care activities, client assessments and findings.

5. **Integrative Experiences** provide opportunities for students to apply all elements of prior learning in a specific clinical context. Rather than students being assigned to particular clients, they are assigned to work with a registered nurse and provide care to her/his assigned patient with and under her/his direction. Students will also attend in-service education and/or committee meetings along with the registered nurse as the student learns the variety of activities registered nurses participate in in the organization. Characteristics of a good integrative practicum include opportunities for students to practice nursing in an organizational context while experiencing the rules, norms, culture and infrastructure of that nursing setting and synthesizing prior learning. Integrative experiences should be of sufficient length to allow students to become immersed in the clinical setting and include 220 hours for students completing the associate degree. In the final terms of the nursing OCNE program, senior nursing students participate in an Integrative Experience of over 450 hours. This expanded experience allows the student to become fully immersed in the clinical area.

The Model elements of intervention-skill-based, case-based and concept-based activities allow learning activities to be carefully designed to ensure opportunities to learn specified competencies. Rather than relying on unpredictable learning opportunities that may present themselves in clinical agencies, deliberate implementation of each learning activity allows the faculty to control for the competencies and for the level of difficulty that students encounter, thus better matching student developmental level to the level of challenge presented in the learning activity. Students are expected to come prepared to each clinical activity, engage fully in the activity and reflect on it to maximize their learning.

For example, one of the OCNE core competencies is effective communication. As communication strategies are introduced in classroom, intervention-skill-based clinical education activities are introduced to support student learning to employ these strategies in conversation with clients. These strategies continue to be refined through cased-based simulation and experiences with patients that involve direct-focused care activities. When students are introduced to strategies to improve communication in the interprofessional team, they again practice these strategies in intervention-skill-based activities and cased-based simulation and extend that learning through direct-focused care and integrative experience as they practice calling a physician for orders and participating in a family care conference. Through careful consideration, faculty connect the Model element with learning outcomes, location in the curriculum and student developmental level. As in OCNE courses, learning activities that illustrate essential characteristics of each element are "spiraled" to link concepts and growth in complexity and difficulty. The curriculum is planned so students are periodically placed in clinical learning experiences that expose them to competencies that they have previously encountered. Students are accountable for previous learning and are expected to fill out and extend their proficiency in each competency as they progress through the curriculum. The deliberate exposure to the competencies multiple times throughout the curriculum and within increasingly complex situations is called "spiraling" (Harden & Stamper, 1999).

In addition to changing the nature of the learning experience, the Model reflects OCNE's emphasis on highly prevalent conditions (such as diabetes and congestive heart failure) across populations and settings, rather than a traditional list of diseases to be studied. New clinical sites, such as neighborhoods, therefore, are identified and developed. Collaborative partnerships among clinical agencies, communities, and nursing education programs support learning using shared language and values to enhance communication and relationships. For example, while schools of nursing teach students about evidence-based practice and clinical agencies employ evidence in developing standards and practice guidelines, nursing staff may not quickly or easily equate a student's question about what evidence the staff nurse is using to support a practice decision with the facilities practice guidelines. Working with nursing staff to make the link between their practices and the student's question mitigates the potential for disruption caused by a simple question. Partners share responsibilities for student learning, faculty and staff development, and the creation and maintenance of nurturing learning environments in which staff, faculty and students learn together. Efficient use of student, faculty and staff time and resources are considered in the design of learning activities to reduce workload and enhance learning outcomes, and interdisciplinary learning is encouraged.

Curricular Considerations — Application of the Five Elements

To apply these five elements of learning experiences in a meaningful way, consideration is given to the curriculum design and goals, as well as to the students' formation of nursing knowledge, skill and ethical comportment. For early experiences, the *Concept-Based, Intervention-Skill-Based*, and *Case-Based Experiences* provide building blocks that facilitate students' abilities required for *Direct-Focused Client Care Experiences*. Learning activities may be a reflection of just one element, but more often represent a blending of more than one of the five elements (see Figure 3.1).

In later courses, the relationship among the elements of the Model shifts to reflect students' ongoing development. When students have developed a larger store of knowledge and skill, the emphasis on *Direct-Focused Client Care Experiences* increases. Other elements of the Model continue to play a role, with *Case-Based Experiences* complementing *Direct-Focused Client Care Experiences*. Since there is more knowledge and skill to integrate, *Integrative Experiences* are extended (see Figure 3.2).

In the final courses, *Direct-Focused Client Care* and *Integrative Experience* merge. Since there is more knowledge and skill to integrate as students near program completion, the *Integrative Experience* is increasingly emphasized, with only periodic use of *Concept-Based* and *Case-Based Experiences* as needed to complete development of competencies that extend beyond direct patient care (e.g., interdisciplinary teamwork). (See Figure 3.3.)

Role Clarification

The OCNE Clinical Education Model relies on a learner-centered approach to clinical learning. Early in the development of the Model, the CERG group recognized the importance of clear delineation of roles for each element of the Model in order to promote collaborative interactions and the creation of optimum, learner-centered environments that assure students focus on learning while engaged in clinical activity. Consequently, an accountability matrix was

Figure 3 – 1
OCNE CLINICAL MODEL FOR EARLY PROGRAM CLINICAL LEARNING EXPERIENCES

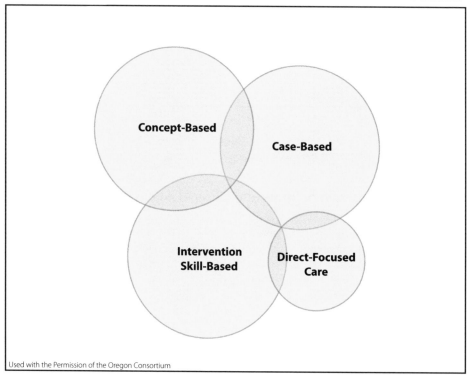

Used with the Permission of the Oregon Consortium

Figure 3 – 2
OCNE CLINICAL MODEL FOR MID-PROGRAM CLINICAL LEARNING EXPERIENCES

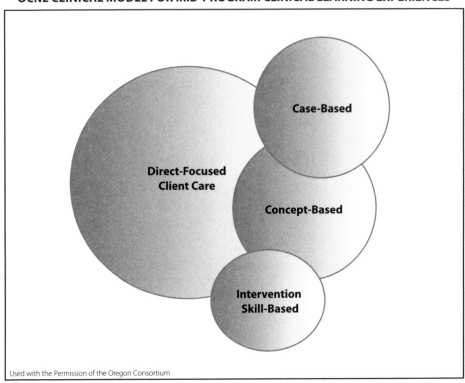

Used with the Permission of the Oregon Consortium

developed to confirm agreed-upon expectations for faculty, students, and clinical staff. This accountability matrix, designed to promote a learning community, is summarized in Table 3.2.

Partnerships Between Schools and Clinical Agencies

The OCNE Clinical Education Model recognizes and accounts for the critical role that clinical agencies play in the education of students and the importance of preparing students to act as nursing professionals employing the full range of nursing competencies in the world of practice. The roles of clinical partners vary within each element of the Model and are influenced by the learning goals for groups of students; for example, clinical partners assume more accountability for teaching and coaching as the student approaches independent practice in the final courses. Clinical partners retain accountability for developing and maintaining a health work environment that facilitates staff, faculty and student learning, and schools engage those clinical partners in discussions of how the Model can be most effectively implemented and evaluated. Finally, clinical agencies are encouraged (by the Consortium) to link orientation and new graduate programs to the Clinical Education Model as a way to enhance the transition of those individuals into the world of practice and foster their continuing learning and development.

Figure 3 – 3
OCNE CLINICAL MODEL FOR LATE PROGRAM CLINICAL LEARNING EXPERIENCES

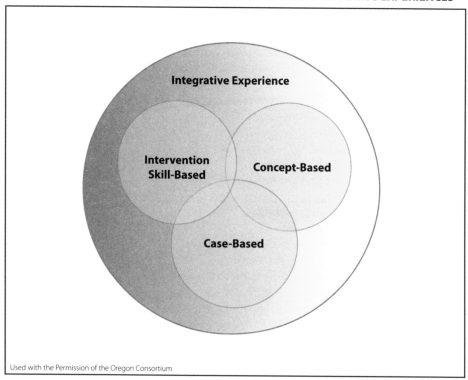

Used with the Permission of the Oregon Consortium

OCNE Demonstration Projects

During the development of the Model, six demonstration projects were funded to explore and test the effectiveness of the new clinical education activities. The projects were directed at designing and implementing case-based and concept-based clinical education, developing new roles for clinical staff mentors, and developing partnerships among academic and clinical agencies. Each project was designed by an academic-practice partnership between either a community college or university partner and one or more clinical agencies. The projects were selected from a variety of sites across the state of Oregon. Clinical agencies included acute care hospitals, skilled nursing facilities, community agencies and neighborhood associations. A brief description of and findings from each of these six demonstration projects is provided.

Community-Based Health Promotion Experiences Across the Lifespan were completed at Lane Community College. This community-based health promotion project was a *Concept-Based* activity that placed students in nontraditional clinical settings in the community. Learning resources (such as self-preparation guides, expectations of the student, and post-experience reflections) were developed and implemented. Individual learning was extended through weekly group discussions, facilitated by nursing faculty so that individual student learning

Table 3 – 2A
Accountability Matrix

Nursing Faculty: Minimum Expectations
- Faculty introduce nursing students to the clinical site and provide the support and functions consistent with the type of learning activity (direct-focused client care, case-based learning, concept-based learning, integrative experience, integrative practicum).
- Faculty are responsible for the design of clinical learning activities.
- Faculty demonstrate knowledge of the clinical facility.
- Faculty initiate and maintain an open dialogue with unit staff and managers regarding the plan and execution of the students clinical experience.
- Promote a climate conducive to learning
- Demonstrate collegial approaches to patient care

Nursing Students: Minimum Expectations
- Prepare for the learning activity
- Are present at the beginning of the learning activity
- Communicate learning needs to faculty and/or care staff
- Communicate to faculty and nursing staff about client safety and condition
- Are fully engaged in all clinical learning activities
- Engage in relationship-centered care
- Reflect on experience to discover and enhance learning related to OCNE competencies
- Engage in ongoing self-reflection and evaluation
- Promote a climate conducive to learning
- Demonstrate collegial approaches to patient care

Clinical Nursing Staff and Management Team: Minimum Expectations
- Seek clarity about the purpose of the student experience
- Communicate with students and faculty within the context of the learning activity
- Welcome the students into the clinical environment
- Provide ongoing formative evaluation and feedback to students and faculty
- Maintain accountability for the patient/client
- Promote a climate conducive to learning
- Demonstrate collegial approaches to patient care

Table 3 – 2B
Accountability Matrix Role Expectations

MODEL ELEMENT	STUDENT ROLE/EXPECTATIONS	FACULTY ROLE/EXPECTATIONS	STAFF NURSE ROLE/EXPECTATIONS
CONCEPT-BASED	Focus on learning expected to use resources to examine the concept(s) being studied prior to learning experience. Responsible for prior learning and ability to construct deeper understanding of the concept. Student is not accountable for delivering care with this type of experience; accountability remains for meeting standards for patient safety and communication of significant observations and findings.	Likely to be on-site with students during learning activity. Communicate expectations regarding student role/activity with staff. Seek feedback from staff regarding effect of student presence and on work flow and patient care. Assure all patient findings related to safety and significant findings are communicated effectively. Provide formative and summative evaluations to students.	Assists faculty in identifying appropriate patients for students learning encounters. Dialogues with students regarding patient problems, assessment findings, plan of care. Retains responsibility for care and assessment of patient conditions and full responsibility for implementing plan of care.
CASE-BASED	Focus on learning expected to use resources to examine the case(s) being studied prior to learning experience. Responsible for prior learning and ability to deepen learning through exploration of the client case.	Guide student exploration of the client case through written, computer or simulated experience. Coach student throughout the case-based experience. Provide formative and summative evaluations to students.	
INTERVENTION-SKILL-BASED	Focus on learning expected to use resources to examine the skill(s) being studied prior to learning experience. Responsible for prior learning and ability to deepen learning and achieve skill proficiency through repetitive practice of the skill.	Coach student throughout the intervention-skill-based experience. Provide formative and summative evaluations to students.	When in the clinical setting, coaches student in skill performance and deepening understanding of the rationale for the skill and practical knowledge.

Used with the Permission of the Oregon Consortium

Table 3 – 2B Accountability Matrix Role Expectations (continued)

MODEL ELEMENT	STUDENT ROLE/EXPECTATIONS	FACULTY ROLE/EXPECTATIONS	STAFF NURSE ROLE/EXPECTATIONS
DIRECT-FOCUSED CLIENT CARE	Applies course outcomes to the pursuit of specific learning activities. Prepares for experience prior to time on assigned unit or agency by studying the specific client (see definition of client in CERG Clinical Model document) prior to the learning experience. Also responsible for rehearsing possible previously mastered interventions and skills that may be performed. Student is responsible for care s/he provides to client. Evaluates own proficiency. Documents client record as directed by faculty. Accountable for patient safety and communicating client assessment findings and the responses to interventions.	Are on site with students during entire period of learning activity. Orient self and student to unit and familiarize self with work flow and unit culture. Assure student assignments for client care are congruent with student proficiency. Assure the student and the nurse assigned to client communicate with each other regarding implementation of the patient's plan of care. Facilitate development of students clinical judgment through coaching, mentoring, cuing. Supervise performance of skills on clients as defined by school and agency policy. In collaboration with staff, may delegate supervision of skills to licensed nurse on unit. Seek staff nurse feedback regarding students performance. Provide summative and formative feedback to students.	Is accountable for all aspects of assuring plan of care is fully implemented, including assessing client and responses to treatment. Assures patient care documentation is complete and accurate. Communicates with student and faculty to assure there is clear understanding regarding care student will be providing. Promotes an environment of learning and offers coaching, prompting, and cuing regarding client condition and problem solving. Offers feedback regarding student performance. May supervise student delivery of psychomotor skills when mutually agreed upon by staff nurse and faculty.
INTEGRATED EXPERIENCE WITHIN OCNE CLINICAL COURSE	Student integrates full set of OCNE competencies into the delivery of client care as appropriate for their level. Assumes responsibility for client care assignment designated by faculty. Client care assignment may be provided by staff nurse if faculty delegates the responsibility. Works closely as a member	Supervision is likely on site throughout the period of learning activity. If faculty are not present during entire period of time students are with clients, frequent site visits are expected. Routine, frequent and extensive time will be spent coaching, cuing, observing and assessing student's performance. Assist student	Works closely with the student as member of the team. Client care assignments are discussed and staff nurse may assume primary role in assigning client care responsibility. Using a collaborative approach with the faculty, staff assumes more oversight of care provided by student and also retains

Table 3 – 2B Accountability Matrix Role Expectations (continued)

MODEL ELEMENT	STUDENT ROLE/EXPECTATIONS	FACULTY ROLE/EXPECTATIONS	STAFF NURSE ROLE/EXPECTATIONS
INTEGRATED EXPERIENCE WITHIN OCNE CLINICAL COURSE (continued)	of the team in collaboration with nurse assigned to clients and as a part of the unit. May participate in facility organizational experiences such as patient care conferences, in-services, unit meetings.	with assuming role of the nurse through instructional strategies. Emphasize helping students organize and prioritize care, and focus on assisting students to integrate the full set of competencies into their client care activity. Retain responsibility for assuring student assignments are congruent with student level and proficiency. Role expectations described in Direct-Focused Client Care are in play.	all accountability and role expectations described in Direct-Focused Client Care.
INTEGRATED EXPERIENCE INTEGRATED PRACTICUM	Assumes roles as defined in the OCNE Guidelines for the Integrative Practicum Including Faculty, Student and Clinical Teaching Associate Roles & Responsibilities document. Student integrates full set of OCNE competencies into the delivery of client care. Assumes responsibility for client care assignment designated by Clinical Teaching Associate (CTA). Works closely as a member of the team in collaboration with CTA assigned to clients and as a part of the unit. May participate in facility organizational experiences such as patient care conferences, in-services, unit meetings.	Assume roles as defined in the OCNE Guidelines for the Integrative Practicum Including Faculty, Student and Clinical Teaching Associate Roles & Responsibilities document. Supervision is off site and includes frequent scheduled visits that emphasize interacting with the student and CTA. Are available for consultation by phone at all times. Faculty role emphasizes coaching and mentoring CTA and facilitating communication between the student and nurse to promote learning. Faculty responsible for formative and summative evaluation and assigning course grade.	Assumes roles as defined in the OCNE Guidelines for the Integrative Practicum Including Faculty, Student and Clinical Teaching Associate Roles & Responsibilities document. Works closely with student and is accountable for client/patient care, but works closely with the student as the student assumes progressive responsibility for all aspects of care. Evaluation of student is a shared responsibility to include faculty, student and CTA.

Used with the Permission of the Oregon Consortium

could be highlighted and shared among the student group with the faculty drawing out critical aspects of the concept among patient population groups. Because of the clinical sites selected (e.g., Women, Infants, and Children nutrition programs, yoga classes, water therapy sessions, and Head Start programs), students had the opportunity to experience a variety of health promotion activities in several different population groups. Post-experience surveys (78% return rate) of these clinical experiences were overwhelmingly positive. Students approached the experience not simply as a task to complete, but as a learning experience to explore, and they reported feeling more engaged and motivated to learn and share their new understandings with each other. At the conclusion of this project, written materials (including a guide for faculty considering similar clinical experiences) were packaged and made available to other OCNE schools.

The *Concept-Based Clinical Learning Activities* project was done at Lane Community College. This project partnered *Concept-Based* learning activities with *Direct-Focused Client Care*, two of the elements of the OCNE Clinical Education Model. First-year students prepared for and completed a *Concept-Based* learning activity such as impaired oxygenation or skin integrity with clients on an acute care unit during the first clinical day. This activity involved collecting data on each patient, completing a focused assessment and analyzing findings. The clinical day concluded with a comprehensive seminar that was facilitated by the faculty. Students were encouraged to compare and contrast their findings and note patterns common among the clients.

Deviations from expected patterns were uncovered and the faculty helped students notice the salient issues that were of concern. On the second clinical day, the students participated in a *Direct-Focused Client Care* experience with one or two of the clients they had studied the day before. This allowed students to first study critical concepts through evaluating the concept across a group of clients, then to further explore the concept and related nursing care activities during the day of focused direct client care. Students and faculty both reported that students were better prepared for the direct care experience because of the extensive preparation day, and faculty reported feeling less burdened by the preclinical work typically associated with prepping themselves and students for direct care activities. Findings from this project confirm one of the assumptions of the Clinical Education Model — that refocusing how clinical education is done can decrease the burden on faculty while improving student learning. Faculty involved with this project created a trifold flyer describing the new Clinical Education Model and the goal for the learning activities, and they shared this flyer with nursing staff on the day students arrived on the nursing unit. The flyer, coupled with a brief verbal explanation, helped the nursing staff understand what was to be accomplished and what their role would be in the experience. Nursing staff reported satisfaction with this method of communication and increasing comfort working with students on the unit.

Nurse Supervision Skills Development, undertaken at Mount Hood Community College, designed and tested a leadership development activity. This *Concept-Based* learning activity included three components: working alongside a charge nurse in a skilled nursing facility; collecting data for a quality improvement activity at the facility; and making patient assignments for a group of nursing staff through a simulated exercise in which the student needed to evaluate client need, match client need to staff qualifications and expertise, and adjust the assignment as circumstances changed throughout the simulation. The project demonstrated that students were able to meet the OCNE competencies in leadership and contributions to the broader health care system, appreciated the effectiveness of different leadership styles, gained a deeper understanding of the role of staff in promoting and delivering quality care, and experienced some of the challenges inherent in the leadership role. A faculty guidebook with student exercises, faculty hints, and evaluation strategies was developed for use by other OCNE schools.

Preparation of Nursing Staff and Their Units for OCNE Students in Clinical Settings, orchestrated by Oregon Health Science University School of Nursing (OHSU), explored strategies to develop a learning environment on an acute care nursing unit that would support students in the OCNE curriculum. Through use of video, printed materials and hi-fidelity simulation, nursing staff on the study unit were introduced to key aspects of the OCNE curriculum and the Clinical Education Model, specifically *Concept-Based* learning. The pilot project supported development of healthy and sustainable partnerships between OHSU nursing faculty and hospital nursing management team members. In addition, surveys of nursing staff demonstrated the positive impact of the activities on staff nurse understanding and excitement for the OCNE Clinical Education Model. As the project progressed, members of nursing management and the clinical staff stepped forward to take the lead in the activities they found particularly interesting. The result was a strong leadership team and the strengthening of working relationships that have outlasted the project itself. Post-intervention, managers, faculty, staff and students have appreciated a more positive learning environment on the study unit.

Preparing Nurses to Assist Patients with Chronic Illness was done at Southwest Oregon Community College/Bay Area Hospital, and surrounding area hospitals. This project illustrated the *Concept-Based and Direct-Focused Client Care* elements of the Model and involved the identification and preparation of nurse mentors in community agencies to support beginning level students engaging with clients in home settings. Students interviewed clients about health and illness issues to understand these conditions as the client experienced them. Students learned about the difficulty accessing resources in rural settings; explored differences in client experiences interacting with the health care team; and prepared and delivered health education for their clients. Sustained contact with clients allowed students to evaluate the outcomes of their teaching. At the conclusion of the experiences, which occurred over the course of the term, students could speak to and give examples of having addressed all OCNE competencies in the course. Nursing faculty noted that students were able to apply their learning to subsequent courses occurring later in the curriculum, such as acute care, as they developed discharge education materials for clients in the acute care setting that addressed discharge issues and health care management in the home setting. In addition to the expected outcomes, students gained insight into the lives of individuals living in poverty and with chronic illnesses and came to appreciate the profound impact of poverty on access to health resources, on an individual's ability to comply with therapy and participate in activities such as traveling across town for a physician appointment. Students expressed a new understanding of the decisions made by persons they had before only seen in an acute care setting. This project also demonstrated the effectiveness of involvement of clinical staff as student mentors, thus extending the faculty role and opening more nontraditional clinical sites in the community.

The *Neighborhood Clinical Experience Model*, done at Oregon Health Science University, School of Nursing, Portland Campus, integrated the *Concept-Based* and *Direct-Focused Client Care* elements of the OCNE Clinical Education Model. Under the direction of course faculty, students developed partnerships with community agencies in the southwest Portland neighborhood, participating in several different population-based health activities, such as Loaves and Fishes, local middle schools, and neighborhood associations. In addition to focusing on student learning related to OCNE competencies, this pilot study demonstrated the feasibility of creating and sustaining long-term relationships with community partners and the efficacy of clinical placements in a nontraditional home health setting. Students had the opportunity to experience clients living in communities outside health care settings, identify resource gaps, and explore the health of populations as well as the health status of individuals. During this experience, students expressed new insights about the isolation of the elderly in the community and appreciated their role in persuading and supporting, but not making health care decisions for, their clients. The neighborhoods were welcoming to the students; however, the Model requires that faculty be willing to engage in a long-term relationship with the neighborhood agencies and ensure consistency of contact while the students come and go over time.

Developing Staff Nurse Mentors— Clinical Teaching Associate Education

In addition to the six funded demonstration projects, OCNE has developed and offered education for staff nurse mentors for the *Integrative Experience*[4]. Staff nurses who serve as nurse mentors are referred to as Clinical Teaching Associates (CTA) in the OCNE curriculum. CTAs attend a one-day workshop to learn about the OCNE curriculum and the Clinical Education Model. They are also introduced to fundamental Model concepts including: the partnership between clinical agencies and academic institutions, the role of the CTA, how to coach for clinical judgment and integrate evidence-based practice, how to provide feedback to students and faculty, and how to create an environment where everyone thrives. These workshops have been well received by participants, and preliminary experience has demonstrated that CTAs are assuming their role as partners in the mentoring of OCNE students with enthusiasm and skill. It is clear that the preparation and support of staff as nurse mentors serves to enhance collaborative partnerships between clinical agencies and academic institutions, which are essential to the success of the new Clinical Education Model.

Next Steps

The next phase of the Model involves full implementation, which will include a systematic and comprehensive evaluation. Fortunately, OCNE has secured a grant through the Robert Wood Johnson (RWJ) Foundation and the Fund for Improvement of Postsecondary Education (FIPSE). The implementation and evaluation phase involves four of the 13 OCNE partner campuses. Two of the campuses include community college partners and two of the OHSU campuses are

---

4 Sponsored by the Ford Family Foundation.

participating. This phase begins in the 2009-10 academic year and will involve a four-year study. The implementation includes development of several measurement instruments and faculty representing each of the four OCNE campuses will refine previously used learning activities. New activities will be designed to assure students have opportunity to develop proficiency in each of the ten OCNE competencies.

Conclusion

The OCNE Clinical Education Model fundamentally changes the way we approach clinical education. Through deliberate sequencing of the five elements into the curriculum, the level of difficulty and challenge presented in the activity can be matched to the level of the student and to course outcomes. Faculty can ensure that certain experiences are always available through simulation and concept-based learning activities. In addition, as students progress through the curriculum, beginning with structured and directed clinical learning activity, faculty can help students learn how to maximize learning from unstructured practice experiences. Through partnerships with clinical agencies and communities, faculty can ensure that students have appropriate opportunities to learn about prevalent populations and health conditions, as well as have a positive influence on the health of individuals, communities, and the organizations in which they learn. Preliminary findings suggest such outcomes are occurring as a result of more deliberately planned clinical learning experiences.

The demonstration projects described here clearly illustrate that the Model is already enhancing both student and clinical staff learning. The projects also illustrate how faculty energy and commitment needed to design and sustain new clinical models can be affected in a positive way. Finally, findings from the pilot projects will shape the design and implementation of the comprehensive OCNE clinical education curriculum.

It is clear that students, faculty and clinical staff need information and support to assume new roles. Students are not always pleased to venture into new learning experiences, and designing new experiences takes a considerable amount of faculty time and creativity. It also is clear that clinical staff must be willing to engage with students and faculty in new ways, and agencies must offer support to their staff to do so. Despite these challenges, however, the OCNE Clinical Education Model continues to be successful. Each demonstration project generates enthusiasm for new learning activities as students, faculty and staff realize the benefits of learning together. Through careful implementation and study, OCNE intends to amass a significant evidence base for the Model, continue to refine and enhance the Model, and view it as an ongoing work in progress.

References

Benner, P. (2004). Using the Dreyfus model of skill acquisition to describe and interpret skill acquisition and clinical judgment in nursing practice and education. *Bulletin of Science, Technology & Society, 24*(3), 188-199.

Cope, P., Cuthbertson, P., Stoddard, B. (2000). Situated learning in the practice placement. *Journal of Advanced Nursing, 31*(4), 850-856.

Ericsson, A. K. (2004). Deliberate practice and the acquisition and maintenance of expert performance in medicine and related domains. *Academic Medicine, 79*(10), S70-S81.

Gaberson, K. B., & Oermann, M. H. (2007). *Clinical teaching strategies in nursing* (2nd ed.). New York: Springer Publishing.

Greiner, A. C., & Knebel, E. (Eds.). (2003). *Health professions education.* Washington, DC: Institute of Medicine, National Academies Press.

Gubrud-Howe, P., Shaver, K., Tanner, C., Bennett-Stillmaker, J., Davidson, S. B., Flaherty-Robb, M., et al. (2003). A challenge to meet the future: Nursing education in Oregon, 2010. *Journal of Nursing Education, 42*, 163-167.

Gubrud-Howe, P., & Schoessler, M. (2008). From random access opportunity to a clinical education curriculum. *Journal of Nursing Education, 47*, 3-4.

Harden R. M., & Stamper, N. (1999). *What is a spiral curriculum? Medical Teacher, 21*(2), 141-143.

Tanner, C. A. (2006). The next transformation: Clinical education. *Journal of Nursing Education, 45*, 99-100.

Tanner, C. A., Gubrud-Howe, P., & Shores, L. (2008). The Oregon Consortium for Nursing Education: A response to the nursing shortage. *Policy, Politics and Nursing Practice, 9*(3), 203-209.

Chapter 4

INNOVATIVE APPROACH TO CLINICAL EDUCATION: DEDICATED EDUCATION UNITS

Joanne Rains Warner, DNS, RN
Susan Randles Moscato, EdD, RN

As nurse educators, we are challenged with the mandate to produce more competent nurses; at the same time, we are limited by certain resources, such as clinical space and faculty shortages. High patient acuity, increasingly complex knowledge work, and nurse burnout also complicate our challenges. Meeting these challenges today requires new thought. Together with our clinical partners, we decided now was an excellent opportunity to look past our time-honored norms and think collaboratively in new ways to create our own preferred future.

The Dedicated Education Unit (DEU) clinical teaching model arose out of two competing issues impacting nursing — the need to increase enrollment and the need to make the best use of the available nursing workforce. These issues were turned into mandates by the Oregon Center for Nursing, a consortium of statewide nursing leadership, whose forward thinking was among the first to develop strategic plans to deal with the nursing shortage (ONLC, 2001).

This chapter tells the story of the University of Portland School of Nursing's innovative clinical teaching model, the DEU. We have used the DEU concept since 2003 and have found it to be a successful way to bridge the gap between academe and service. It uses the diploma education model of long-term student mentoring by expert nurses, and it connects working nurses with the scholarly characteristics of the university. In essence, the DEU concept, developed out of need, embodies best practices and thrives in partnership.

Definition

A DEU is a client unit that is developed into an optimal teaching/learning environment through the collaborative efforts of nurses, management, students, and faculty. Its purpose is to provide students with a positive clinical learning environment that maximizes the achievement of student learning outcomes, uses evidence-based teaching/learning strategies, and capitalizes on the expertise of both clinicians and faculty. Adapted from the clinical education model at Flinders University in Australia, the DEU reorganizes the roles of nurses and academic faculty to increase both the quantity and quality of faculty supervision and mentoring experiences that are available to students and to increase the capacity of the nursing education system (Moscato, Miller, Logsdon, Weinberg & Chorpenning, 2007).

In the DEU model, practicing nurses, not university faculty, are the primary teachers of the students. Selected, oriented, state board-approved staff nurses become clinical instructors (CI) and participate in the education of students as part of their normal work routine. Staff nurses who serve as DEU clinical instructors are prepared for their teaching role through a one-day workshop at the University of Portland, during which they learn about the concept of the DEU, review the curriculum, understand the program outcomes, and practice effective teaching strategies. Afterwards, two student nurses of the same preparation level are assigned to work with each staff nurse/CI for an entire 6-week rotation, a faculty-to-student ratio well below the Oregon State Board of Nursing (OSBN) 1:8 ratio requirement. This increased ratio and consistency of relationship allow the students and clinical instructor to develop an ongoing mentoring relationship. Participants have reported that because the CIs become familiar with the abilities and development of each student, they are able to provide students with more opportunities to practice their nursing skills and use critical thinking in real clinical situations. In addition, daily contact provides greater opportunity for students to improve and for instructors to intervene when performance problems are discovered. In a DEU model, university faculty are no longer directly responsible for the day-to-day supervision of students; instead, academic faculty focus on coaching the clinical instructors to increase their clinical teaching skills.

All staff on a DEU commit to putting teaching first and making workplace adjustments in staffing, scheduling, and time allocation to achieve the teaching goal. Partnership with one school of nursing, ongoing relationships with clinical faculty coordinators, and commitment to collaborative problem-solving are components that make the DEU concept highly successful. In this model, the work group or unit becomes a "village" working together and contributing talents to support student learning. Not all nurses on the unit serve as CIs, but all contribute their own special talents and skills to support the learning environment. Anecdotal evidence from the DEUs shows that secretaries, physicians, physical therapists, clergy and other personnel embody this village spirit and contribute to the pride and identity of an optimal teaching environment.

Describing Our DEUs

The first DEUs were opened in two different medical centers in 2003. Because of staff interest, Chief Nursing Officer (CNO) requests and opportunity, the number of our DEUs has grown to seven acute-care units in three medical centers:

- Providence Portland Medical Center — 8S (neuro) and 5G (medical)
- Providence St. Vincent Medical Center — 9E (neuro), 9E Tower (med/surg), and 9W (ortho)
- Portland VA Medical Center — 6D (med/oncology) and 5C (psych)

Each DEU has 24-26 beds, and on a typical DEU shift, there are three CIs working in triads with six students (the 1:2 ratio mentioned above). For some DEUs, students are on the clinical unit both day and evening shifts: other units have students on day and night 12 hour shifts. The placement of the student on shifts other than days depends on the needs of the unit, the student learning goals and the interest and qualifications of the CIs on that unit.

Students complete a minimum of one-third, and up to one-half, of their clinical practice hours on DEUs. In fact, for most students, all of their medical-surgical experience occurs on a DEU, which has had a significant impact on the school's clinical teaching capacity. Before implementing the DEU model in 2002, 227 University of Portland students had clinical rotations on 14 medical-surgical units in these three agencies. Six years later, the number of students placed in clinical rotations at these three agencies has increased to 388 and only six medical-surgical DEUs are used. More than 1,050 students have graduated from the program since we began using the DEU model, and the overall mean first-time NCLEX pass rate of the 2005, 2006, 2007 and 2008 graduates is 95 percent.

DEUs are extremely versatile and can be developed in any care setting. Colleagues in New Zealand and Australia have DEUs in clinics and community health centers. Indeed, an entire hospital can be a DEU. We have continued to explore with our clinical partners the development of additional DEUs, especially in non-acute-care settings. Currently, a DEU is being developed in a long-term care facility that is staffed by a number of our graduates who remember the value of their own DEU experience and who want to serve in the CI role with students.

Creating a DEU

Creating a DEU is a choice that involves multiple layers in both the academic and service organizations. Understanding the concept and agreeing to its tenets (see Table 4.1) at each level are key components of successful DEU operation in health care facilities. For example, nurse administrators are called upon to provide vision and support for a new way to meet professional obligations to educate students. Our development efforts have received unwavering support from administrative nurse leaders in Oregon, despite the cost implications, because they believe this is an appropriate way for nurses to contribute to the future of our profession and because they see the potential benefits of a robust pool of competent graduates.

In several instances, nurse administrators have opened new units with the DEU design; in others, existing units have been targeted and asked to consider adopting the DEU model. Administrative support is needed for flexible budgeting, unit-controlled staffing, and release

Table 4 – 1
Tenets of the Dedicated Education Unit

- Exclusive use of the DEU by one school of nursing

- Efficiency of model requires fewer units of clinical instruction for the school

- Clinically expert staff nurses as the primary clinical instructors of the students

- Clinically expert staff nurses who want to teach are oriented to clinical teaching role

- Continuity of students with clinical instructor over the length of the clinical rotation

- Patient assignment for staff nurses when they are teaching varies with skill level of students

- Students may be placed around the clock

- Use of faculty expertise as educators to support the development and comfort of the CIs in the teaching role

- Commitment of all parties to work together to build an optimal learning environment and cultivate mutual respect for each other's skills and knowledge

Source: Moscato, Miller, Logsdon, Weinberg, & Chorpenning, 2007.

time to participate in the CI training. The increased success with recruitment, increased professionalism, and increased staff satisfaction and retention has rewarded administrative support. In addition, each of our three partnering clinical facilities has earned Magnet designation, and in each case the DEUs were cited for commendation by the reviewers. Many nursing indicators for Magnet hospitals (e.g., job satisfaction, low staff turnover, strong leadership, collaborative problem-solving, and an emphasis on advanced training and education) are outcomes promoted by the DEU concept, so partnering institutions are able to achieve two valuable goals — Magnet status and quality patient care — through the design and implementation of DEUs.

Support for the DEU concept at the nurse manager level is also essential. Nurse managers serve a key role in providing the framework and support for developing the unit culture that supports the DEU's optimal teaching/learning environment, and they serve as role models for the collaboration that makes the model work. DEUs benefit from nurse managers who are strong leaders, create healthy working relationships with their staff, and commit actively to quality care. A unique feature of the DEU model is that each unit develops its own character and style of operation. Thus, as DEU model concepts are applied to match the culture of the unit, staff have a sense of ownership as they design their own DEU within the parameters of the clinical teaching/learning model. The nurse manager works in collaboration with the university's clinical faculty coordinator (CFC) to develop the positive clinical learning environment that maximizes the achievement of student learning outcomes, uses evidence-based teaching/learning strategies, and capitalizes on the expertise of both the clinicians and faculty in alignment with the model's intent.

In some cases, nurse managers have been asked by their administrators to open DEUs. In others, nurse managers, on behalf of their staff, have requested that their units be developed into DEUs. The work of developing the DEU is collaborative between the university and the agency/unit, since designation as a DEU comes with the expectation that there will be strong "buy-in" to the concept on the part of management and staff. Thus, planning sessions, relationship-building, orientation to the concept, pilot launch rotations, summative and formative evaluation, and continuous and ongoing communication are all important strategies in the development of a DEU.

One nurse manager intentionally applied his knowledge of change theory as he led his unit through the development phase. He knew the transition of becoming a DEU meant change in the practice, culture, environment, and organization of his unit, and he worked collaboratively with the nurses on the unit to create such change. He credits the early adapter, innovator registered nurses who facilitated change as the key to initial success, and his continued attention to each of the change areas noted above (Weinberg & Moscato, 2006) ensures ongoing success.

When a unit decides to become a DEU, the nurse manager recruits and/or hires baccalaureate-prepared nurses who want to assume the role of clinical instructor. Existing units that convert to the DEU model already employ nurses with varying levels of advanced training and varying willingness to be part of a DEU. In these instances, nurse managers then identify staff nurses who are interested in teaching and willing to take on the added responsibility of orienting themselves to and serving in the CI role. The other unit nurses who are not CIs are mentored by the nurse manager and the CFC regarding ways in which they can provide support for the CI and lend their valuable expertise or special skills to the learning environment.

The university provides a one-day orientation for new CIs to prepare them for the teaching role. During this program, the dean welcomes them to the faculty and provides a university overview, and the associate dean and various faculty present the curriculum, our clinical reasoning tool and paperwork, and the DEU model. Those preparing to be CIs also receive a clinical teaching handbook that provides guidance on important issues like establishing student relationships, asking higher order questions, dealing with overwhelmed students, and empowering the student as learner (Kaakinen, 2007). CIs learn best practices in clinical teaching through a faculty-created DVD entitled Clinical Faculty Development Scenarios, and after viewing and discussing the DVD, they participate in a clinical teaching simulation scenario during which student nurses are used as actors scripted to make errors at the bedside. This creative use of simulation produces positive results as these staff nurses explore their role in clinical instruction (Krautscheid, Kaakinen & Warner, 2008). All materials used in the orientation and further information on the Clinical Faculty Development Scenarios and Teaching Guide are available on our school's website (http://nursing.up.edu/).

A value-added feature of the DEU is the inclusion of all health care disciplines in the clinical learning of nursing students. Physicians, social workers, occupational and physical therapists, pharmacists, and chaplains learn that the DEU is a teaching place, and they incorporate the students and their CIs in rounds, activities, and communications. For example, physicians learn to expect SBARR (Situation-Background-Assessment-Recommendation-Repeat) style calls from students, stroke rounds include reports from students as the primary care providers for their clients, social workers consult with students for discharge plans, and students are included as members of interdisciplinary teams on a DEU psychiatric unit.

Start-Up Costs and Needed Resources

Any model of clinical teaching requires financial and human resources. Developing and sustaining the DEU model, in our experience, does not require more resources, but it does call for rethinking, reorganizing, and reallocating existing resources. The main categories of resources, discussed below, are human, financial, and partnership infrastructure.

Human resources include the staff nurses, faculty, and a university-based advocate or DEU coordinator. Staff nurses are already employed by the hospitals to provide nursing care to patients, but their role is reframed to also include serving as a clinical instructor to two students for a six-week interval. Such reframing gives fuller expression of their professionalism through role modeling, mentoring and teaching, and it is embraced by the staff nurses. Teaching two students has been reported to be manageable within the clinical responsibilities of the RNs. By utilizing the staff nurses' current clinical expertise and experience in the pursuit of student learning, the university bears less of a burden in clinical faculty recruitment and hiring, especially important in an era of faculty shortage. The academic faculty also have an opportunity to reframe their role to coach, support, and mentor the staff nurse CIs, thereby easing the issue of supply since fewer academic faculty are needed in the CFC role. The university does need to designate a DEU coordinator or advocate to provide oversight as to the quality and processes involved in the teaching/learning and partnerships, and we have found that a senior faculty member who can adeptly represent the university in partnership conversations best serves in this role. The CFC is not expected to be on the unit at all times students are there, but is available electronically at all times.

The financial efficiency of this model is seen through the CFC to student ratio, as well as the CFC to CI ratio. In the traditional model, faculty to student ratio is mandated by state regulation and is usually 1:8. Our state regulation was modified to allow a faculty to student ratio of 1:24 for those working in a DEU environment, thus a CFC to CI ratio can be 1:12. But the efficacy of the model is seen at the bedside where the typical CI to student ratio is 1:2 in a consistent relationship over the length of the entire clinical rotation. The finances of a DEU align closely with the human resources. Salaries of the clinical instructors are paid by the hospital. Hospitals also pay for release time for the CIs' orientation and development, and they also provide supplemental pay (an additional $1.25/hour), which is what preceptors had been being paid. In general, the staff costs for the DEUs are higher at the beginning of the rotation when students' learning curves are steep, CIs need to be trained, and the relationship is being established. Staffing costs are found to decrease, however, as the collaboration progresses and the students' abilities expand. Hospital managers have reported that these fluctuations "balance out the bottom line."

Our university pays the salary of the CFCs and the DEU coordinator. The university also provides CIs with adjunct faculty privileges, most of which involve a modest cost: for example, reduced cost athletic tickets, continuing education related to clinical teaching skills (our Lunch and Learn program), health and wellness appreciation activities, quarterly meeting expenses, and orientation sessions. University personnel also provide scholarly mentoring to hospital nurses in the form of assistance in preparing abstracts, refining presentations, and critiquing articles for publication.

In the university budget, the nursing dean calculates and includes the replacement cost of CIs so that our budget reflects the true cost of the education of the nursing students. The hospitals are credited with in-kind contribution to the school at year's end and given appreciation for their contribution to the partnership. This budget tactic positions the school with resources to reallocate if the DEU model needs to be altered.

The most unique resources that are required involve building and sustaining the partnership infrastructure to align multiple agencies, sites, and missions. While hospitals and schools both are concerned with promoting health, they operate with different schedules, budgets, cultures, and reward systems. Thus, success of the DEU model hinges on resource allocation of both tangible and intangible rewards. Tangible rewards include items like promotional cups, T-shirts and bags, but they also include more creative things like appreciation activities, seated-chair massages brought to the staff units, meals for the CI development activities "Lunch and Learn," and remembrances on special days and at the end of each school year. Our university hosts a quarterly dinner meeting, including a healthy menu and wine, for senior hospital administration, nurse managers, university deans, and faculty. The 25 people who attend this dinner/meeting enjoy networking and jointly shaping the partnership, and participants see it as a visible marker of our collaboration and commitment to the DEU, as well as a recurring thank-you to those involved.

The intangible rewards that people contribute to the DEU model are similar to those features that sustain any partnership: patience; commitment to clear, transparent communication; an ability to see the long view; respect for the unique expertise, contribution, and demands of each partner; and buy-in on the shared vision. It is these traits that have carried our partnership over the academic-service gap, mission differences, and busy demands of professional nursing. With these, and all the resources discussed above, we conclude that our return on investment is worth every expense of time, money and human effort.

Successes And Challenges

Evaluating the outcomes of an innovative clinical teaching model is a political and scholarly challenge. First of all, the "black box" of clinical learning is a challenge to understand. In addition, the DEUs themselves have many stakeholders as well as unique characteristics and intangibles that are difficult to measure and quantify. We can, however, present the successful outcomes and the accompanying challenges that are emerging from our formative and summative evaluations as well as the lived experience of the past six years. Those outcomes include the impact of the DEU model on student enrollment and teaching capacity, faculty work-life and satisfaction, and nurse recruitment and retention.

As a result of the clinical placements and CIs on the DEUs, we have tripled our school's enrollment in the last five years. More importantly, our graduation rate has quadrupled, with 2009 seeing just under 200 individuals eligible to sit for the licensing exam. Our first-time NCLEX pass rates continue be at 95 percent. We have an increased number of clinical placements per core university faculty member, a lower overall faculty-to-student ratio, and higher student satisfaction with their clinical education.

Our partnering DEU clinical facilities are all credentialed by the American Nurses Credentialing Center (ANCC) and have received Magnet designation. In all cases, the Magnet evaluation visitors cited the DEUs for commendation when they awarded this esteemed designation. In addition, our clinical partners have reported increased DEU staff retention, enhanced recruitment to these units, and a shorter orientation time that translates into cost savings. We now have clinical instructors we are calling second-generation DEU, staff nurses who learned as student nurses on the DEU and who are now delighted to complete the cycle and give back to the profession through this clinical teaching.

Early on, we noticed a change in the professionalism of the staff nurses. The CIs showed a greater involvement in their clinical unit, and they showed the use of creative student-centered teaching strategies. Interestingly, nurses who had vowed they would never return to school were seeking certification, upgrading their clinical knowledge, and sometimes actually returning to school for another degree. We saw so many CIs being recruited and taking their DEU knowledge, experiences, and passions to new positions within the organization that we coined the phrase positive turnover to describe what was happening. The agencies, of course, see this as a plus.

Nurse managers have described the DEU model as cost-neutral. We found that most units had one extra RN on duty at the beginning of each rotation, and RNs serving as CIs had to put one day into their training orientation, but these costs are being more than recovered by lower orientation costs for resulting new hires and lower attrition rates.

The close, collaborative and committed relationships with our clinical partners are a significant part of the success of the model. These service colleagues give the university feedback and suggestions about curricular changes through several communication venues: our quarterly meetings, representation on our curriculum committee, or informal conversations between CIs and CFCs. In turn, the university brings new documents and resources to the clinical units through our scholarly experiences. The partnership, therefore, creates a win-win for all.

There is one key challenge: communication. The model requires clear, consistent, and transparent communication and continual nurturing at all levels. We find the model design and implementation also needs continual nurturance, modification, and enlivenment. When key players at any of the organizations change, information about background, history, abiding assumptions, and shared commitment needs to be provided or updated. One effective strategy is the development of partnership assumptions that are jointly written, reviewed and revised periodically (University of Portland, 2009).

We are being challenged now to think of applying the DEU model on other than medical-surgical and psychiatric nursing units, and we are challenged to create cooperative relationships within our community to share resources. Initially, when other local nursing schools heard that the model allowed students from only one school of nursing to participate in a facility's DEUs, we were accused of "aggressive hoarding." We needed to explain the purpose of the design and how by using existing resources differently, we were actually making more clinical units available for their use. Fortunately, our fellow schools of nursing understand, and are now developing DEUs with their close clinical partners. The sharing of clinical units in specialties beyond medical-surgical requires more delicate negotiations among all schools seeking clinical placements, because of the scarcity of those units. We are committed to the ethical sharing of our community resources, and not merely meeting our own needs.

The successes as reported from both the service and academic perspectives have outweighed the challenges in our DEU implementation and maintenance. All partners contribute resources, all receive their unique benefits, and all are committed to the success of this transformative model of clinical nursing education.

Research Questions

Two desired outcomes of the DEU model are to expand teaching capacity and improve clinical education. Preliminary findings suggest improvements in available clinical placements; increased satisfaction of students, nurses, and faculty; and perceived improvement in educational outcomes. Interest in the DEU continues to grow, and a number of schools around the United States and internationally have begun to implement the model.

Rigorous evaluation has been a challenge. For those involved in the development and implementation of DEUs for nursing students, the benefits of this approach seem obvious. However, the extent to which the intended benefits of DEUs have been realized has been difficult to quantify, as have the costs associated with making the transition to this clinical education model. Both benefits and costs are distributed across multiple organizations, each of which must weigh these factors in deciding whether to expand or contract their participation in traditional or DEU approaches to clinical placements. In addition, like many sites involved in the development of a new program, the available DEU sites were not built with the intention of creating the conditions necessary for a rigorous evaluation of the effectiveness of the DEU approach.

Recently, a feasibility study was conducted to a) clarify the research questions that should be the focus of such an evaluation, b) identify data sources and research design features that could be used to address these questions, and c) make recommendations about the most appropriate and cost-effective approach to conducting evaluation research that would provide useful knowledge about the effectiveness of the DEU approach. The results helped us identify questions of interest to our DEU partners as a whole, as well as questions that are important to individual partners. These evaluation questions explore the value of the DEU model along four lines of inquiry: a) nurse education system capacity; b) perceptions and outcomes for DEU participants (i.e., students, clinical instructors, and nurse managers); c) effectiveness in preparing students for nursing careers; and d) implementation, sustainability, and replication considerations. A multisite evaluation plan has been developed that will use qualitative and quantitative data to compare teaching capacity and productivity, faculty work-life satisfaction, and the quality of the clinical learning environment of DEUs and traditional clinical education placement systems. We are currently negotiating the funding needed to conduct the study.

Conclusion: Encouragement Toward Innovation

What is the risk of innovating? How can we achieve different outcomes by continuing to use the same processes and models? What does it take to change nimbly within the intractable cultures of academe and health care delivery? The story of the DEU at the University of Portland in collaboration with its clinical partners is a tribute to the courage of innovation and several other factors.

First, the academic leadership embodied a feisty and bold sense of confidence in something new. University faculty are generally prone to resist change by waving the "quality flag," especially in nursing, where the stakes of human safety are so high. Yet with a constant eye to quality improvement, innovation is possible and, frankly, requisite in today's environment. With the backing of a dean who was willing to see less-than-perfect pilot projects that would be refined for the next round, faculty were emboldened to step out.

A campus administration that admired innovation also fueled the DEU efforts. Then and now, the provost cherishes the model for the way it softens our hiring needs, aids our salary budget line, and produces quality student outcomes.

Innovation is encouraged when a partnership built out of mutual respect can be pursued, ensuring that everyone benefits. When we refer to the advantages of the model, we often describe a win-win-win situation, meaning the multiple agencies, individual nurses and faculty, our student learners, and the patients who are recipients of our nursing care all benefit. Efforts to assure that all participants reap benefits support and sustain innovation.

A spirit of innovation becomes contagious, and innovation begets more innovation. Our faculty feel the successes of prior risks and then dare to try others. We are marching off into new applications of simulation, creating another DVD to equip our CIs for best practice in clinical teaching, considering a DEU in long-term care, and developing new and interesting Lunch and Learn topics and teaching strategies.

Within our program and nursing community, the DEU model of clinical teaching has been a fitting solution to several challenges. It was born in the spirit of innovation and developed out of our need for expanded clinical placements and more clinical faculty. It utilizes best practices in clinical and didactic teaching, and it thrives under the continual nurturing of strong, respectful partnerships between service and education.

References

Kaakinen, J. R. (2007). *Clinical teaching handbook for the faculty instructor.* Unpublished manuscript, University of Portland, Oregon.

Krautscheid, L., Kaakinen, J., & Warner, J. R. (2008). Clinical Nurse Leader faculty development: Using simulation to demonstrate and practice clinical teaching. *Journal of Nursing Education, 47,* 431-434.

Moscato, S., Miller, J., Logsdon, K., Weinberg, S., & Chorpenning, L. (2007). Dedicated Education Unit: An innovative clinical partner education model. *Nursing Outlook, 55*(1), 31-37.

Oregon Nursing Leadership Council [ONLC]. (2001). *ONLC strategic plan: Solutions to Oregon's nursing shortage.* Portland, OR: Author.

University of Portland (2009). *Assumptions about Dedicated Educational Units.* Unpublished manuscript, University of Portland, Oregon.

Weinberg, S., & Moscato, S. (2006, June 19-21). *Dedicated Education Unit: Partnering education and practice.* Podium presentation at Bridging Education and Practice, 8th Annual Nursing Education Institute Conference at OHSU: Portland, Oregon.

REFLECTIONS ON CLINICAL EDUCATION: INSIGHTS FROM THE CARNEGIE STUDY[1]

Lisa Day, PhD, CNS
Patricia Benner, PhD, RN, FAAN
Molly Sutphen, PhD, RN
Vickie Leonard, PhD, RN, FNP

1 This Chapter draws heavily from the forthcoming book: Benner, P., Sutphen, M., Leonard-Kahn, V., & Day, L. (in press). *Educating nurses: A call for radical transformation*. San Francisco: Jossey-Bass and The Carnegie Foundation for the Advancement of Teaching.

Introduction

The Carnegie Foundation for the Advancement of Teaching is completing an ambitious program of research, entitled Preparation for the Professions, that includes comprehensive national studies of the education of the following five professions: clergy, engineering, law, medicine, and nursing. This large program of research is a comparative study of professional education that also seeks to examine and recover civic professionalism in response to current threats to professional work organization and ethics (Sullivan, 2004). One hundred years after the highly influential Flexner Report (1910) — which called for increased education in basic sciences and increased standardization of medical curricula and which influenced the education of all professions, including nursing, even though it focused on medical education — the time is again right to examine professional education (Benner & Sutphen, 2007; Shulman, 2004; Sullivan, 2004).

Current research on the education of practitioners for professional fields (Dunne, 1997; Dunne, 2004; Eraut, 1994; Grossman & McDonald, 2008; Shulman 2004; Sullivan, 2004; Sullivan & Rosin, 2008) has raised new lines of inquiry about teaching and learning a professional practice. As part of the Carnegie Foundation for the Advancement of Teaching's Preparation for the Professions series, the National Study of Nursing Education was designed as a comprehensive evaluation of the state of nursing education in the United States using multiple methods, including interpretive ethnography (Benner, 1994a) and web-based surveys. The site visits to each of the nine schools of nursing that had been selected for in-depth study were designed using general guidelines and data collection instruments taken from the earlier Carnegie for the Advancement of Teaching Professional Studies (clergy, engineering, and law) with adaptations and additional interview questions designed specifically for nursing. The nursing schools were chosen to represent excellence in teaching, based on the receipt of teaching awards from the National League for Nursing and/or the American Association of Colleges of Nursing, or by reputation from within state organizations, standing of the school by national and by state reputation. Each type of program offering prelicensure nursing education was represented — bachelor's degree, accelerated bachelor's degree, master's entry, associate degree, and diploma education — as were different geographical locations in the United States. The medicine and nursing studies were conducted simultaneously and in dialogue with joint visits to two universities that offered both medical and nursing education.

The purposes of the Preparation for the Professions study were to determine the signature pedagogies of professional education, compare and contrast educational methods across professions, determine how to educate for both competence and integrity, and determine best practices for imparting professional judgment and teaching complex skills. Because the nursing study is embedded in the larger comparative project, some of the methods were dictated by previously completed studies in order to develop comparisons across the professions. However, each study was also shaped by discipline-specific concerns and the nature of the particular professional practice (Benner, Sutphen, Leonard-Kahn, & Day, in press).

Teaching and learning in each of the apprenticeships identified in previous studies (i.e., cognitive, practical, and ethical) were explored during visits to the participating schools through interviews, observations, and document review. Based on the analyses of these site visit data, the nursing research team developed and pilot-tested three web-based surveys for faculty and students, all of which focused on teaching and learning. One of the faculty surveys was done in collaboration with the National League for Nursing (Carnegie-NLN Survey), another was done in collaboration with the American Association of Colleges of Nursing (Carnegie-AACN Survey), and the student survey was undertaken collaboratively with the National Student Nurses Association (Carnegie-NSNA Survey). Each survey was sent via email to all members of the particular collaborating organization, and the questions on each were designed to help the researchers confirm or disconfirm site visit findings. Faculty members and students were asked about the educational effectiveness of their programs, pedagogies used most often, challenges and rewards of nursing education, and school-to-work transition experiences. The National Study of Nursing Education (i.e., the site visits, two faculty surveys, and one survey of students) resulted in recommendations for revisions of the current system to better prepare student nurses for contemporary nursing practice. In this chapter, we describe the demands of nursing practice and discuss ways current clinical education does and does not address the preparation of new nurses to confront these demands. We end by suggesting four shifts in nursing education we think are necessary in order adequately to prepare nurses for professional practice.

Demands Of Professional Nursing Practice: Practical Reasoning

"Critical thinking" has become the predominant understanding of good nursing. To be a good nurse means one is able to think critically. Sullivan and Rosin (2008) note that the critical thinking agenda in higher education seeks to help students disengage from context-bound, concrete knowledge to what is considered a "higher" form of knowledge that is explicit, formal, operational, and more abstract and general:

> Virtually all educational programs to develop critical thinking imagine their aim as teaching students to abstract general rules from specific contexts and thereby to inculcate the priority of analytical over concrete or intuitive thinking. This agenda overlooks the embodied, often tacit knowledge present in skillful judgment. Knowledge is reduced to formal or representational modes exclusively" (Sullivan & Rosin, 2008, pp. 99-100).

Nurse educators' use of "critical thinking" as an umbrella term may be a way they have adapted to comply with this higher education mandate. By placing all forms of thinking under this one label, whatever they teach meets the requirement to teach "critical thinking." But the strategy of combining all kinds of thinking under the rubric of critical thinking unwittingly overlooks the multiple ways of thinking actually required of nurses. In addition to formal analytical thinking, such as diagnostic rule-in/rule-out strategies and identifying when to apply standard guidelines to a practice situation, nurses use multiple forms of critical, creative, and imaginative thinking.

Nursing practice requires relational skills, skills of involvement, technical skills, problem-solving, teaching, and communication with people from a wide range of cultures, education and socioeconomic backgrounds, and who have multiple points of entry to health care. Thinking critically about these issues is important for nurses. But most importantly, because nursing, like all professional practice disciplines, requires practitioners to use their knowledge in practice situations, nurses must use practical reasoning in real time.

Nurses are required to think flexibly, depending on the demands of the situation, and to appraise the current situation based on experiences with past, similar situations. Thus, situated cognition — thinking about the particular in a real-time changing context, reasoning through changes in the patient's condition or concerns and/or changes in one's own understanding of the patient's clinical condition or concerns, and responding based on past, similar experiences — is an essential form of practical clinical reasoning for nurses. Situated cognition in nursing has also been described as reasoning-through-transitions or through changes across time as situations unfold, which requires familiarity with what is common as well as involvement in the situation and attentiveness to the particular (Benner, 1994b; Benner, Hooper-Kyriakidis & Stannard, 2000; Taylor, 1993). This kind of thinking is essential to nursing practice and is not captured adequately by the term "critical thinking."

Clinical reasoning is a form of situated cognition and, like all types of practical reasoning, demands engagement in the patient's situation in order to yield necessary knowledge that the abstract, detached analysis used in critical thinking cannot. For example, nurses monitor and respond to the patient's evolving condition and adjust therapies based on an interpretation of the patient's physiologic responses. To respond appropriately to these demands, the nurse might draw on abstract, decontextualized knowledge from such fields as theoretical science, mathematics or philosophy, but also, and most importantly, must be able to engage in situated cognition and exercise clinical reasoning through transitions over time as the patient's situation and condition changes.

Demands of Nursing Education: Formation of Professional Nurses

As noted, nursing education needs to teach for practical reasoning. Unfortunately, academia holds a hierarchical view of knowledge, such that abstract knowledge of theoretical science, mathematics and philosophy is highly valued while the knowledge of the technical and applied disciplines is devalued. The Carnegie studies of professional education call for a change from this emphasis on abstract and formal knowledge to broader academic agendas that also focus on formation, social learning, and practical reasoning, all of which are required for adequate education in any practice discipline (see Foster, Dahill, Golemon, & Tolentino, 2005; Sheppard, Macatangay, Colby, Sullivan & Shulman; 2008; Sullivan 2004; Sullivan & Rosin, 2008; Sullivan, Colby, Wegner, Bond, & Shulman, 2007).

All the Carnegie Foundation studies of professional education (Cooke, Irby, & O'Brien, in press; Foster et al., 2005; Sullivan et al., 2007; Sheppard et al., 2008) were framed by an understanding of what Carnegie scholars call the "professional apprenticeships" that all professional education should provide. The first apprenticeship in the Carnegie framework is the *cognitive*; that is, the theoretical knowledge base required for practice that occurs in all learning settings, but is typically the focus of classroom teaching. In nursing, this knowledge base is broad and encompasses natural sciences, social sciences, and the humanities. The second apprenticeship is the *practical*: the skilled know-how required for competent clinical practice. In nursing, this typically takes place in clinical settings and skills labs. The third apprenticeship is the *ethical*: the inculcation, infusion or instantiation of the responsibilities, concerns and commitments of the profession that show up in what we call the professional's "ethical comportment."

By "apprenticeship" is meant the embodied, skillful, cognitive, and ethical experiential learning that takes place as part of the preparation required for any complex practice discipline. Apprenticeship does not mean "on-the-job training" or learning that occurs only in actual clinical settings, nor does it refer to the historical apprenticeship model of learning that characterized diploma school education that existed until the early 1970s, before nursing moved into the academy. In the older hospital training programs, students provided the major portion of care to patients. The hospital nursing administrator directed the school and relied on students to work; students were seen not as engaged in a program of education, but primarily as an extra pair of working hands. In the service-driven diploma programs of forty years ago, classroom instruction and planned, tutored clinical experiences were in short supply and subordinated to hospital service demands for an inexpensive, and relatively unskilled, labor pool to care for patients.

Apprenticeship should also not be misconstrued as a contrast to simulation as in "on-the-job training," since simulation and actual experience in ambiguous, open-ended real clinical situations are both necessary as formative and clinical practice pedagogical strategies for nurses. The pedagogy of simulated clinical experiences used in the classroom or skills lab — when done well — is an enactment and integration of all three apprenticeships and, therefore, represents quality teaching.

While the framework for professional education is articulated as a three-fold apprenticeship, it is important to emphasize that when the apprenticeships are taught separately or in isolation from one another, it is very difficult to help students integrate them in their practice. In the best educational practices observed during this study, the three apprenticeships were intertwined and taught in integrative ways.

The Cognitive Apprenticeship: Learning to Think Like a Nurse

The cognitive apprenticeship consists of theoretical and factual content. It is where the cognitive and conceptual training occur that enables students to think in ways typical of and important to the profession; for instance, learning how to "think like a nurse." Subjects in the cognitive apprenticeship for nursing include microbiology; the interpretation of laboratory results; the ways in which culture and health practices intersect; or the influences of family and community on individuals' illness experiences.

Nurses need a rich educational background in many areas. In addition to general liberal arts education, they need education in natural sciences, social sciences, and humanities that are specifically relevant to nursing practice. For example, student nurses need good communication skills for writing, speaking and listening. They must master reflective and interpretive skills in order to identify changes in patient and family needs, clinical conditions and concerns. Training in syntax and grammar is crucial to educating nurses who can communicate effectively with patients and other members of the health care team as well as create institutional directives and contribute to shaping policy on all levels.

Beyond abstract facts and theories learned in isolation, however, nurses must be able to use their knowledge in particular practice situations and according to particular patient care concerns, demands, resources and constraints. Thus, even classroom teaching, to be effective, must approach theories, facts and concepts in terms of their relevance to patients and clinical situations. As Barab and Roth (2006, p. 3) argue,

> When educators fail to engage students in meaningful relations and instead impart core ideas as isolated facts or abstract concepts, these facts and concepts are no longer connected to the situations that allow them to be powerful tools in the world. The core disciplinary formalisms (facts, concepts, practices, methods, principles) run the likely risk of becoming disembodied and effectively disconnected from any meaningful use in the world.

The ability to reason through changes in a particular patient's condition is a core skill for nurses. Such situated use of knowledge is an essential feature of the cognitive apprenticeship, and the integration of knowledge for the sake of practice must be accomplished in classroom teaching as well as clinical teaching. This is true in schools of nursing and in continuing education for practicing nurses, since a field like nursing, whose research and knowledge base are expanding exponentially, requires even seasoned, expert professionals to continually develop and update the knowledge they use in practice (Benner, Tanner, & Chesla, 2009; Malloch & Porter-O'Grady, 2006). This is an ethical mandate of many professions, including nursing: those who practice must stay engaged in the cognitive apprenticeship throughout their professional lives.

The background in natural sciences relevant to nursing practice has grown more complex, and in many ways nursing education programs have not kept pace with these changes. In order to practice competently, today's nurses require a sophisticated understanding of chemistry, microbiology, physics, and genetics. But to be most effective these areas of study must be made relevant to nursing practice. Clinically focused and upgraded science teaching and learning in nursing draws on natural science fields in ways different from what nursing education required a decade ago.

For example, nurses need clinically focused learning in normal physiology and pathophysiology, particularly in the interactions of living human systems. Many therapeutic interventions that nurses deliver and manage require that they be able to draw on knowledge of acid-base balance, electrolytes and solutions, and biochemical cascades like inflammation, coagulation and fibrinolysis. Another example is cellular energy production and its use in living systems, which is an essential area of chemistry that typically is not taught at the level necessary for nurses in basic, general education chemistry classes. It is no longer sufficient for nurses to have a basic understanding of gas exchange in the lungs; they must also gain knowledge in integrated, clinically relevant physics in order to understand respiratory dynamics and gas exchange at the cellular level. Essential for nurses practicing in acute care and many home and community settings is a solid knowledge of microbiology, human-pathogen interactions, appropriate use of antibiotics, and the worldwide problem of antibiotic resistance.

Nurses must now know more about the interpretation of laboratory findings than simply normal and abnormal ranges. Nurses are expected to practice safely and effectively in administering an increasing array of pharmaceuticals, many of which must be carefully monitored and titrated, and that are often prescribed for unlabeled or investigational uses. Nursing practice in the 21st century requires a sophisticated knowledge of pharmacokinetics and pharmacodynamics that requires nursing students to do more than memorize lists of drugs, possible side effects, and simple teaching points. For practice in all clinical units of the acute care hospital, nurses must be better prepared to administer, monitor and evaluate a wide range of pharmaceutical therapies.

On the horizon lies the increased use of genomic medicine. In order to follow the ongoing research on both genetic markers and gene therapies for multifactorial diseases, nursing students will need to have a background understanding of the basic scientific knowledge of medically relevant genomics. As genomics becomes more prevalent in everyday health care, there will be an increasing need for dedicated, well-educated genetic counselors. But nurses will need to be prepared to provide patient education for informed consent, assist patients to engage in self-care, and convey the goals and risks of genetic therapies for patients with chronic illnesses. As medicine begins to use research from genomics, such as adjusting and tailoring medications to a particular patient's genetic profile, nurses will be expected to have at least a general understanding of the field of pharmacogenomics. Other topics in human genomics will also be increasingly important for nurses to learn, since they will be called upon to offer patient education about genetics related to diseases, alterations at birth, and later life onset diseases that have multiple genetic markers.

Of equal importance to the natural sciences in nursing are the social sciences and humanities. Because nurses must do extensive patient and family teaching and work with a variety of health care team members, they must be able to articulate practical clinical knowledge and what they have learned from their practice and from caring for particular patients. This requires that nurses be able to elicit and interpret patient illness narratives (stories of illness) as well as formal medical histories of injury and disease. To this end, nurses require skills of social interpretation, understanding of the social contexts of disease and illness, and good written and oral communication skills in order to grasp and use narratives of patient-family illness experiences and concerns. A narrative understanding is also essential for the patient's experience of care. Patients who feel known, whose stories inform the care they receive from nurses, experience better care than those who feel objectified and unknown (Benner & Wrubel, 1989). In addition, nurses need to learn how to make a clinical case to their physician colleagues by synthesizing patient and family information from many different sources and reporting changes in or concerns about the patient's condition in ways that convey the relative urgency of the situation.

In sum, the introduction to natural science, social science, and humanities that students typically get in prerequisite courses is no longer adequate to prepare new nurses to understand and respond appropriately to the complex health and illness phenomena they will encounter in practice. General education classes in areas like anatomy, physiology, psychology, philosophy and history are necessary but not sufficient. Nursing students need rigorous training in these fields that is specific to their practice. Bringing rigorous sciences and humanities to classroom, clinical, and skills lab settings in schools of nursing will call for collaboration between nursing faculty and teachers of other disciplines. For example, we see great value in a philosophy professor co-teaching an advanced medical-surgical nursing class; or a scholar of history co-teaching a class in public health nursing.

The Apprenticeship of Skilled Know-How and Clinical Judgment

The second apprenticeship encompasses the ways that students are inducted into the practice of the discipline. In this apprenticeship, students are taught how to integrate the theoretical knowledge gained in the classroom into the real-world practice setting. In the apprenticeship of skilled know-how, students learn to "read" a patient's condition over time; manage time and resources; know what the pathophysiology of chronic obstructive pulmonary disease, for example, actually looks like in a patient; and learn technical skills such as inserting a urinary catheter on an actual patient who needs one. In this apprenticeship, students also learn relational and communication skills required for providing patient care and for being effective health care team members; for example, learning "to make a case" to professional colleagues on behalf of a patient.

Most clinical nursing practice requires a flexible and nuanced ability to interpret a not-yet-defined practice situation as an instance of something salient that should call forth an appropriate response. Once a clinical situation is understood or grasped by the student, the teacher must then guide that student toward recognizing the relevant research, possible interventions, and other possibilities available in the particular situation. How does the student nurse come to recognize possible good and less-than-optimal ends in actual clinical situations? The teacher must help the student see both the medical and nursing implications of a situation, the latter always requiring an understanding of the pathophysiological and diagnostic aspects of the patient's clinical presentation and disease, as well as an understanding of how best to strengthen the patient's own physical, social and spiritual recovery resources.

In the process of learning the skills required for a complex practice such as nursing, students must be allowed to try out aspects of the practice in safe and directed ways. At the same time, it is important that students also be allowed to feel the burden of what is at stake in the practice: the health, well-being and safety of a patient, family, and/or community. As part of their clinical education, novices are expected to act like nurses before they feel like they are nurses. On the way to fully embodying and internalizing the practice, students will ultimately be required to shift from detachment and "acting like" a nurse to being and responding like a nurse in a real situation.

The requirements of the skills-based apprenticeship speak to the need for solid, high quality clinical experiences that are integral to nursing education. Simulated situations are useful and even essential, but simulations actually feel "real" only in isolated moments during the exercise. No matter how seriously they are enacted, the players in a simulation always know that the risks are confined to their own performance and do not really impact the actor patient or high-tech manikin. In clinical settings, students grasp what is at stake for both nurse and patient as they learn how to respond practically and ethically to errors.

The Apprenticeship of Ethical Comportment and Professional Values

This apprenticeship involves the appropriation and elaboration of the commitments, concerns and values required for ethical comportment. It is through the ethical apprenticeship that the novice is introduced to the meaning of a practice that integrates all the dimensions of the profession in the service of achieving the "goods" defined by the practice. Nurses need a good grasp of everyday ethical comportment (e.g., responding to a patient's needs with attentiveness and respect) as well as ethical decision making and problem solving skills for dealing with situations of breakdown or disagreement. Nurses need critical reflective skills to discern ethical dilemmas and injustices created by inept or incompetent health care providers, by an inequitable health care delivery system, or by the competing claims of family members and/or other members of the health care team. What the study of clergy education (Foster et al., 2005) came to call "formation" describes the integration of the three apprenticeships. That is the common end in clergy education and all professional education, including nursing.

Ethical comportment in everyday nursing care provides the basic structure upon which all of practice is built. To this end, nurses need to learn nursing practice ethics and develop moral imagination from their practice and everyday relational ethics and the ethics of care and responsibility as well as a range of ethical theories that will enable them to cope with difficult ethical problems or quandaries. These problems include high-profile dilemmas as well as less conspicuous problems of "everyday ethics," such as substandard care. As the research team observed students in clinical settings working with patients and in postclinical conferences describing their care, we were particularly struck by the compelling narratives of care they provided that were suffused with ethical concerns. Yet students did not describe these concerns as "ethics"; they described their concerns and the resulting actions as nursing, underscoring how thoroughly nurses ground their practice in the ethical. Nurses in all health care settings also face cultural level ethical problems such as the impact of violence on health; environmental injustice; pollution; and the socioeconomic, racial or ethnic disparities in health and health care. Nurses need to be educated about their role in health policy and to be armed with knowledge that contributes to their developing a sense of their own agency, capability and power to act in the face of everyday ethical notions of good practice and ethical dilemmas in order to demand their rightful place in the policy making arena.

Integration of the Three Apprenticeships in Clincal Nursing Education

Nursing practice demands rich background knowledge, high-level skills and ethical comportment. These three apprenticeships must be integrated in nursing education in order to produce nurses who are capable of integrating their practice. All practice disciplines face the challenges of teaching students to use skills informed by complex knowledge and professional ethics in open-ended, underdetermined situations that cannot be made fully explicit by methods of empirical science or by gathering together a collection of predetermined discrete facts. In nursing education, there is a rich tradition of clinical teaching and learning that requires students to engage in real (or as close to real as possible) practice situations. Experiential clinical learning and using knowledge in practical clinical situations are central to nursing education. Clinical education in high-stakes learning environments, which begins early in nursing programs, is ripe for integration of the three apprenticeships as students confront new skills, witness suffering and resilience, and form new relationships with patients and families.

Nursing education encounters unique challenges for faculty and students in clinical settings, including some impediments to integration that the best clinical teachers are able to overcome. For example, teachers who seek to both integrate and coordinate classroom and clinical learning find they have little or no control over what patients will be available to students on the clinical unit at any particular time. Consequently, students may be exposed to patient care that they have not yet studied in class. Thus, the clinical teacher must be ready to seize learning opportunities when they are available and not just when they are planned. This kind of flexible teaching requires confidence and comfort, not just with clinical nursing, but also with the teaching of a practice.

Another element that can derail integration is the student nurse's preoccupation with technical and procedural skills. Learning to perform new skills and procedures safely is vital to nursing practice, but integrating these technical skills with the skill of clinical judgment, theoretical knowledge and ethical comportment is also vital. Early in their clinical education, students who are focused on following the steps of a procedure may be unable to identify why the procedure is necessary or why the steps occur in the sequence they do. In addition, the novice student is unable to sense what the patient's concerns are and may have difficulty communicating with the patient or responding to the patient's needs while performing a new skill. The clinical teacher must be ready to coach students toward integrating all of these concerns.

Student anxiety often disrupts learning in high-stakes clinical environments. To mediate student anxiety, the best clinical teachers coach students in what to expect and how to prepare for new situations, sights, sounds and smells. Through role modeling, clinical teachers help students expand their zones of comfort and develop new sensibilities and responses to injuries, illnesses, patient fears, wounds, and disfigurement. This formation is vital to the development of ethical comportment in the new nurse. Theoretical nursing and medical knowledge are not sufficient if interpersonal relational and communication skills are not developed. To this end, the teacher coaches the student in confronting and coping with patient vulnerability and suffering, as well as developing skills of interpersonal involvement. Attunement and openness to the patient's mood is a key skill of involvement that allows patients to feel comfortable in communicating concerns to the student. In nursing practice, these skills are complex and guided by the patient's clinical needs and concerns.

Early in their education, students are too inexperienced to appreciate the subtle distinctions in complex, open-ended and changing clinical situations. Clinical faculty must be prepared to coach students toward developing a grasp and getting a feel for what is more or less important in the situation. This is called helping students develop a *sense of salience* in particular clinical situations, so that they recognize what is most and least important, and what is most and least urgent. Clinical teachers typically rely on rich coaching pedagogies that allow them to address students' thinking and knowledge use within a particular situation as it unfolds over time. They pull students along with carefully chosen questions that fit the most salient aspects of a situation and guide students to pay attention to the right things in ordering their approaches and interventions. In this way, the teacher guides students in ongoing experiential, situated learning and instills a sense of how to stay open, curious and reflective, so that experiential learning becomes a lifelong habit.

Learning nursing practice is cumulative, requires synthesis, and depends upon knowledge and skills introduced throughout the nursing program. As one student put it, "You are not free to just learn something and then forget about it after you have taken the test. You have to carry it with you to the next class." This student's insight captures the feeling of high-stakes learning.

Yet, what nursing students learn in the classroom is often not connected enough to what they learn in the clinical setting, and vice versa. When the cognitive apprenticeship is addressed primarily in the classroom, and the skills-based apprenticeship and apprenticeship of ethical comportment are addressed primarily in skills lab and clinical practice settings, integration of the three apprenticeships is most difficult. The changes called for in the next section are intended to move nursing education toward integrated teaching and learning in clinical, lab and classroom settings.

Four Essential Shifts for Integration

The examples that inform the recommendation that nursing education strive for deeper, more effective integration of the three professional apprenticeships came from teachers who changed their assumptions about teaching and their approach to fostering student learning (Benner, Sutphen, Leonard, & Day, 2008). There is no reason to doubt that other nurse educators, at whatever point they are in their careers, also can change their thinking about and approach to teaching, particularly by making the following shifts:

1. From a focus on covering decontextualized knowledge to an emphasis on teaching for a sense of salience, situated cognition and action in particular clinical situations

2. From an emphasis on critical thinking to an emphasis on clinical reasoning and multiple ways of thinking that include critical thinking

3. From a sharp separation of classroom and clinical teaching to integrative teaching in all settings

4. From an emphasis on socialization and role-taking to an emphasis on formation

From a Focus on Covering Decontextualized Knowledge to an Emphasis on Teaching for a Sense of Salience, Situated Cognition, and Action in Particular Clinical Situations

Nursing schools have created curricula with what many call "threads" that are designed to expose students to ideas, practices, or theories in different courses with a built-in plan for continuity. The idea is that students will grasp the need to draw on these threads of knowledge and skills in different situations. For example, the role of the family in the care of patients might be a thread in a nursing school curriculum, and content related to family care is included in several courses. Most curricular attempts to integrate knowledge have been focused on integrating threads or strands of nursing content or process in all courses across the curriculum. We recommend a shift to deliberately integrating the three high-end professional apprenticeships: cognitive, skills, and ethical comportment.

With the three high-end apprenticeships taught in both clinical and classroom settings, teachers can also shift away from highly abstract theoretical classroom teaching, which takes the form of presenting information about physiology, disease categories, signs, symptoms, interventions, and outcomes as layered taxonomies to be memorized. Of all strategies for presenting theories and clinical knowledge, taxonomic naming systems are the most abstract, and they create the least demand for clinical imagination. Few students can imagine how the classification systems can be used in their actual direct patient care. But even more troubling in classroom teaching is the tenacious assumption that the student learns an abstract theory and then applies that theory in practice. This is a narrow rational-technical view (Schön, 1983) of theory and practice. Practice itself is underdetermined and covers a wide and diverse range of theoretical and scientific areas. No one abstract theory can be directly applied, except the most technical physiological theories about things like laboratory values, pulmonary pressures and hemodynamics. Instead, knowledge use in a complex practice discipline calls for a dialogue between theory and practice, between the particular and the general, and between the evidence base for care and the fittingness of that evidence for a particular patient/family. These dialogues can happen in the classroom through the use of unfolding case studies and real clinical practice examples.

Although taxonomies, or classification systems, are integral to information systems, and are required for information retrieval (Bowker & Starr, 1999), the use of precious classroom time for introducing students to flat representations of multiple taxonomic structures must be called into question, as it is little more than "cataloguing." Nursing students do use classification systems, but the classroom is not the best setting in which to learn these. Classification systems are more easily learned in computer-based exercises as students learn various nursing documentation and care planning strategies. Those classification systems should then be made a topic for critique, prompting students to update and improve them and not simply memorize them.

For effective professional practice, students need to develop a sense of salience about what is relatively important and unimportant in any particular clinical situation. As Bourdieu (1990) points out, the heart of practical reasoning is understanding the nature of the situation. The teaching-learning implications of the need to recognize what is most urgent, most important, and what is less urgent in particular practice situations is a demand shared by all practice disciplines. Practice situations are never fixed; always change over time, and cannot be broken down into a collection of discrete elements. Clinicians must first grasp the nature of the situation as a whole before they can act intelligently and prudently. The instructor must coach novice nursing students to recognize what must be addressed during care of a particular patient/family, and must teach and coach them to develop their own situation recognition capacities. Simulating this process in the classroom is essential, since it is not possible for the student to build up a holistic grasp of the situation element by element in actual, complex practice situations. The most effective way for teachers to reduce and simplify the clinical setting (where things play out in real time) is to assign patients who are not in crisis and who require relatively straightforward, simpler interventions. Continued situated coaching is required for students to grasp the changing relevance, demands, resources and constraints in particular situations. Eraut (1994) calls this productive form of knowledge use and Lave and Wenger (2006) have called it a form of situated cognition.

The National Study of Nursing Education reported here revealed that students had too little opportunity in a clinical setting to titrate or adjust therapies based on patient responses. This is a complex skill, the development of which requires the opportunity to practice reasoning across changes in the patient's condition, and changes in the clinicians' understanding of that condition. Experience with this kind of clinical reasoning, informally known as following the patient's clinical trends and trajectories, can happen in the classroom and skills lab as well as in the clinical setting if teachers move away from teaching content by cataloging and instead embed content in simulation of patient care situations that change over time. Such an approach does not require high-tech simulators or costly technology; it can be done using unfolding case studies in the classroom. This kind of teaching calls on students to actively imagine a patient situation, think in multiple ways, and think and talk about how to respond to changes as they occur (Benner, Hooper-Kyriakidis, & Stannard, 2000).

This study also revealed that students had little opportunity to practice making a case to physicians for a change in therapy. This, too, calls for situated cognition and is often difficult to teach in live practice settings. Practice in making a case to physicians can be effectively taught using high-fidelity simulations and can be supported by systems such as the SBAR reporting strategy. The acronym SBAR stands for Situation, a brief statement of the problem; Background relevant for the situation at hand; Assessment, a summary of what the clinician believes is the underlying cause and its severity; and Recommendation, what is needed to resolve the situation (Pope, Rodzen, & Spross, 2008). The SBAR tool is useful for making a clear, concise case and is especially useful for helping nursing students organize significant clinical information in order to best advocate for a change in medical orders. Students also need to be taught how to go up the chain of command when they need a second opinion when they do not get the response they believe the patient's situation demands.

From an Exclusive Emphasis on Critical Thinking to an Emphasis on Clinical Reasoning and Multiple Ways of Thinking

As already described, "critical thinking" has become a catch-all phrase for all forms of thinking required in nursing practice. This use of "critical thinking" needs clarification, so that teaching and learning can focus on multiple ways of thinking and greater emphasis can be placed on clinical reasoning. A broader and more rigorous rationality that can address the practical reasoning required in all practice disciplines — particularly the endemic form of practical reasoning for nurses, that of clinical reasoning or phronesis (Dunne, 1997) — is needed.

Critical reflective thinking is essential for deconstructing situations of practice breakdown. Critical reflection is also essential for questioning received ideas, including outmoded, inept theories and practices that need reform. But critical reflection cannot be the only or even primary focus in learning a professional practice. Nurses — like physicians, lawyers, engineers and clergy — have to have some areas of solidified evidence-based knowledge to ground their understanding in order to take action. For example, upon confronting a patient in acute respiratory distress with low blood pressure and an extremely slow pulse, the nurse must take quick action based on a well-established scientific understanding of the functioning of the cardiopulmonary system, and possible causes of bradycardia and hypotension. Definitive action and therapeutic interventions require evidence-based knowledge that is not "up for grabs" in the moment when quick action is required.

Cynicism and excessive doubt that is often the by-product of overuse of critical thinking will not help the professional nurse draw on appropriate knowledge and act in particular situations, nor will it help the nurse develop perceptual acuity or clinical imagination about well-defined, discipline-specific practical knowledge. Thinking like a nurse requires clinical reasoning as well as critical, creative, scientific and formal criterial reasoning. Nurses need to be able to use clinical imagination in clinical situations and to generate their own narratives of clinical experiences and encounters with patients, families and co-workers. Also important to nurses is an ability to elicit and interpret patient narratives of the illness experience in order to grasp the nature of patients' clinical needs as they change over time.

From Separating Clinical and Classroom Teaching to Integration in All Settings

With a shift in approach to teaching that integrates the three apprenticeships in all settings can come a much needed reform in unifying knowledge acquisition and use. With the integration of clinical and classroom learning as a seamless whole, nurse educators can repair the fragmentation and information overload students currently experience. Therefore, the apprenticeships must be taught in an integrated way in all teaching and learning settings — clinical settings, classrooms, and skills or simulation laboratories. This form of curricular integration would take some of the burden off students and faculty who struggle to bring their unwieldy and often poorly coordinated curriculum into a more coherent whole. It also would simplify and aid in reducing the overloading that ineffectively tries to introduce too much content in abstract ways.

From Socialization and Role-Taking to Formation

While much of social theorizing about roles, role taking, role making and role performance are useful in a practice discipline that must coordinate and link role functions with other disciplines and team members, nursing must go beyond a mere role enactment view to a more constitutive view of transformation and formation. Formation is a term borrowed from the Carnegie Foundation for the Advancement of Teaching Clergy Study, because it addresses the kind of transformation and reformation of senses, aesthetics, perceptual acuities, relational skills, knowledge and dispositions required by students of any practice discipline. Margaret Mohrmann (2006) uses the metaphor of dance to describe formation. Especially in nursing and medicine, where ethical formation occurs through learning in particular situations, the metaphor of dance is more apt than imagining static shapes or forms that the learner becomes:

> Formation refers to the method by which a person is prepared for a particular task or is made capable of functioning in a particular role. One forms, as well as educates, priests, soldiers, nurses, and doctors in a process that moves beyond the knowledge content of those crafts to the moral content of the practices — the obligations entailed, the demands imposed — and thus to the moral formation of the practitioners. Moreover, it is generally the case that one is formed toward something, some telos, some ideal shape or condition. …A better metaphor [for being true to form] is dance: having and displaying integrity is more a matter of being able to move in ways that are consistent with the originating and developing themes of our lives. Teachers, guides, and practice make us better dancers because they help us listen more carefully and follow the music we hear more confidently. We learn which movements fit the rhythms and which do not (pp. 93, 95).

Formation occurs in every formal and informal learning setting, in the formal curriculum and the hidden curriculum. Deliberative and nondeliberative learning forms the aspiring clinician's identity, self-understanding and character, as it instills skilled capacities and new aesthetic perceptual acuities related to recognizing key signs and symptoms in actual patient situations.

Nursing students interviewed for the National Study of Nursing Education provided many accounts of experiential learning that transformed their sense of identity. Eight themes emerged from senior nursing students' stories of significant experiential learning that speak of transformation:

Formation stories were often a major singular theme in the senior's narratives and themes of formation were woven into many of the stories senior nursing students told during the interviews that did not have formation as the overriding theme; for example, as they related how a particular learning experience had changed their perspective, their capacities to act in future similar situations and their self-knowledge and understanding, or how another experience reassured them that they were on the right path and that they were going to be good at their chosen profession.

The fear of making a mistake, the recognition of the level of responsibility of nursing practice, that a nurse's actions could cause serious harm or even death, were major formative themes of nursing students. The students' lay expectations of "nurses as helpers" had not included the high-precision knowledge and skill actually required by nurses. Student nurses told stories of making mistakes, reporting their errors, and experiencing terror at the possibility of making a more dangerous mistake.

Learning technical skills was a major theme in most of the narratives; however, many of the students' stories took the form of telling their anticipatory fear of inserting an IV, assisting with hemodialysis or inserting a naso-gastric tube, and their relief over successfully accomplishing the technical feat and then having it recede in the background with more experience.

Meeting and treating the patient as a person rather than as a patient or object of care also emerged as a theme. These stories of learning were the most frequent themes for nursing students who were preoccupied in the beginning of their practice with technical interventions, patient safety, and knowledge and skills of patient assessment and responses to therapies. In their stories, it was as if the patient as a person suddenly claimed their attention and reframed their ethical comportment. They responded with a mixture of discovery and chagrin over their prior overfocus on the technical.

Recognizing the patient first as a person led students to efforts of *preserving the patient's personhood and dignity in the face of the ravages of injuries, illness, and the influence of many medications.* The students learned to highlight the person's social and family identity, often using pictures from the patient's life, humor, and stories of outside everyday life.

Stories of *effective staff nurse or teacher coaching in difficult clinical situations* that enabled the student to take responsibility and experience independence while performing a difficult clinical intervention were also told as stories of formation through taking on the identity of "nurse" in actual clinical settings. Students were relieved when their teachers protected their sense of professional identity in front of the patient. They also appreciated teachers' preparatory coaching outside the room as well, because it provided them the opportunity to take up and feel responsible for the patient.

Confronting substandard care in hospital settings and the ethical challenges to report substandard care were major themes for students, who hold a low status position in a rigid hospital hierarchy. Students usually went to their nurse educators for support and correction and were then met with a range of satisfactory corrective responses, or less satisfactory advice "not to make too many waves" since students are precarious guests in the hospitals and clinical placements are hard to find.

Difficulties in making the transition to work loomed large for all the senior students. When one student told of her concerns about the first job, other students chimed in and agreed adding their own fears. Many stories focused on fear of not being prepared to move competently into the work role. Seniors wanted to find good institutional cultures and hoped to find residencies or specialized training for newly graduated nurses.

Formation of student nurses occurs within the context of skilled practices and highly relational work that literally transform their ways of perceiving and acting in situations. A shift to a focus on students' reflections of their transformation through formative experiences in nursing school is essential, as such a focus will enrich each student's sense of identity and self-understanding as a nurse.

Conclusions: Strengths and Challenges in Clinical Teaching

The Carnegie Foundation for the Advancement of Teaching National Nursing Education Study (Benner et al., in press) found that, currently in schools of nursing, clinical teaching is stronger and more advanced in content than is classroom teaching. Much of the cognitive apprenticeship for practicing nursing is currently being taught primarily in clinical settings. This statement is not as optimistic about clinical teaching and learning as it may seem, since the current state of classroom teaching is so badly in need of a radical upgrade and transformation. Classroom, skills labs and simulations need to move beyond a narrow technical approach to nursing education toward a much more integrative approach to acquisition of knowledge by using that knowledge in particular clinical situations. Classroom instruction also needs a stronger foundation in clinically relevant natural and human sciences and humanities.

The study reported here revealed that clinical instruction often suffers from staff nurse preceptors or clinical instructors who are not given any formal preparation for their teaching role, and who are not involved in, or even familiar with, larger teaching and learning goals or class content. Often the clinical teacher did not even know the learning goals of the week for the student. Only one of the nine schools visited gave extensive formal instruction to their clinical teachers and preceptors, and then incorporated those teachers into bi-weekly course meetings.

The Carnegie/National Student Nurse Association Survey results showed that student nurses still feel unwelcome and are often verbally abused in many of their clinical settings. It is obvious that teachers and students need to collaborate with health care institutions to upgrade the clinical environments for teaching and that nursing administrators need to usher in a new age of zero tolerance for horizontal abuse and toxic communications in clinical settings. This is a good in its own right, but has the further moral force of evidence that interpersonal conflicts and abusive communication patterns threaten patient safety (Hesketha et al., 2003; Long, 2003).

It was evident throughout this study that many clinical nursing teachers are excellent clinical coaches. Indeed, situated coaching clearly emerged as a signature pedagogy in nursing education. Situated coaching is best if the teacher is a skilled questioner who coaches students to enhance their sense of salience in particular clinical situations, recognizing what is most and less important in that situation. Recognizing the nature of the clinical situation is at the very heart of clinical reasoning, which is a subset of practical reasoning through the many transitions that occur in clinical situations (Benner, 1994b; Bourdieu, 1990; Taylor, 1993). For novice nursing students to recognize the nature of a situation, they need coaching and exposure to extensive situated learning in ambiguous, open-ended clinical situations. This is at the center of situated coaching as a central nursing pedagogy.

Reflecting on the essence of clinical teaching and learning, the research team (Benner et al., in press) offers the following questions to guide future research:

- What are key recurring successful patterns of integration of classroom and clinical teaching of natural sciences, social sciences and humanities in nursing education?

- What strategies do students use to integrate classroom teaching with clinical practice?

- How is quality of care and patient safety currently being learned by students in clinical assignments?

- What is the learning impact on disparities between classroom-taught formal assessments systems, such as Nursing Diagnosis, Interventions and Outcomes and actual practice in clinical practice assignments?

- How can clinical performance assessments be improved in clinical teaching in undergraduate education?

- To what extent is the development of clinical imagination being fostered in clinical assignments?

- How can situated coaching be improved in clinical teaching?

- What impact does having different or same clinical and classroom faculty impact students integrative learning in clinical settings?

The Carnegie Foundation for the Advancement of Teaching National Study of Nursing recommends a radical transformation of nursing education in order to overcome the current practice-education gap. Nursing has fallen behind in research and development of teaching and learning for the complex practice of nursing. Nursing education is under a great deal of strain due to work overload, inadequate preparation for teaching, limited number of graduate programs focused on teacher preparation, salary shortfalls (in comparison to clinical practice salaries), and gross underfunding at the state and federal levels. It is little wonder that nurse educators have fallen behind the current clinical practice found in major university medical centers and community hospitals. Schools of nursing have a central role to play in upgrading and transforming the education of nurses, including creating a better articulated and more rational system that ensures students learning experiences do not vary dramatically in quantity and quality across programs.

On a more optimistic note, this study made it clear that nursing faculty and students have a tremendous commitment to and zeal for self-improving practices. There was little cynicism and much genuine commitment to teaching and learning to be safe and effective nurses.

This is a great moral source that could be squandered if schools of nursing are not able to meet the challenges of upgrading their programs and if practice environments are not able to improve the working environments of nurses. But American society depends on nurses acting proactively and being engaged in policy level discussions that will lead to the needed transformation of nursing education, so that it becomes and remains equitable and excellent.

References

Barab, S. A. & Roth, W. M. (2006). Curriculum based ecosystems: Supporting knowing from an ecological perspective. *Educational Researcher, 35*(5), 3-13.

Benner, P., & Wruble, J. (1989). *The primacy of caring.* Menlo Park, CA: Addison-Wesley.

Benner, P. (1994a). The tradition and skill of interpretive phenomenology in studying health, illness, and caring practices. In P. Benner (Ed.), *Interpretive phenomenology: Embodiment, caring and ethics in health and illness* (pp. 99-127). Newbury Park, CA: Sage.

Benner, P. (1994b). The role of articulation in understanding practice and experience as sources of knowledge. In J. Tully & D. M. Weinstock (Eds.), *Philosophy in a time of pluralism: Perspectives on the philosophy of Charles Taylor* (pp. 136-155). Cambridge, UK: Cambridge University Press.

Benner, P., Hooper-Kyrikides, P., & Stannard, D. (2000). *Clinical wisdom and interventions in critical care: A thinking-in-action approach.* Philadelphia: W. B. Saunders.

Benner P., & Sutphen, M. (2007). Learning across the professions: The clergy, a case in point. *Journal of Nursing Education, 46*(3), 103-108.

Benner, P., Sutphen, M., Leonard, V., & Day, L. (2008) Formation and ethical comportment in nursing. *American Journal of Critical Care, 17*(5), 173-176.

Benner, P., Sutphen, M., Leonard, V., & Day, L. (in press). *Educating nurses: A call for radical transformation.* San Francisco: Jossey-Bass.

Benner, P., Tanner, C., & Chesla, C. (2009). *Expertise in nursing practice: Caring, clinical judgment and ethics.* New York: Springer Publishing.

Bourdieu, P. (1990). *The logic of practice.* (R. Nice, Trans.). Stanford, CA: Stanford University Press. (Original work published in 1980)

Bowker, G. C., & Star, S. L. (1999) *Sorting things out: Classification and its consequences.* Cambridge, MA: MIT Press, Inside Technology Series.

Cooke, M., Irby, D., & O Brien, B. (in press). *Educating physicians.* San Francisco: Jossey-Bass.

Dunne, J. (1997). *Back to the rough ground. Practical judgment and the lure of technique.* Notre Dame, IN: University of Notre Dame Press.

Dunne, J. (2004). Arguing for teaching as a practice. In J. Dunne & P. Hogan (Eds.), *Education and practice: Upholding the integrity of teaching and learning* (pp. 170-186). Oxford: Blackwell.

Eraut, M. (1994). *Developing professional knowledge and competence.* London: Washington, Falmer Press.

Flexner, A. (1910). *Medical education in the United States and Canada (The Flexner Report).* Princeton, NJ: The Carnegie Foundation for the Advancement of Teaching.

Foster, C. R., Dahill, L. E., Golemon, L. A., & Tolentino, B. W. (2005). *Educating clergy: Teaching practices and pastoral imagination.* San Francisco: Jossey-Bass.

Grossman, P., & McDonald, M. (2008). Back to the future: Directions for research in teaching and teacher education. *American Educational Research Journal, 45*(1), 184-205.

Hesketha, K., Duncanab, S. M., Esabrooksa, C. A., Reimerc, M. A., Geiovanettia, P., Hyndmande, K., et al. (2003). Workplace violence in Alberta and British Columbia Hospitals. *Health Policy, 63*(3), 311-321.

Lave, J., & Wenger, E. (2006). *Situated learning: Legitimate peripheral participation.* New York: Cambridge University Press.

Long, B. (2003). Psychologic aspects of the hostile workplace: Harassment and bullying. *Clinics in Occupational and Environmental Medicine, 3*(4), 803-820.

Malloch, K., & Porter-O Grady, T. (Eds.). (2006). *Introduction to evidence-based practice in nursing and healthcare.* Sudbury, MA: Jones and Bartlett.

Mohrmann, M. E. (2006). On being true to form. In C. Taylor & R. Dell Oro (Eds.), *Health and human flourishing: Religion, medicine, and moral anthropology* (pp. 89-102). Washington, DC: Georgetown University Press.

Pope, B. B., Rodzen, L., & Spross, G. (2008). Raising the SBAR: How better communication improves patient outcomes. *Nursing, 38*(3), 41-43.

Schön, D. A. (1983). *The reflective practitioner: How professionals think in action.* New York: Basic Books.

Sheppard, S., Macatangay, K., Colby, A., Sullivan, W. M., & Shulman, L. S. (2008). *Educating engineers.* San Francisco: Jossey-Bass.

Shulman, L. S. (2004). *The wisdom of practice: Essays on teaching, learning, and learning to teach.* San Francisco: Jossey-Bass.

Sullivan, W. M. (2004). *Work and integrity: The crisis and promise of professionalism in America* (2nd ed.). San Francisco: Jossey-Bass.

Sullivan, W. M., Colby, A., Wegner, J. W., Bond, L., & Shulman, L. (2007). *Educating lawyers: Preparation for the profession of law.* San Francisco: Jossey-Bass.

Sullivan, W. M., & Rosin, M. S. (2008). *A new agenda for higher education: Shaping a life of the mind for practice.* San Francisco: Jossey-Bass.

Taylor, C. (1993). Explanation and practical reasoning. In M. Nussbaum & A. Sen (Eds.), *The quality of life* (pp. 238-231). Oxford, UK: Clarendon.

6

Chapter

EVALUATION OF CLINICAL PERFORMANCE

Karen J. Saewert, PhD, RN, CPHQ, CNE
Suzanne S. Yarbrough, PhD, RN

Nursing is a practice-based discipline and a large portion of the preparation for this practice has historically been achieved through an apprenticeship model. Apprenticeship learning is best facilitated through collaborative and trusting relationships between the teacher and apprentice, and its goal is the preparation of an individual who can perform the role competently. In nursing, the goal of this model has been to produce a competent clinician who is ready to assume responsibility for patient care across all levels of care and in all types of care environments.

The term *competent* infers that the clinician possesses the knowledge, skills, and attitudes necessary to enact the role. Competence is demonstrated within the context of a clinical situation (Tanner, 2001). To be fully competent, the graduate must understand and be able to integrate the complex components of care — making sense or meaning of the interplay between knowledge, skills and attitudes; performing tasks safely and effectively; and embodying the values of the profession (Axley, 2008).

The Institute of Medicine's [IOM] report on the education of health professions, however, called the apprenticeship model into question and suggested that graduates of health professions programs are not as competent as they need to be to practice in today's complex environments (IOM, 2003). This report cited the need for improved assessment of clinical proficiency in nursing and other health professions' education to assure adequate preparation to provide the highest quality and safest care possible.

The IOM's challenge was reinforced by Holaday and Buckley (2008), who called for educators to address how outcomes deemed essential for safe and competent patient care by professional organizations are incorporated into clinical assessment and evaluation of nursing students, what drives instruction and evaluation practices, how outcomes are assessed and evaluated, and what evidence supports the way we do clinical evaluations (i.e., evidence-based education). This chapter provides an overview of clinical evaluation studies, formative and summative evaluation, rubrics for clinical evaluation, challenges to conducting clinical evaluations, pitfalls to avoid, diversity considerations, and building the science of nursing education.

Overview of Clinical Education Studies

In 1982, Wood conducted a comprehensive review of literature published during the 1960s and 1970s to identify practices that would assist both educators and students manage the many challenges associated with clinical evaluation, not the least of which was the problem of subjectivity in evaluation. The practices identified ranged from rating scales and guidelines to clinical evaluation forms and attempts to develop acceptable and effective grading schemes.

Although the practice of clinical evaluation has advanced and improved since Wood's 1982 analysis, the identified underlying difficulties of past decades inherent in clinical evaluation have remained. Examples of these difficulties include the following:

- clinical evaluation is based on direct observation, which brings inherent bias and subjectivity;

- clinical evaluation is a performance-based process situated in the authentic or simulated
- clinical environment and, therefore, subject to the influence of the clinical milieu, actions of other health care professionals, and responses of patients;
- clinical evaluation is based on only a sample of students' clinical performance, since the faculty member cannot be with every student during every moment of her/his practice;
- learning and clinical evaluation occur simultaneously; and
- the ever-changing clinical milieu creates different learning and clinical evaluation situations for each student, thereby making it nearly impossible to evaluate each student in the same way, on the same bases, or under the same circumstances.

The history of evaluation of clinical performances was well documented by Krichbaum, Rowan, Duckett, Ryden, and Savik (1994), who emphasized that the problems faculty face in making clinical evaluations mirror difficulties faced when doing evaluations in general. Despite repeated documentation of the challenges associated with clinical evaluation, only a limited number of studies on clinical evaluation have been reported (Bourbonnais, Langford, & Giannantonio, 2007; Dolan, 2003; Oermann, 2004), thereby making this a fertile area for pedagogical research.

Elements of Effective Clinical Evaluation

An effective clinical evaluation system supports student learning and is multifaceted and dynamic. Clinical evaluation involves making a judgment regarding the competency of an individual. It integrates all learning domains — cognitive, affective, and psychomotor — and results in an inference about a student's performance ability and her/his readiness to move forward or need for remediation. Assessment of students' knowledge, skills and attitudes in the clinical environment, as well as their patterns of behavior in that setting, must be the foundation for determining their clinical competence.

Effective clinical teaching results from the alignment of learning outcomes and objectives, instructional activities, and assessment and evaluation strategies. An *outcome* defines the behavior or standard of performance that is the expected "end product" of learning (AACN, 2008; Billings & Halstead, 2009). Outcomes are stated more broadly than *objectives*, which are used to provide a more precise description of the expected behaviors and the conditions under which the behaviors are to be observed. Observations of student performance in the authentic or simulated clinical environment should serve as core assessment data for making judgments regarding an individual's progress in meeting expected clinical course outcomes and objectives and achieving clinical competence across all learning domains.

Effective clinical evaluation must be integrative and include aspects of all three learning domains (see Figure 6-1). Knowledge must be possessed to be applied, values internalized to be demonstrated, and skills practiced if they are to be executed (Billings & Halstead, 2009). Evaluation of knowledge acquisition within the cognitive domain is most readily associated with the classroom setting; however, its evaluation is essential in the clinical environment. This can take the form of purposeful discussion, guided reflection, care plan development, concept mapping, reflective journals, and other oral or written discourse associated with clinical practice learning experiences that make evident students' abilities to articulate knowledge development and its relevance and contribution to professional development.

Figure 6 – 1
Integrative Clinical Evaluation

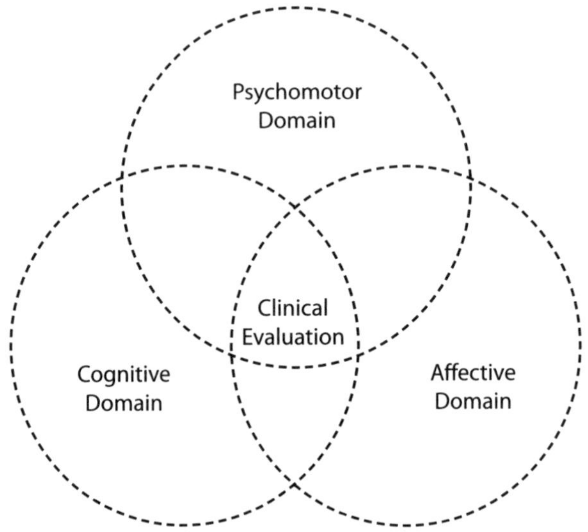

Evaluation within the affective domain encompasses attitudes, beliefs and values, and feelings and emotions, and requires attention to the progressive nature of the valuing process over time (Billings & Halstead, 2009). Even though the primary focus in the clinical learning environment may be on cognitive processing and psychomotor functioning, affective learning is an important part of the clinical educational experience (Bastable & Doody, 2008) and crucial to professional development. Although not insurmountable, the less overt and observable nature of affective behaviors contributes to its evaluation challenges. Selection of evaluation strategies associated with clinical learning activities aimed at eliciting affective responses (e.g., case studies, role-playing, clinical simulation, gaming, synchronous or asynchronous discussion, clinical debriefing) provides the opportunity for successful affective learning and development. The psychomotor domain, by contrast, is a familiar focus of the clinical learning environment, where overt and clearly identifiable performance of skills is conducted and observed. The use of both formative and summative evaluation strategies is essential to determining progress and engaging students meaningfully in their own learning and professional development across these interrelated learning domains.

Formative Evaluation

Formative evaluation is used as a means of providing feedback to students regarding progress (Oermann & Gaberson, 2006). Through the use of formative evaluation, the clinical educator can identify areas of strengths and weaknesses, and then formulate a plan with the student to build on the strengths and overcome the weaknesses. Thus, the clinical educator must develop acumen for assessing student progress, ensuring that assessment reflects the learning outcomes specified for the course, and identifying strategies to enhance continued growth.

The clinical educator should collaborate with the student to identify activities that will address clinical deficiencies and take full advantage of the student's strengths. Such personalization enhances the experience for both faculty and students (Diekelmann & McGregor, 2003; Poorman, Mastorovich, & Webb, 2008). When faculty partner with students in this way, clinical evaluations move from being a "cold" judgment about whether or not the student is in danger of failing to a collaborative effort designed to help the student meet clinical competency objectives (Oermann & Gaberson, 2006). Rather than focusing only on the deficits, clinical educators who strive to understand the learning experience from the student's perspective can use assessment data to formulate an individualized approach to clinical education and continued professional growth.

Summative Evaluation

Summative evaluation is the form of evaluation that reflects an inference or conclusion about whether or not a student has achieved stated learning outcomes (Oermann & Gaberson, 2006). It results in assigning a pass/fail or graded summation. A summative evaluation notes whether the student has demonstrated the ability to consistently integrate relevant knowledge, skill and attitudes expected for the course; provide safe, quality care to patients; interact collaboratively with nursing colleagues and other members of the health care team; and so on. When formative evaluation is effective, the summative evaluation outcome should not be a surprise to the student. If the evaluation process is fair, focused, appropriate, and consistently applied, even the failing student should be prepared to accept the news (Boley & Whitney, 2003; Brown, Neudorf, Poitras, & Rodger, 2007; Diekelmann, & McGregor, 2003; Poorman et al., 2008).

Rubrics as Tools for Clinical Evaluation

Clear communication about expected clinical behaviors and performance are essential if the evaluation is to be fair and relevant. Despite faculty efforts to clarify these expectations, however, students often claim to not understand the basis for clinical evaluations or grading methods, and they expend energy trying to figure out the implicit criteria that may be used instead of using that energy to learn (Bondy, 1983; Burghart & Panettieri, 2009). Thus, faculty must find ways to eliminate uncertainties regarding the bases for clinical evaluation.

The use of observation to evaluate clinical competence has long been considered subjective, inconsistent and a stubborn problem not readily ameliorated by new approaches and concepts (Wood, 1982). The use of a criterion-based schema, or rubric, is coming to be used by many educators to help assess and evaluate a wide range of students' academic performance both in the classroom and clinical environments, and it has promise in clinical evaluation in nursing. Rubrics provide the clinical educator with a standardized framework within which to observe students' clinical behaviors while facilitating communication among students and providing students, preceptors and clinical educators with language to foster feedback and discussion (Bondy, 1983; Burghart & Panettieri, 2009; Lasater, 2007).

A rubric is an assessment tool, not a checklist, that serves (a) as a template to explicate a standard of quality and (b) as an effective tool for taking what may seem like "guesswork" out of grading (for students and educators) while guiding the learning process for students (Burghart & Panettieri, 2009; Truemper, 2004). When a concept or clinical behavior and evidence of its understanding and expected performance are clearly described, students and clinical educators are able to recognize and agree about ability when the behavior is actually performed.

Clinical evaluation rubrics may be holistic (i.e., consider overall clinical performance) or analytic (i.e., consider individual or separate components of clinical performance). The design of clinical evaluation rubrics may vary, but they usually are organized in a matrix format that includes (a) the clinical behavior or task description, (b) the scale of achievement or quality rating, (c) the dimensions or evaluation criteria, broken down into specific skills or knowledge to be demonstrated, and (d) a description of the dimensions or level of performance for each of the evaluation criteria (Burghart & Panettieri, 2009). Careful design, content development, and use consistent with the intended purpose can make clinical evaluation rubrics effective and efficient and help diminish some of the challenges faced when evaluating clinical performance.

Maximizing the Effectiveness of Clinical Evaluation

Despite extensive work, competence remains an ill-defined concept (Axley, 2008). However, it is the expected outcome of clinical teaching, and clinical faculty are expected to make judgments about a student's progress toward or accomplishment of practice competence goals. This evaluative judgment is based upon assessment of data evidencing a student's ability to integrate and apply knowledge in patient care situations, while performing skills and exhibiting professional nursing values as outlined in course material (Oermann & Gaberson, 2006).

Most often evaluative judgments are made by clinical educators while they are enacting the teaching role. Thus, clinical educators often find themselves being both teacher and gatekeeper at the same time (Mahara, 1998). Likewise, students are judged or evaluated while they are in the midst of learning. The enactment of these dual roles can be problematic for both faculty and students (Diekelmann & Scheckel, 2004).

The clinical educator must have sufficient and relevant evidence of a student's clinical competence to make fair and equitable decisions about her/his ability to provide safe, quality patient care (Axley, 2008; Boley & Whitney, 2003; Brown et al., 2007; Oermann & Gaberson, 2006). Thus, the evaluation tools used in making competency judgments must be closely aligned with the school's mission and values, program outcomes, conceptual framework, and course objective. It is expected that these documents are informed by professional standards, accreditation and licensure requirements, national standards for health care, essentials of education, and core areas of knowledge/skills/values articulated by nursing education leaders and professional associations (Billings & Halstead, 2009; Oermann & Gaberson, 2006). The individual faculty working with each student is responsible for interpreting these guidelines and standards, and using them to judge a student's performance and make a valid clinical evaluation. This is a challenging process rife with potential perils and pitfalls (Brown et al., 2007; Poorman et al., 2008).

Pitfalls to Avoid

Students have the right to an education, but they also have a responsibility to engage actively in the learning process (Boley & Whitney, 2003; Oermann & Gaberson, 2006). The right of a clinical educator to make evaluative decisions is accompanied by an obligation or responsibility to follow professional standards and college or university policies and processes. Thus, a positive, respectful relationship between the clinical educator and student and a well-articulated process for making evaluative decisions form the cornerstone for optimal outcomes of clinical evaluation.

Effective evaluation requires a consistently applied, systematic approach (Boley & Whitney, 2003; Brown et al., 2007). Some would equate the evaluation process to the research process regarding the use of valid and reliable assessment/measurement tools and consistent use of those tools (Mahara, 1998). However, time-tested tools do not exist for the evaluation of nursing students' clinical performance, and it is difficult for faculty to consistently apply the tools that are available due to the changing nature of clinical environments (Axley, 2008; Mahara, 1998; Woolley, 1977). Boley and Whitney (2003) recommend knowing and developing policies and processes for grading that address those areas, such as attendance policies and grievance procedures, where there may be room for disagreement. Legal questions may surface when there is concern that a failing grade was given arbitrarily or capriciously. Grading decisions are more likely to be supported when policies are clearly articulated in course syllabi and consistently applied by clinical educators.

When developing curriculum documents, clinical educators should articulate a clear and consistent conception of the core knowledge, skills, values and behaviors expected of students at various points in the curriculum while allowing latitude for the vagaries of clinical experiences. This conceptual document should address professional practice standards, values or attributes of professionals, and the need for adaptability in professional practice environments that change constantly (Axley, 2008; Brown et al., 2007).

A good clinical evaluation process must provide opportunities for students to learn and develop professionally. Students need consistent and clear feedback from faculty regarding their performance, as well as guidance regarding best approaches to competence development. Current literature points toward more student-centric approaches to nursing education, including evaluation (Diekelmann & McGregor, 2003; Diekelmann & Scheckel, 2004), and faculty are well advised to consider how to maintain such an approach when conducting evaluations of students' clinical performance.

Focusing exclusively on clinical performance deficits will not serve the intended developmental purpose of clinical evaluation (McGregor, 2007). Wilson (1994) found that students' goals in nursing school were to do no harm, to help, to learn, and to make a good impression. A student's sense of self or dignity can be negatively impacted when the evaluation process overly emphasizes deficits, and this is likely to interfere with the educational process.

When students sense that faculty comments are unfair or subjective, or that the focus is only or primarily on weaknesses or problems, they may become fearful, which in turn may impede or halt the learning process (Clark, 2008). Students perceive the evaluation process as unfair or subjective when policies and processes are not followed or are altered during the unfolding of a particular course. In one study (Clark), changes or violations were perceived as bias or differential treatment and reflected micro-inequities in the evaluation process, making students feel powerless and helpless and, in some cases, determined to withdraw from the nursing program. Obviously, this is not the outcome educators hope for.

Our classrooms and clinical environments increasingly reflect the diversity of our global community. This diversity of students' backgrounds and lived experiences challenges faculty to consider student needs even more carefully when creating positive teaching-learning environments (Malek, 1988; Williams & Calvillo, 2002). Consideration of these differences is additionally warranted for their potential impact on the selection of assessment and evaluation strategies.

Student Diversity Considerations in Clinical Evaluation

A positive teaching-learning environment — which is important for all students, but particularly so for those who are in a minority — must include evaluation practices that acknowledge the unique learning needs of each student, respond to the broad diversity of learners, and incorporate a variety of formats and techniques to help students know their strengths and limitations regarding clinical practice. This added dimension warrants attention and consideration given the strong link between lack of diversity in health care providers and health disparities (Sullivan, 2004). In order to meet the health care needs of a multicultural population, nursing programs are enrolling increasing numbers of individuals from diverse cultural and ethnic backgrounds (Rew, Becker, Cookston, Khosropour, & Martinez, 2003). Diversity often is interpreted to mean only ethnicity, race and language, and ethnic minority success often means the student must change her/his behaviors to fit the dominant culture of nursing education (Lancellotti, 2008). A more inclusive view of diversity also incorporates factors such as a place of birth, immigration status, age, gender, life style, life experiences (including academic, family, and work), individual learning style, socioeconomic status, and family situation. Such factors impact on learned, shared, and transmitted beliefs, norms, and life style practices that guide thinking and action (Williams & Calvillo, 2002), and they, therefore, must be considered when planning teaching and evaluation strategies.

A perception of cultural insensitivity has been shown to generate barriers to seeking health care and create uncomfortable health care experiences (Rew et al., 2003). In nursing education, perceptions of cultural insensitivity can generate barriers in the educational process, create uncomfortable educational experiences, and ultimately influence (in a negative way) student retention and success. Clinical educator competence regarding diversity (i.e., values, sensitivity, knowledge and behaviors), therefore, must be considered as fundamental and essential in the clinical teaching-learning environment and evident in evaluation practices.

Building Evidence for Nursing Education

Insufficient research-generated evidence exists to guide our education practices in many areas of program development, teaching and evaluation in nursing (Oermann, 2007). Significant efforts are needed to build an evidence base for nursing education that would lead to increased retention of students and faculty, responsiveness to diversity, and excellence in nursing education, including clinical evaluation. Table 6–1 proposes questions that can serve as a catalyst for further discourse and scholarship that will generate evidence-based practices for the clinical evaluation of nursing students.

Table 6 – 1
Questions for Clinical Evaluation Scholarship and Educational Research

1. How does the use of integrative clinical evaluation strategies affect the outcomes of clinical learning in the cognitive, affective and psychomotor domains?

2. How does student diversity impact outcomes of clinical practice learning as related to the use of specific evaluation strategies?

3. What clinical learning outcomes are directly or indirectly associated with specific evaluation strategies?

4. What evaluation strategies are most effective when used in the authentic clinical environment? In the simulated clinical environment?

5. What is the relationship between faculty pedagogical knowledge and selection of clinical evaluation strategies?

Conclusions

Learning in the clinical environment is complex. Students are expected to acquire and integrate vast amounts of information, develop a set of complex psychomotor skills and comport themselves as caring and compassionate professionals. While clinical evaluation is about assessing the students' ability to meet clinical milestones and determining their readiness to progress to more complex patient care situations, it will be most successfully accomplished when all elements of the process are attended to carefully and consistently. The ultimate goal, after all, is to provide an accurate assessment of the student's ability to provide the highest quality and safest care possible.

References

AACN [American Association of Colleges of Nursing]. (2008). *The essentials of baccalaureate education for professional nursing practice* [Brochure]. Washington, DC: Author.

Axley, L. (2008). Competency: A concept analysis. *Nursing Forum, 43*(4), 214-222.

Bastable, S. B., & Doody, J. A. (2008). Taxonomy of objectives according to learning domains. In S. B. Bastable, *Nurse as educator: Principles of teaching and learning for nursing practice* (3rd ed., pp. 393-406). Sudbury, MA: Jones and Bartlett.

Billings, D. M., & Halstead, J. A. (2009). *Teaching in nursing: A guide for faculty* (3rd ed.). St Louis, MO: Saunders.

Boley, P., & Whitney, K. (2003). Grade disputes: Considerations for nursing faculty. *Journal of Nursing Education, 42*(5), 198-203.

Bondy, K. N. (1983). Criterion-referenced definitions for rating scales in clinical evaluation. *Journal of Nursing Education, 22*(9), 376-382.

Bourbonnais, F. F., Langford, S., & Giannantonio, L. (2007). Development of a clinical evaluation tool for baccalaureate nursing students. *Nursing Education in Practice, 8*, 62-71.

Brown, Y., Neudorf, K., Poitras, C., & Rodger, K. (2007). Unsafe: Student clinical performance calls for a systematic approach. *Canadian Nurse 103*(3), 29-32.

Burghart, G., & Panettieri, R. C. (2009). Faculty guide to rubrics. *Radiologic Technology, 80*(3), 266-268.

Clark, C. M. (2008). Student voices on faculty incivility in nursing education: A conceptual model. *Nursing Education Perspectives, 29*(5), 284-289.

Diekelmann, N., & McGregor, A. (2003). Students who fail clinical courses: Keeping open a future of new possibilities. *Journal of Nursing Education, 42*(10), 433-436.

Diekelmann, N., & Scheckel, M. (2004). Leaving the safe harbor of competency-based and outcomes education: RE-thinking practice education. *Journal of Nursing Education, 43*(9), 385-388.

Dolan, G. (2003). Assessing student clinical competency: Will we ever get it right? *Journal of Clinical Nursing, 12*, 132-141.

Holady, S. D., & Buckley, K. M. (2008). A standardized clinical evaluation tool-kit: Improving nursing education and practice. *Annual Review of Nursing Education, 6*, 123-149.

IOM [Institute of Medicine]. (2003). *Health professional education: A bridge to quality.* Washington, DC: National Academies Press.

Krichbaum, K., Rowan, M., Duckett, L., Ryden, M. B., & Savik, K. (1994). The clinical evaluation tool: A measure of the quality of clinical performance of baccalaureate nursing students. *Journal of Nursing Education, 33*(9), 395-404.

Lancellotti, K. (2008). Culture care theory: A framework for expanding awareness of diversity and racism in nursing education. *Journal of Professional Nursing, 24*(3), 179-183.

Lasater, K. (2007). Clinical judgment development: Using simulation to create an assessment rubric. *Journal of Nursing Education, 46*(11), 496-503.

Mahara, M. S. (1998). A perspective on clinical evaluation in nursing education. *Journal of Advanced Nursing, 28*(6), 1339-1346.

Malek, C. J. (1988). Clinical evaluation: Challenging tradition. *Nurse Educator, 13*(6), 34-37.

McGregor, A. (2007). Academic success, clinical failure: Struggling practices of a failing student. *Journal of Nursing Education, 46*(11), 504-511.

Oermann, M. H. (2004). Reflections on undergraduate nursing education: A look to the future. *International Journal of Nursing Education Scholarship, 1*(12), 1-13.

Oermann, M. H. (2007). Approaches to gathering evidence for educational practices in nursing. *Journal of Continuing Education in Nursing, 38*(6), 250-255.

Oermann, M. H., & Gaberson, K. B. (2006). *Evaluation and testing in nursing education* (2nd ed.). New York: Springer Publishing.

Poorman, S. G., Mastorovich, M. L., & Webb, C. A. (2008). Teacher's stories: How faculty help and hinder students at risk. *Nursing Education Perspectives, 29*(5), 272-277.

Rew, L., Becker, H., Cookston, J., Khosropour, S., & Martinez, S. (2003). Measuring cultural awareness in nursing students. *Journal of Nursing Education, 42*(6), 249-257.

Sullivan, L. W. (2004). *Missing persons: Minorities in the health professions. A report of the Sullivan Commission on Diversity in the Healthcare Workforce.* Battle Creek, MI: W. K. Kellogg Foundation. Retrieved from http://www.aacn.nche.edu/Media/pdf/SullivanReport.pdf

Tanner, C. A. (2001). Competency-based education: The new panacea? *Journal of Nursing Education, 40*(9), 387-388.

Truemper, C. M. (2004). Using scoring rubrics to facilitate assessment and evaluation of graduate-level nursing students. *Journal of Nursing Education, 43*(12), 562-564.

Wood, V. (1982). Evaluation of student nurse clinical performance: A continuing problem. *International Nursing Review, 29*(1), 11-18.

Woolley, A. S. (1977). The long and tortured history of clinical evaluation. *Nursing Outlook, 25*(5), 308-315.

Wilson, M. E. (1994). Nursing student perspective of learning in a clinical setting. *Journal of Nursing Education, 33*(2), 81-86.

Williams, R. P., & Calvillo, E. R. (2002). Maximizing learning among students from culturally diverse backgrounds. *Nurse Educator, 27*(5), 222-226.

7
Chapter

STUDENT PERSPECTIVES
ON CLINICAL LEARNING

Beth Phillips Cusatis, MSN, RN, CNE
Kathleen Blust, MSN, RN-BC

The clinical experience in an undergraduate nursing program is a time for students to strengthen and solidify the skills, assessments, and procedures they learned in the classroom and the laboratory. Anxiety often prevails when students first begin the clinical experience. Some have fears that they will not know what to do, others fear the unknown and are extremely anxious, and yet others are concerned about the possibility of hurting a patient. Cooke (1996) addressed nursing students' perceptions of difficult or challenging situations and noted situations in which anxiety and stress were created. Initial exposure to the clinical setting, evaluations of self, interpersonal communication involving staff and patients and dealing with certain patients are examples of the situations students find difficult or anxiety provoking. High levels of anxiety can affect students' clinical performance, presenting a clear threat to success in a clinical rotation (Moscaritolo, 2009). Students, therefore, would benefit greatly from a variety of strategies faculty could use to decrease this anxiety, enhance their learning, and contribute to their development as nurses. For the purposes of this chapter, the term faculty refers to full-time faculty, clinical instructors, and part-time instructors.

This chapter examines students' perspectives of clinical education and faculty as described in the literature, as well as through students' narratives. The narratives shared throughout this chapter were offered by students currently enrolled in baccalaureate and associate degree nursing programs and are threaded throughout the chapter. Students were asked to "Describe your ideal clinical faculty" and "What do faculty members do to enhance or negatively impact your learning experiences?" In addition, students were asked, "What is your perspective on clinical learning based on your ethnicity, gender, culture, and background?" and "What was the most remarkable thing about your clinical experiences?" Questions were posed informally by the authors, and no attempt was made to conduct a research study or analyze responses to identify themes in student responses. The authors wish to thank the 170 students of Duke University and Collin College who helped us better understand student perspectives on clinical learning.

Student perceptions of effective clinical learning are determined by a variety of factors deemed important to each student, and those perceptions often are the basis for assessing faculty effectiveness (Berg & Lindseth, 2004). Since the characteristics students think the ideal clinical faculty should have are related to many factors, including the generation in which students are raised (Pozo-Munoz, Rebolloso-Pacheco & Fernandez-Ramirez, 2000), faculty must understand that "one size does not fit all" and that different students may want, need, and expect different things from faculty.

Clinical Learning Experiences

Clinical learning experiences involve many elements that are essential to students' success. Two of the most important elements are *enhancement of student learning and faculty support*.

Enhancing Student Learning

Enhancement of student learning is achieved in many ways. When faculty help students integrate knowledge learned in the classroom with real-life clinical experiences, their learning is enhanced. When faculty collaborate with clinical partners to create positive learning environments in the clinical setting, student learning is enhanced. And when students and faculty focus on providing quality patient care, student learning is enhanced.

Before placing students in clinical settings, many nursing programs "front load" content and skills in the classroom and laboratory. The rationale for this is that students are "armed" with an arsenal of knowledge and skills they can use as they begin to care for patients. Students often want to perform skills and complete hands-on procedures in order to feel prepared, to feel a sense of accomplishment (by checking things off their "to do" list), and feel like nurses. Students often learn best by kinesthetic methods, and they do need to learn how to perform various skills and procedures. But faculty also need to help them think critically, prioritize care, and manage their time. Combining the skill performance with this more conceptual learning enables the students to realize the full potential they will have as nurses. For example, inserting a nasogastric (NG) tube is a step-by-step process that can easily be memorized and performed well. But understanding the potential complications related to the gag reflex, aspiration and anatomy is essential for the nurse to effectively manage the care of a patient with an NG tube. Thus, integration of knowledge and skills is critical to practice (AACN, 2008).

Students appreciate the opportunity to contribute to the care of patients in clinical settings, but they also appreciate being accepted and acknowledged by members of the health care team in those settings. Dunn and Hansford (1997) completed a research study consisting of 229 undergraduate nursing students, examining factors that affected student perceptions of their clinical learning environment. They found that staff-student relationships were crucial to the development of a positive learning environment for the students. This included staff nurses, physicians, nurse managers and other ancillary personnel. Recently, a first semester nursing student was in her patient's room checking vital signs when the physician and team of residents entered the room. Her initial reaction was terror, especially when the physician asked about the patient's vital signs and other findings from her assessment. But when the physician recorded this information in the chart and thanked the student, that terror changed to excitement and surprise. Knowing that the team valued what she had to say increased her confidence and helped her feel as if she were part of the team. Her learning, therefore, was greatly enhanced.

Student learning is enhanced in the clinical setting when staff nurses acknowledge and encourage the students. Fostering the relationship between the staff nurses and the students may help establish closer bonds (Windsor, 1987) and ultimately improve the students' introduction into the profession as a graduate. As one student noted, "It is helpful when nurses on the units are receptive to students." It will also benefit the clinical agency by helping to produce well-educated registered nurses who are part of the team and have the knowledge and skills to provide safe and cost-effective patient care (Dunn & Hansford, 1997).

Diverse Student Populations

Millennial Students

Generational change impacts student perceptions of faculty effectiveness. Howe and Strauss (2000) contend that the millennial generation, those born between 1982 and 2002, comprise the majority of current college students today and have unique qualities that influence the students' perception. Among the traits of this population, identified by Howe and Strauss, are the following: they are structured rule followers, cooperative and team-oriented, and talented achievers. According to these experts on generational change, millennial students have mastered the ability to multitask through their access to and use of cell phones, computers, and technology; and they have been raised under the close eye of their parents as overprotective advocates of the student's success. These traits influence students' perceptions of effective clinical learning by expecting the same from the clinical faculty.

Millennial students, as structured rule followers, respect policies and procedures. Therefore, course material, expectations of the program, rules and regulations, syllabi, and guidelines must be specific and fairly enforced (Elam, Stratton, & Gibson, 2007). They also prefer that guidelines be presented in multiple formats, including printed booklets and on the Web.

As team-oriented individuals, millennial students like to collaborate with others and work together on community projects, and they often expect to receive a group grade (Elam et al., 2007). Accustomed to being engaged in numerous service projects, millennial students are socially networked and organized. They work well in groups, preferring this to individual endeavors.

Pressured throughout their education to excel in their actions, millennial students have clearly defined objectives and high expectations of their own success. As talented achievers, they actively seek help to accomplish their goals and are accustomed to being assessed, receiving focused feedback, and being goal-directed (Howe & Strauss, 2000).

Elam and colleagues (2007) note that the challenges presented by millennial students are a result of the unique qualities they possess. Being over reliant on communication technology, millennial students may have become stunted in interpersonal, face-to-face skills. Routinely engaging in multitasking, they may also develop a shortened collective attention span. Being accustomed to supervision from parents, students are used to being told what the best decision is and tend to avoid "owning" their decisions. The talented achiever is accustomed to being rewarded for "attempting" an assignment and expects a satisfactory grade that reflects that attempt; millennial students therefore, may be dissatisfied with a grade that reflects the quality of the product of their work rather than one that reflects merely the effort itself.

Students from Different Cultures and Backgrounds

Today's generation of college students is different from previous generations in terms of demographics, racial and ethnic diversity, and attitudes toward diversity issues (Broido, 2004). According to the 2000 United States census, 39.1 percent of people under 18 are people of color, compared with 28.0 percent of people over 18, and 20 percent of this generation of college students has at least one parent who is an immigrant (Howe & Strauss, 2000). The US Census Bureau (2000) confirms the influx of immigrants and notes half of those living in the United States who are foreign-born are from Latin America and Asia. As expected, with a rising percentage of students with immigrant parents, the level of English language proficiency is different than prior generations of students. As noted by Livingston and Wirt (2003), six percent of this population was identified as able to speak English less than very well. These unique qualities in today's generation of students challenge instructors to ensure that an educational path toward self-fulfillment is as direct and accessible as possible (Elam et al., 2007).

Personal and academic barriers may be challenges for ethnically diverse students and may hinder their success. With an increased percentage of minority students entering college, nursing faculty are compelled to address some of these barriers. Vasquez noted, as early as

1976, that, in the absence of supportive relationships, the minority student may be unable to share their perceptions or clarify clinical expectations. Buckley's (1980) well-known study showed that the key ingredient to success was faculty commitment. Buckley confirmed the importance of faculty commitment by noting that, even if there are no organized programs to address the ethnically diverse student, when faculty is committed to student success, students are more successful. Campbell and Davis (1996) also noted that the primary factor in promoting success is the commitment and increased involvement of nursing faculty.

Mann (2001) wrote that students disconnected from their familiar cultural experiences may feel tension because the beliefs and values of their new environment are likely to be very different from their previous experiences. An ethnically diverse student, commenting on the disconnection she felt, stated, "For me, nursing school and the clinical experience is like learning a foreign language while living in a foreign country at times!" Mann further noted that the consequence of disengagement may be poor outcome performance or potential withdrawal and/or failure to complete the course. Another student, remarking on the tension she felt, stated:

> It's a little awkward sometimes to take care of hygiene needs of the opposite gender. During clinical experience, I have to force myself to deal with the situation professionally. My background didn't prepare me to take care of other people's basic human functions. Having to do this in the beginning of first semester is [a] good reality check (student survey).

Clinical faculty can reach out to culturally diverse students by being conscientious about making themselves available to serve as role models and sources of support. The faculty-student relationship can be as simple and informal as providing encouragement, or as formal as using specific strategies for achievement. In serving as role models, faculty can show understanding, insight, and comfort to students in the clinical setting as well as show support to students in the didactic setting. Students may feel accepted versus estranged, develop security versus insecurity, feel capable versus incompetent, and feel superior versus inferior with positive role modeling and support (Campbell & Davis, 1996). An Asian-American student expressed her feelings regarding faculty support by saying,

> The faculty helped me a lot when I was in nursing school by helping me with my decision making, planning, nursing process, personal problems, and others. I am glad that my instructors provide[d] help for me and I hope the instructors will continue to help other students (p. 302).

Enhancing engagement by fostering closer student-faculty and student-student relationships encourages students to have a "sense of belonging," according to Kemper, Lee, and Li (2001). Those with a sense of belonging found their education a more fulfilling and enjoyable process than those without a sense of affiliation. Today's generation of students is team-oriented; they are individuals who like to collaborate with others and work together. Culturally diverse students, who are encouraged to form study groups, share a common learning environment, which helps develop their confidence in their ability as a student. Feeling more connected to the institution, students may be able to persist and succeed (Campbell & Davis, 1996).

Gender

A significant challenge facing nursing today is increasing the diversity of a profession that provides care to a diverse population (Roth & Colman, 2008). Although, historically, men were discouraged and denied entrance into nursing, they want to go into the profession for the same reasons as women: to care for sick and injured people, in a challenging profession that provides reasonable job security and good wages. To recruit more men, however, the image, culture, and language of nursing should be reviewed and changed (Tranbarger, 2003). Males cited numerous barriers experienced in nursing school, including: the imagery of nursing as presented to the public; the feminine image in nursing texts; the difficult balancing of school and family; and the fundamental gender communication differences.

The public's perception of nursing is generally positive, but is primarily viewed as a traditional feminine career (Lusk, 2000). Roth and Coleman (2008) contend that this perception of femininity strongly stereotypes the profession, and may be reflected as a barrier in male students' perspective on nursing. As noted by a male student, "The public view of a nurse would probably be female." Textbooks also promote the feminine image of nursing with the repeated use of the pronoun she and an absence of historical male contributions to the profession. Tranbarger (2003) reported that prior to the 20th century, more than half of those offering nursing services to the ill were male, but there is little recognition reflected in nursing textbooks.

Perceptions concerning the rigor of the nursing program may overwhelm some male students. Smith (2006) relayed the anxiety that was felt by some men who have multiple responsibilities concerning family, work, and school. One student summarized his greatest challenge this way, "When you consider working 30-40 hours, going to class and clinical, and trying to keep up with the readings, you realize there are not enough hours in the day." Male students perceived some challenges in meeting the academic demands of college and balancing family responsibilities and schoolwork, because men and women are acculturated differently in society, with different expectations imposed by family and friends (Ellis, Meeker, & Hyde, 2006). "Survival" or "Just getting through" were predominant views in interviews conducted by Smith (2006). Male students agreed that nursing school was tiring, stressful, busy, and intellectually difficult. Recognizing the rigors of the nursing program, one male student commented,

> I believe the curriculum warrants being demanding due to the level of responsibility, clinical competencies, and knowledge expected of RNs [Registered Nurses]. Unfortunately, many students have family responsibilities that conflict with the program's time requirements (p. 266).

Smith (2006) offered recommendations that might assist some male students with the rigors of balancing their multiple responsibilities. A major consideration for students is flexible times for support and services. Nursing programs could review office hours for advising, tutoring, and clinical practice times and consider more flexibility in scheduling. Comprehensive orientation programs, specifically outlining the time constraints of the program, are also suggested. Programs could explore the development of peer supports with older and diverse male students, study groups, or informal networks consisting of linking freshman-level male students with senior-level male students. Intercessions that address the challenges for male students may ease the transition into nursing programs.

In addition to addressing the feminine image of nursing and the difficulty of balancing school and family, fundamental gender communication differences also affect some male students and can be a barrier in the student perception of nursing. Villeneuve (1994) revealed men often had trouble fitting in with dominant groups of women. Many felt frustrated by what they perceived as test questions, classroom discussions, and whole courses "set up by women for women," as they felt unable to understand nursing from women's point of view. Male students felt female instructors lectured differently than male instructors and preferred male instructors because they "get to the point" (Ellis et al., 2006). This view is reflected in the comment by a male student, "On occasion, I have encountered test questions that assume the nurse is female, where the correct answer would have been inappropriate for a male to have chosen that action." Nursing faculty who review their lecture content, test questions, and written course material for gender-biased language may decrease some of the frustration of male students.

Okrainec's (1994) comparison of male and female nursing students' perceptions of nursing education showed that male respondents had a preference for science and technical nursing courses. Ellis and colleagues (2006) also determined similar perceptions in their literature: male students considered the more difficult side of nursing — the technical skills and the hard science, such as pharmacology — to be the easier content.

Nursing programs should examine the language and examples used in classes to determine the extent to which they represent both men and women in the field. Modifying class activities or adopting texts that refer to men in nursing might recognize the role of men in the profession (Smith, 2006). Thus, interventions addressing the stereotypical feminine image of nursing, flexibility in scheduling, and communication differences of male and female students may promote positive student perceptions of clinical nursing.

Characteristics of Effective Clinical Faculty

Supportive

Students want knowledgeable and competent clinical instructors (CIs) to guide, direct, and support them, and they appreciate clinical instructors who provide individualized attention and feedback while taking the time to work with them. Clinical instructors often are the first nursing role models students see, so it is important that they uphold standards of practice and are professional while enabling students to learn in safe, positive environments. It is crucial for clinical nursing faculty to foster a supportive learning environment conducive to undergraduate nursing student learning (Moscaritolo, 2009). When CIs are kind and patient, students learn more. When CIs are supportive and encouraging, student learning is enhanced. When CIs give challenging assignments and ask questions that stimulate their thinking, students grow professionally. In the authors' experiences, questions such as the following help students develop their thinking and skills as clinicians:

> What are your priorities of care for this patient…and how did you determine those to be your priorities? What else do you need to know to care for this patient…and where will you get that information? What is the most important point you want to help this patient and his family learn before being discharged to home?

These questions stimulate student critical thinking and help them connect concepts they have learned in order to plan and deliver quality care to the whole patient. Educating critical thinkers is more than developing critical thinking skills. A complete approach to developing good critical thinkers includes nurturing the disposition toward critical thinking, which includes inquisitiveness, systematicity, analyticity, truth-seeking, open-mindedness, critical thinking self-confidence, and maturity. (Facione, Facione, & Sanchez, 1994). The goal is that ultimately students will develop expert clinical judgment as professional nurses.

Being part of the pains and joys experienced by patients and their families enhances student learning and strengthens their confidence. Such experiences help students realize the trust patients and families have in them, help them appreciate how they can make a difference in patients' lives, and help them be more confident. As one student said after his first clinical rotation, "I didn't realize the intimacy in the nurse-patient relationship." Oftentimes, however, students hesitate to proceed with care for fear of hurting the patient: "I have a fear of walking in the room for the first time" …"It is frustrating that I can't do that much to help and I need to move past my fear." Part of the goal of providing support, then, is for faculty to allay students' fears and hesitancies and build their confidence as nurses.

Students need to be acknowledged for the things they do know and encouraged and guided in the areas where they are deficient. Thus, faculty need to help students mesh their previous experiences with their new role. For example, an engineer who is now enrolled in a nursing program can be encouraged to use her/his knowledge to develop new devices that will enhance the practice of nursing and improve patient care. Encouraging such thinking enables the student to be creative and innovative and can, ultimately, improve nursing practice.

As noted, a most important element in clinical education is the faculty member who designs the experience with clinical partners, teaches students in the clinical setting, and evaluates students' clinical performance. Students have defined the effective clinical instructor in terms of interpersonal relationships, evaluation, teaching ability, nursing competence, and personality (Knox & Mogan, 1985).

Establish Positive Interpersonal Relationships

Knox and Mogan (1985) asserted that an interpersonal relationship includes the faculty member's communication capabilities, empathy, motivation, availability, and understanding. Berg and Lindseth (2004) also identified similar qualifications in students' perspectives of effective and ineffective nursing instructors. Although students perceive all of these components to be important; communication may be one of the most important features, as noted by this student:

> The instructor should be organized and good at communication. The program is so stressful, that a lack of communication greatly increases my stress. Good communication puts me at ease from the beginning so that I can focus on learning, even from my mistakes, rather than fearing I have to be perfect when I'm so new at this. Communicate the rationales of why I am to do things in a specific way so I can understand (Berg and Lindseth, p. 567).

Negative communication for millennial students can be perceived when the technology used in delivering instruction is not as technologically advanced as they have become accustomed to using. As one student states, "I need to be challenged to think during lecture. Using pictures in PowerPoint® and games instead of reading from slides will allow me more participation."

Empathy toward students is also necessary. Students want faculty to appreciate them when they do well, and added that this appreciation would motivate them (Elcigil & Sari, 2008). A student said, "Instructors acting as cheerleaders can enhance my learning experience. When instructors lead by example, I am motivated to learn. I would say this is one of the biggest factors in a student's positive learning experience." Another student noted:

> An ideal clinical instructor is someone who verbalizes they are there to help me learn and succeed without pressuring me to perform. Someone who is down to earth and remembers what it's like to be a student is helpful. I think it's important for the instructor to remember they have passed this way before me and will take my hand in theirs and show me the way (student survey).

Availability and understanding are also considered significant components of the interpersonal relationship. Students expect understanding from faculty, especially if the workload is intense (Elcigil & Sari, 2008), as noted by this student:

> Mentors should have understanding. In fact, when I have a problem or when I get confused, they should help me and give sound advice. Further, mentors should not stop communication when we ask for help. Actually, they are the source of information during practice hours and when we need information about something, they should offer it (p. 120).

Fair and Encouraging with Evaluation

Students often perceive evaluations to be little more than judgments about their performance. They note, however, that evaluations should also be encouragement. One student suggested:

> Let me know what I can do better or more efficiently. Explain rationales in detail as I am going through my lab practice. Give examples of how to plan and organize my clinical day and discuss care plans individually as a teaching tool, rather than a grade (student survey).

Positive evaluations encourage students to learn more, and they enhance self-respect and self-confidence. Students note that feedback is important but believe that faculty should not be overly critical when providing feedback (Elcigil & Sari, 2008). As one student stated: "Critique me honestly when I am doing something wrong and help me make corrections." "Guide and advise me in a non-overly, judgmental manner" was what another student desired.

As noted earlier, millennial students are accustomed to supervision by their parents, therefore, taking responsibility for their own decisions may be difficult. A student commented that, "I cannot be responsible for developing myself as there is so much new material to absorb, just to meet the basic demands of the faculty." The following comments by students exemplify their hesitation to think critically in an independent way: "My instructor should be with me in the hospital to help me make the difficult decisions"; "Tell me how to plan and organize my clinical day"; "I should be observed and guided through every procedure at the hospital. It is the responsibility of the instructor to develop my individual learning experience."

Student engagement in the learning process may help in developing independent critical thinking, and assist in the evaluation process. Accountability for their decisions may be more likely if the teaching methods employ student engagement, problem-solving, and cooperative learning (Ramsden, 2003). Taking an active role in their learning may enable the student to recognize, as stated by Mann (2001), that a personal stance in the learning process will enable them to take on the role of an active agent. This promotes self-sufficiency in the student and less dependency on the instructor. Therefore, a continuum of engagement using teaching methods in a way that the student is likely to understand may promote independent critical thinking and student ownership of their learning experiences during the evaluation process.

This generation of students is accustomed to receiving a satisfactory grade merely for attempting an assignment, but their perceptions of the quality of their work may be naïve. Having been nurtured to expect praise with each effort, the student may be dissatisfied with a grade that appropriately evaluates their performance. Sensitivity to a student's sense of expectation appears to be a key element in creating a more conducive environment for teaching and learning. Faculty need to explicitly acknowledge the effort students are making and offer praise where it is due as well as constructive criticism and encouragement where further progress is required (Bryson & Hand, 2007).

Competent

Nursing competence is also a characteristic of an effective clinical instructor. Nursing competence encompasses faculty experience in the field, knowledge of clinical situations, and proficiency in their specialty. Students expect faculty to offer information and insights that are not available in textbooks (Elcigil & Sari, 2008). As one student remarked, "I like someone who is very experienced, knowledgeable and has high standards for me; someone wanting me to be the best a nurse can be." Another noted:

> I appreciate the wealth of experience faculty have to share. Faculty that are very knowledgeable and are able to answer my questions well enhance my learning experience. I am fascinated listening to some of the stories from the faculty and hope one day I'll be as knowledgeable as they are (student survey).

And yet another student shared this thought: "When an instructor gives personal stories they had as a nurse, it really helps me learn."

Able to Teach Effectively and Display Positive Personal Traits

Characteristics of an effective clinical instructor include teaching ability and several personal traits. Students expect faculty to be advisers who guide and offer information or explanations about clinical practices, and sources of knowledge who answer their questions and provide them with resources. They believe faculty should demonstrate new skills and help the student practice those skills (Elcigil & Sari, 2008). As one student noted, "I like to see something performed and then be able to practice it as someone walks me through it, giving me rationales and practical tips throughout. I learn by seeing and following examples." Another student said, "I think the faculty should be supportive, providing guidance in the situation when the student is not sure what to do." Simply stated by one student, "Repeat, repeat, repeat."

In addition to being competent, knowledgeable and self-confident as nurses, students also value enthusiasm for nursing and teaching, the ability to admit mistakes honestly, patience, approachability, caring, and flexibility (Elcigil & Sari, 2008). This is evidenced by the student who commented that, "The ideal clinical faculty is approachable and knowledgeable; someone who listens and answers the question I am asking, not the question they think I am asking and someone who is calm, encouraging, and supportive to me."

Additional traits include clarity, preparedness, and consistency in their teachings. A student's comment, "It's definitely the lecturer that can really make it interesting or can almost destroy a subject" illustrates this point. Applying these teaching skills and traits can enhance student engagement, active participation, and understanding of the material (Bryson & Hand, 2007).

When faculty members view students as capable individuals with much to offer, students become more confident in their own abilities. But faculty, too, need to be prepared and confident in their own abilities and expertise as clinicians and as teachers. They must maintain clinical skills, understand changes in how the clinical environment functions, and be technologically savvy. They play a key role in building the relationships between the staff nurses and the students. The CI is invaluable to negotiating the acceptance of the students onto the clinical unit. The relationship between the unit administration and the CI also influences the attitudes with which the staff approach and address the students (Dunn & Hansford, 1997). Finally, faculty must help students critically analyze the many time-honored practices still in effect today to determine which need to remain because they are based on sound evidence, and which need to be challenged, questioned, or changed.

Conclusion

In conclusion, sound, effective clinical learning is essential for nursing students to become independent, qualified nurses, and students value the role that clinical instructors play in their development and growth. They recognize the benefits of linking the classroom to the clinical setting. They value a supportive, challenging experience to help them achieve their goals and learn how to organize and prioritize care. They benefit from the willingness of patients and families to share their personal health struggles with them in the name of education. When students are considered part of the team, they feel more valued and accepted. Combining student perspectives with excellence in clinical instruction provides a valuable learning environment for growth and success in the profession.

Students' perspectives of effective clinical learning are related, in part, to their culture, previous experiences, and upbringing. Instructors need to understand the perspectives and unique expectations students bring to clinical experiences and respond positively to this diversity. They also would do well to appreciate that students value clinical proficiency, positive interpersonal relationships, helpful evaluations, patience, clear communications, and sensitivity to individual learning needs.

Recommendations for future research include a perspective study, using a questionnaire given in the beginning of the student's first semester and completed in their last semester, to evaluate if the student's perceptions of nursing faculty change over time. Using the same format, another study could evaluate the student's perception of the ideal clinical instructor to determine if there are changes over time. Repeating the study again, using a more broadly based sample of schools to validate the findings, could also be considered.

To review, a study asking the following questions might be given to graduates and faculty:

- Are the students' perspectives of clinical learning in tandem with the purpose and objectives of the course and program? If not, what needs to change?
- Are the students adequately prepared for the rigors and realities of the nursing profession?
- Are faculty members proactive in the role as facilitator amongst staff and students?

A qualitative study, using survey or interview, to determine role-strain of male nursing students is suggested. Sex-role characterizations of both male and female students can also be explored in a qualitative study. Finally, future studies, including clinical observations of male nursing students as compared to female students, may be beneficial.

References

AACN (American Association of Colleges of Nursing). (2008). *Essentials of baccalaureate education for professional nursing practice*. Washington, DC: Author.

Berg, C., & Lindseth, G. (2004). [Research brief]. Students' perspectives of effective and ineffective nursing instructors. *Journal of Nursing Education, 43*, 565-568.

Broido, E. (2004). Understanding diversity in millennial students. *New Directions for Student Services, 106*, 73-85.

Bryson, C., & Hand, L. (2007). The role of engagement in inspiring teaching and learning. *Innovations in Education and Teaching International, 44*, 349-362.

Buckley, J. (1980). Faculty commitment to retention and recruitment of black students. *Nursing Outlook, 28*, 46-50.

Campbell, A., & Davis, S. (1996). Faculty commitment: Retaining minority nursing students in majority institutions. *Journal of Nursing Education, 35*(7), 289-303.

Cooke, M. (1996). Nursing students' perceptions of difficult or challenging clinical situations. *Journal of Advanced Nursing, 24*, 1281-1287.

Dunn, S., & Hansford, B. (1997). Undergraduate nursing students' perceptions of their clinical learning environment. *Journal of Advanced Nursing, 25*, 1299-1306.

Elam, C., Stratton, T., & Gibson, D. (2007). Welcoming a new generation to college: The millennial students. *Journal of College Admission, 195*, 20-25.

Elcigil, A., & Sari, H. Y. (2008). Students' opinions about and expectations of effective nursing clinical mentors. *Journal of Nursing Education, 47*(3), 118-123.

Ellis, D. M., Meeker, B., & Hyde, B. (2006). Exploring men's perceived educational experiences in a baccalaureate program. *Journal of Nursing Education, 45*(12), 523-527.

Facione, N., Facione, P., & Sanchez, C. (1994). Critical thinking disposition as a measure of competent clinical judgment: The development of the California Critical Thinking Disposition Inventory, *Journal of Nursing Education, 33*(8), 345-350.

Howe, N., & Strauss, W. (2000). *Millennials rising: The next great generation*. New York: Vintage Books.

Kemper, D., Lee, K., & Li, N. (2001). Cultivating a sense of belonging in part-time students. *International Journal of Lifelong Education, 20*(4), 326-341.

Knox, J., & Mogan, J. (1985). Important clinical teacher behaviours as perceived by university nursing faculty, students, and graduates. *Journal of Advanced Nursing, 10*, 25-30.

Livingston, A., & Wirt, J. (Eds.). (2003). *The condition of education 2003 in brief*. Washington, DC: U.S. Department of Education, Institute of Education Sciences, NCES. Retrieved April 4, 2009, from http://nces.ed.gov/pubs2003/2003068.pdf

Lusk, B. (2000). Pretty and powerless: Nurses in advertisements, 1930-1950. *Research in Nursing and Health, 23*, 229-236.

Mann, S. (2001). Alternative perspectives on the student experience: Alienation and engagement. *Studies in Higher Education, 26*(1), 7-9.

Moscaritolo, L. (2009). Interventional strategies to decrease nursing student anxiety in the clinical learning environment. *Journal of Nursing Education, 48*(1), 17-23.

Okrainec, G. D. (1994). Perceptions of nursing education held by male nursing students. *Western Journal of Nursing Research, 16*, 94-107.

Pozo-Munoz, C., Rebolloso-Pacheco, E., & Fernandez-Ramirez, B. (2000). The "ideal teacher." Implications for student evaluation of teacher effectiveness. *Assessment & Evaluation in Higher Education, 25*, 253-64.

Ramsden, P. (2003). *Learning to teach in higher education* (2nd ed.). London: Routledge Falmer.

Roth, J., & Coleman, C. (2008). Perceived and real barriers for men entering nursing: Implications for gender diversity. *Journal of Cultural Diversity, 15*(3), 148-152.

Smith, J. (2006). Exploring the challenges for nontraditional male students transiting into a nursing program. *Journal of Nursing Education, 45*(7), 263-269.

Tranbarger, G. (2003). Where are the men? *Nursing, 33*(9), 56-57.

U.S. Census Bureau. (2000). Profile of the foreign-born population in the United States: 2000. Current population reports: Special studies. Retrieved January 16, 2009, from http://www.census.gov/prod/2002pubs/p23-206.pdf

Vasquez, J. A. (1976). *Locus of control*. Hillsdale, NJ: Lawrence Erlbaum.

Villeneuve, M. J. (1994). Recruiting and retaining men in nursing: A review of the literature. *Journal of Professional Nursing, 10*, 217-228.

Windsor, A. (1987). Nursing students' perceptions of clinical experience. *Journal of Nursing Education, 26*(4), 150-154.

Chapter 8

EDUCATOR PERSPECTIVES ON TRANSITIONING CLINICIANS TO THE ACADEMIC FACULTY ROLE WITH EMPHASIS ON CLINICAL TEACHING

Marsha Howell Adams, DSN, RN, CNE

Impacting the nursing shortage crisis and the future of nursing education itself is the shortage of nursing faculty. It is the major factor affecting how many qualified nursing students are admitted to nursing programs and consequently added to the nursing workforce. The National League for Nursing (NLN) has identified faculty aging, increased numbers of part-time faculty and a decrease in the number of doctoral prepared faculty as significant factors affecting nursing education (2005a) — by 2019, 75 percent of presently employed nurse faculty are expected to retire; the number of part-time faculty has increased from 29 percent to 39 percent over the last 10 years; and only 50 percent of faculty in baccalaureate and higher degree programs, 6.6 percent of those who teach in associate degree programs and five percent of the faculty in diploma programs possess doctoral degrees (NLN, 2005b).

Data from the American Association of Colleges of Nursing (AACN) show a national faculty vacancy rate in baccalaureate and higher degree programs of 7.6 percent, which is approximately 1.8 vacant faculty positions per school (AACN, 2008). Nurse clinicians are being heavily recruited into nursing academe in an effort to fill the vacant faculty positions evident in nursing programs across the country. In addition, clinical agencies are collaborating with nursing programs to creatively design positions for clinicians who are interested in teaching.

Transitioning from the role of expert clinician to a full-time or part-time faculty role can be an arduous but very rewarding task. The NLN has developed competencies for nurse educators (Halstead, 2007; NLN, 2005b) that articulate the complexity of the role and guide educators as they develop expertise in the role. These competencies address eight crucial areas: a) facilitate learning, b) facilitate learner development and socialization, c) use assessment and evaluation strategies, d) participate in curriculum design and evaluation of program outcomes, e) function as change agents and leaders, f) develop the educator role, g) engage in scholarship, and h) function within the educational environment.

This chapter addresses the key components associated with transitioning from a clinician role to a faculty role as described in the NLN's nurse educator competencies. Emphasis will be placed on clinical teaching, including preparation, implementation and evaluation as major expectations of the faculty role. Benefits and barriers to transitioning are discussed as well as strategies for success. Lastly, research areas are identified that have the potential to provide evidence to inform the development and implementation of successful transition programs for new/novice faculty members.

Key Components in Transitioning to the Faculty Role

Level of Education

Educational preparation for the faculty role has always been a debated issue. In the early 1900s, the baccalaureate degree was considered acceptable in some academic programs, such as licensed practical nursing programs and associate degree programs. Today, the master's degree (MSN) is required as the minimum level of education for full-time nurse faculty. The National Council of State Boards of Nursing (NCSBN) states that nursing faculty in both Registered Nurse and Practical Nurse programs should have either a master's or doctoral degree (2008). However, while there are an increasing number of master's programs designed to prepare educators, the majority of MSN programs focus on preparing advanced practice nurses for a clinical specialty area.

Bartel (2007) voices concern over the number of MSN nurse educator programs emerging across the country in an effort to address the nursing faculty shortage and notes that (a) most focus only on the teaching aspect rather than the entire tripartite mission of teaching, research, and service and (b) individuals completing such nurse educator preparation programs bring only baccalaureate level clinical skills to their teaching. This author asserts that for faculty teaching in baccalaureate and higher degree programs, it is imperative that the doctoral degree serve as minimal preparation for the nurse educator.

In contrast, the NLN (2002) has asserted that preparation for the educator role appropriately takes place at either the master's or doctoral level. However, such preparation must include a focus on advanced practice as well as teaching skills. While the focus on advanced practice does not necessarily mean that one must also prepare as a nurse practitioner or clinical nurse specialist to be a nurse educator, it does suggest that one must possess advanced knowledge and skill in assessment, pharmacology, pathophysiology, and clinical problems. Such an assertion would lead one to conclude that, like Bartel (2007), master's programs that focus only on teaching are inappropriate preparation for the complexity of the educator role.

Most nurse clinicians entering the academic arena have an MSN with a clinical focus. While clinical knowledge and skills are important for the faculty role, they are not sufficient for assuming the role of a full-time nurse educator in an academic environment. The transition from a clinical to an academic role, then, is difficult and involves more than just practicing in a different setting. For individuals transitioning to a part-time faculty position or as an adjunct faculty, level of education requirements may vary based on role expectations of such part-time clinical instruction versus classroom instruction. For example, baccalaureate-prepared nurses in some states can serve as part-time clinical faculty, but cannot be hired as full-time faculty for classroom and clinical instruction.

Faculty Appointments

Academic appointment may vary depending on the type of nursing program, the institution's and school of nursing's missions, and employment status (i.e., full-time or part-time). There are different tracks for faculty appointment — tenured, nontenured/contract, and clinical — and each has specific role expectations and responsibilities. Tenured track appointments usually emphasize teaching, research and service; clinical track appointees typically focus on teaching and clinical practice; and while a nontenured/contract track can vary from one institution to the next, teaching and/or clinical is usually the main focus of such roles. Expectations for scholarship differ for various types of appointments, but all faculty are expected to remain current in their areas of teaching responsibility, contribute to the profession, and grow professionally. Within each track, individuals can be appointed or promoted to the rank of Instructor, Assistant Professor, Associate Professor and Professor.

Individuals transitioning to the academic environment need to have a clear understanding of the implications of their appointment status (full time versus part time), track, rank and responsibilities (Billings & Kowalski, 2008; Penn, Wilson, & Rosseter, 2008). Knowledge about this issue is crucial, since it is also connected to advancement and success within the organization.

Clinical Teaching

The clinical setting allows students the opportunity to apply theory to practice, and the clinical instructor guides students to meet clinical objectives and develop clinical competencies. While clinicians transitioning to the educator role will find a certain "comfort level" being back in the clinical setting, the knowledge and skills one needs to teach in such a setting are quite different from those needed to practice there. Faculty and student success in the clinical environment requires the new/novice faculty to approach clinical teaching in phases: a) preparation of the clinical environment; b) implementation of students' clinical experience; and c) evaluating the clinical environment.

Preparation of the clinical environment. There is a great deal of preparation that must be done prior to taking students to the clinical area. The process for *securing a clinical site* may vary by institution. Usually this process is carried out by an administrative person, particularly if a new contract is required between the clinical agency and the college of nursing. But one must realize that in some nursing programs securing a clinical site is performed by the individual faculty member. Several considerations must be made when securing a clinical site, including agency philosophy (whether it is congruent with the nursing program's mission, vision and core values), agency requirements and policies (background checks, drug testing, costs, etc.), course objectives, students' level of knowledge and skills to provide safe patient care (general medical surgical unit versus critical care unit), staff attitudes toward working with nursing students and faculty, physical size of the clinical area (whether the site can accommodate the number of students) and clinical site opportunities available to promote a strong learning environment.

Faculty orientation to the clinical site is an important component to be considered. The new/novice faculty needs to be allotted time to fully orient to the clinical site prior to the students' arrival for the semester. Contacting the individual responsible for the clinical site, such as the nurse manager, and setting up a meeting to discuss a collaborative approach to orientation is the first step. Shadowing nurses at the site to learn the true "ins and outs" of the area will provide great insight for the faculty member to clinical site practices, staff relationships, patient population, and potential student learning experiences. It is very important that the staff understand their role and the faculty's role when students are in clinical. The students are there in the role of the learner and are not present to replace staff, but can be available to assist staff when needed.

The *development of positive relationships with the staff* is a "must" for success. The staff needs to understand that they are a valued commodity to the enhancement of student learning experiences. Staff can alert faculty to learning opportunities occurring on the clinical site at any given time and can serve as a preceptor to the student when the faculty member is working with another student. Therefore, the faculty needs to demonstrate to the staff that you are organized when working in the clinical area with students and that you value the staff's knowledge, expertise and time. Providing the staff with positive feedback and thanking them each week for their help and support for student learning can assist the cultivation of these relationships throughout each semester.

Implementation of the students' clinical experience. The clinical experience is where nursing students are provided opportunities for application of knowledge and validation of psychomotor skills based on specific student outcomes. Students need to be provided experiences that enhance their critical thinking abilities and position them for making sound clinical decisions that support patient safety and quality patient care. The faculty member serves as the facilitator of students' learning. The number of clinical hours allocated in each clinical nursing course is a contract, in a sense, between the faculty member and the students. It is the faculty member's responsibility to provide students with a positive clinical learning environment within the designated time frame of clinical hours. Another responsibility of the faculty member is to provide students with as many "hands on" experiences as possible. Don't forget what Confucius said in 450 BC, *"Tell me, and I will forget. Show me, and I may remember. Involve me, and I will understand."* The use of observational experiences and their value to student learning have always been a faculty concern. Some state boards of nursing specify a specific and limited percentage of clinical time allocated to observation. For the observational experience to be valuable, there needs to be specific objectives related to the experience, and it is recommended that a written assignment detailing the experience be required. For example, using the operating room as an observational experience can be beneficial to student learning, particularly if nursing students are able to follow patients through preoperative, intraoperative and postoperative stages of surgery.

Throughout the clinical experience, faculty should keep "anecdotal notes" on each student in the clinical group. These notes are a descriptive record of student actions that have occurred during the clinical day. Anecdotal notes should be written in a timely manner in order to prevent omission of pertinent information about the clinical experience. Students' strengths and areas needing improvement should be addressed in the notes. Anecdotal notes can be used when providing formative and summative evaluation to students.

Student orientation to the clinical portion of the course and the clinical site is very important. Prior to going to the clinical site, the faculty can meet with the students to discuss overall clinical expectations, such as how to prepare each week for clinical, specific agency policies that affect student performance when providing patient care, paperwork (concept maps, drug cards, etc.) due dates, how a typical day may flow, and how technology will be used on the site, including computerized charting, electronic medication administration records, and the use of portable electronic devices such as PDAs. A thorough clinical orientation to the institution and the actual clinical site usually occurs on the first day of clinical. Students need to acclimate themselves to the clinical site. Some faculty use a "scavenger hunt" approach to orienting students to the clinical site.

Making clinical assignments is an important component of clinical teaching. Based on clinical objectives and specific student learning needs, the faculty member will assign patients whose care allows the student to meet or expand those objectives. The staff can also be helpful in determining which patients are most suitable for the students. Another important aspect of making assignments is that it allows students to make more focused preparation for the clinical day, and it enables faculty to hold the students responsible for that preparation. Based on the level of nursing student, faculty can determine when it is appropriate for nursing students to make their own patient assignments. This can occur based on semester or course progression.

As stated earlier, faculty serves as facilitators of student learning, not supervisors or overseers. During clinical teaching, the faculty *facilitates the students' learning activities*. Throughout the clinical experience, faculty need to serve as professional role models, identify individual student strengths and areas needing improvement, design additional learning activities for students who need it, promote students' critical thinking abilities by asking questions, and make sound decisions about students' clinical performance. In addition to asking questions throughout the clinical day, faculty can hold pre and postclinical conferences with students. Preclinical conferences can be held with the entire clinical group or individually. This time is used to assess the students' knowledge base in preparation for performing safe, quality nursing care. Postclinical conference allows students' time to reflect on their actions and decisions made throughout the day. In both situations, the faculty needs to clarify with the students that asking questions and receiving answers is an important component to the teaching/learning process and to the development of critical thinking.

Evaluation of students' clinical performance is an integral part of clinical teaching. Formative evaluation occurs throughout the semester as faculty observe students' performance and progress toward meeting the stated clinical objectives and competencies. Faculty identify students' strengths and areas of improvement and share this information with the students throughout the semester, enabling them to grow and make necessary behavior changes that position them for success. Summative evaluation occurs at the end of the clinical experience. The evaluation reflects what has been learned by the students and whether clinical objectives and competencies have been met.

Evaluating the clinical environment can be accomplished at the end of each semester or annually. Most colleges of nursing have developed a set of criteria used to evaluate the clinical area. Once the evaluation is completed, the faculty member needs to set up an appointment to discuss the evaluation with the nurse manager/staff. During this time, the nurse manager/staff has an opportunity to discuss their perception of how the clinical experience went and if any changes need to be made.

Teaching Responsibilities in the Classroom and Online

For the clinician transitioning to a faculty role, teaching responsibilities have been found to create the highest level of concern or stress (Penn et al., 2008; Siler & Kleiner, 2001). Typically this is due to a lack of background or experience with academic teaching. While the new/novice faculty member may be an expert clinician, the role of teacher is viewed as a path untraveled.

To further complicate the situation, the focus of teaching has evolved from teacher-centered to student-centered learning, and today's faculty must engage students to facilitate learning using collaborative and active learning strategies such as gaming, case studies, and simulation experiences. Since most nurses have not been educated in such an environment themselves, learning how to teach this way is even more challenging. In addition, faculty need to understand and develop strategies to meet the learning needs of an increasingly diverse student population, including the multigenerational students now known as Traditionalists, Baby Boomers, Generation Xers, and Millennials, each of whom has their own unique traits and behaviors. Gibson (2009) recommends taking the basic principles of adult learning, such as motivation, level of engagement, and life experiences, and applying them to each generation's core values of life, work, authority, and relationships in order to enhance learning.

In addition to knowing and being able to use a variety of strategies to meet the learning needs of diverse students, new/novice faculty need to be knowledgeable in many other areas that are part of their responsibility:

- *Course Design and Development of a Course Syllabus*: When designing a course, it is important to keep in mind the level of student being taught, as well as what students "need to know" versus what is "nice" for them to know or "nuts" for them to know (Ignatavicius, 2009). Increasingly, it is becoming apparent that it is more important for students to master a smaller amount of information than it is to simply or superficially be exposed to a larger amount.

- *Instructional Design: Onsite and/or Online Courses*: The instructional design of a course refers to the incorporation of a wide range of teaching/learning strategies that will most effectively enhance student learning. New/Novice faculty will need to become knowledgeable about how to integrate technology into teaching, and those teaching online will need to know how to use course delivery modalities such as Blackboard, WebCT, or other systems.

- *Evaluation of Student Learning*: One of the most intimidating areas for new faculty is that of evaluating what students have learned, including the creation of tests. Test development involves creating a blueprint based on content covered, writing test items with the majority at an application level, ensuring the test items are valid and reliable, and analyzing test questions to confirm validity and reliability…all areas where new faculty typically have little expertise. In addition to testing, faculty must know how to design and effectively use a number of other methods to evaluate student learning, including portfolios, formal papers, clinical logs, presentations, and clinical performance. The latter is complex but critical to assure that student learning outcomes are met and that students deliver safe, quality patient care; evaluation can be accomplished through the use of an established list of critical behaviors the student will be expected to demonstrate in the clinical area.

- *Course Evaluation*: Individual evaluation of courses is used to determine whether a course was successful in achieving specified outcomes and in facilitating student learning. Such evaluation allows students to participate in the teaching/learning process and provides them with a unique opportunity to describe their experiences in working to meet course objectives; it also is part of a quality improvement process that contributes to continual refinement and enhancement of the educational process.

- *Technology Integration*: Integration of technology has become an important aspect of student learning. Most nursing courses are either web-supported or totally online. New faculty will need development on creation of web-supported or web-based courses. Also, nursing education programs across the country are moving toward the requirement of portable electronic devices such as a Personal Digital Assistant (PDA) or iPod Touch for nursing students and faculty to be used in the classroom and clinical area. The devices allow quick retrieval of important reference information about medications, laboratory values, disease processes, pathophysiology, etc. New faculty may need to complete tutorials and hands-on practice to become proficient with these devices. Human patient simulation is another area in which a clinician transitioning to the faculty role will need faculty development. Simulation is a teaching strategy that can be used in the theory or clinical portions of courses. The learning curve for faculty acquiring competence in simulator operation, scenario development and implementation, and debriefing expertise can be a rewarding but challenging one.

- *Dealing with Student Concerns and Disciplinary Issues*: Student concerns primarily revolve around grades, exams, and excuses. New/Novice faculty need to be open, approachable, and "good listeners." Discussing student concerns should always be done in private. Policies focusing on attendance, grading scales, makeup exams, and absenteeism from both class and clinical should guide the faculty when making decisions; one should always follow the policy. Most students want to be provided an environment where they can voice their concerns and feel that they have been heard, no matter what the outcome. Students should be familiar with the line of communication regarding resolution of concerns. For example, if a concern is directly related to a nursing course, the student should start with the course/clinical faculty and then the course leader. If the concern is not resolved at that level, the student may seek resolution through a conference with the director of the program, associate dean, or the dean, respectively. In addition, each college of nursing has a grievance policy. Students need to be made aware of this policy. A student complaint can lead to an academic grievance when the student deems an academic action unfair. Examples include allegations of unfairness in grading, alleged violation of written or oral agreement with the student, and alleged inconsistent application of existing policies. Faculty should consult the college of nursing's code of academic conduct and the academic misconduct disciplinary policy when dealing with students' disciplinary issues.

Faculty Role Responsibilities

While teaching and clinical expertise are two areas that are very important in the transitioning of clinicians to the academic environment, there are other responsibilities inherent in the faculty role. Siler and Kleiner (2001) found that novice faculty viewed academia through the eyes of the student they had been, and their perceptions did not include a realistic look at the complexities of the academic environment or the demands of faculty role responsibilities. To make a successful transition to the faculty role, individuals will need to be knowledgeable regarding the following areas:

- *Mission, Vision and Core Values*: These serve as the guiding framework for the institution and the school of nursing. They reflect the institution's and school's purpose and give shape and direction to their future.

- *Strategic Plan*: This reflects the key goals for the parent institution and the school of nursing. It describes where the institution/school of nursing is going over the next three to five years and how it plans to get there. For each goal, outcome measures, specific objectives, action plans, and timelines are articulated. In addition, the plan often identifies the individual or office expected to provide leadership in achieving the goal.

- *Organizational Chart*: This chart reflects the formal relationships within the organization based on job responsibilities or position, and it is helpful to the new/novice faculty when questions about formal lines of communication arise.

- *Service to the School of Nursing and the Parent Institution*: This area involves expectations of attending faculty organization meetings or hearings/open forums, serving on committees, advising students, serving as an adviser to student groups, participating in the community through volunteerism and service/learning opportunities, and so on.

- *Faculty Handbook*: This resource contains the policies and procedures of the organization and usually addresses the major areas of administration, faculty, curriculum, students, academic support systems, college organizations, and descriptions for major organizational positions, all of which are important for both full-time and adjunct faculty to know.

- *Faculty Evaluation System*: This provides the faculty with an ongoing mechanism to (a) document accomplishments and performance, which often are used to determine merit increases; (b) evaluate progress toward attainment of the goals that were set in the previous year; and (c) establish goals for the upcoming academic year.

- *Legal and Ethical Issues*: All faculty must be familiar with the Family Educational Rights and Privacy Act (FERPA), which was designed to "protect the privacy of student educational records" (US Department of Education, 2008). When an individual student becomes 18 years of age or attends a college (any school beyond high school), she/he has the right to determine who has access to any information related to her/his educational record. The student must provide permission in a written format to allow parents to have access to her/his academic record or discuss her/his performance with faculty.

- *Program Evaluation and Accreditation*: Program evaluation is performed to determine the extent to which the academic program has helped students achieve intended outcomes and to assess the satisfaction of graduating students, alumni, faculty, and employers with the nursing program in preparing graduates for the practice setting. Accreditation is a voluntary process that guides faculty to conduct a critical review of the nursing program and determine its strengths and areas in need of improvement, assess the resources (faculty, technology, library, etc.) available to implement the program, the effectiveness of policies, and so on. The two accrediting bodies in nursing are the National League for Nursing Accrediting Commission (NLNAC) and the Commission on Collegiate Nursing Education (CCNE), both of which are approved by the US Department of Education. The NLNAC accredits all types of nursing programs, while CCNE accredits only baccalaureate and higher degree programs (NLNAC, 2008; CCNE, 2008). Components of the accreditation process are a self-study of the program by the faculty, an onsite evaluation of the program by external certified evaluators, and a determination by one's peers whether accreditation standards have been met and accreditation should be recommended.

Benefits and Barriers to Transitioning to the Faculty Role

The faculty role in the academic environment has both benefits and barriers that an individual needs to consider prior to taking a faculty appointment (Culleiton & Shellenbarger, 2007; Penn et al., 2008). Benefits include the following:

- Experiencing the best of both worlds, working with students in the academic setting and remaining connected to the clinical environment
- Witnessing the "aha" moments students experience, and knowing you were part of making such insights happen
- Engaging in significant work with individuals who share one's goals and expectations
- Enjoying a stronger sense of freedom and flexibility than in the practice setting
- Being able to access a variety of resources (e.g., library, technology) and faculty development opportunities (e.g., workshops, conferences)
- Enjoying a more flexible schedule and work hours, with holidays off and summer work often optional
- Continuing to practice, particularly if on a nine-month contract
- Being rewarded for professional contributions such as presentations, consultation, and manuscript development
- Receiving encouragement and support to continue one's education, publish, conduct research, and write grants

Barriers to successful transitioning include:

- Earning a lower salary than one would receive in a practice setting
- Experiencing a "mismatch" between one's value of teaching and clinical practice and the institution's value of research, publication, and obtaining external funding

  Carrying a workload that requires taking work home at night, grading student assignments/papers with short turnaround time, preparing for clinical experiences, classroom preparation, answering emails in a timely manner, and preparing student evaluations
- Balancing all components of the faculty role, including scholarship and practice, and still having a personal life

Strategies for Successful Transitioning to the Faculty Role

Despite barriers like those mentioned above, there are several strategies that can promote successful transitioning into the faculty role. Some of these strategies still remain untested and need to be researched to document their value, but they hold promise nevertheless.

Mentoring Programs

Mentoring in nursing encompasses "a guided, non-evaluated experience, formal or informal, assigned over a mutually-agreed-on period of time that empowers the mentor and mentee to develop personally and professionally within the auspices of a caring, collaborative, and respectful environment" (Grossman, 2007, p. 2), and it has been identified as the single most influential method to successfully develop new/novice faculty into the academic role (Durham-Taylor, Lynn, Moore, McDaniel, & Walker, 2008). The NLN (2006) has developed a position statement on mentoring of nursing faculty that advocates this strategy to promote healthful work environments and facilitate ongoing career development of nurse faculty. The position statement recommends that new/novice faculty be assigned a senior faculty member with extensive experience in the faculty role to serve as the mentor. The senior faculty should be approachable, positive and caring toward the mentee.

Smith and Zsohar (2007, p. 185) identified components of a successful mentoring program for new faculty. Those components are as follows:

- Positive mentor qualities, such as good interpersonal skills, commitment to the relationship, caring, and competence
- Focus on more than just career development
- Knowledgeable about the elements of a mentoring relationship — Relating, Assessing, Coaching, and Guiding (Portner, 1998)
- Mutual trust
- Understanding that a relationship changes over time
- Development of a collegial relationship
- Development of a mentor relationship with a senior faculty as well as a peer
- Cultural and gender sensitivity
- Knowledgeable about current mentorship literature

Orientation Programs

The orientation of new/novice faculty to the educational institution and college of nursing is fundamental to the effectiveness of the nursing program. Hand (2008) stated that a formal orientation program provides support to new/novice faculty as they experience change in the individual, organization and society. *Individual change* involves the opportunity to reflect on personal values and beliefs in relation to those of the institution and school of nursing. *Organizational change* relates to policies and procedures that influence overall operations, and societal change involves strategies for positive student interaction and classroom management.

An effective orientation program should have two foci: the overall institution and one's specific discipline. Usually part-time/adjunct faculty receive only a discipline-specific orientation, but part-time faculty need to understand the context for their teaching, so an institutional orientation also is important. The time frame for the orientation program varies from one day to a full week to sessions spread over an entire semester. Also, it is not uncommon for web-based orientation materials to be available for the new faculty, allowing them to access it anytime, anywhere. The orientation should address the institution's and school's mission, vision and core values; organizational structure; administrative support team responsibilities; tutorials for learning about eLearning courses and other technology; overview of the curriculum and the objectives of the specific course(s) that the new faculty member will be teaching; and information about characteristics of the student body. When orienting new faculty to individual course assignments, extensive detail should be given about the relationship between overall student outcomes/objectives for the program and specific student course objectives. Faculty expectations for the theory and clinical portions of the course should be explicit.

Ongoing Faculty Development

Since the transition to the nurse educator role does not occur overnight, some nursing programs elect to provide ongoing faculty development throughout the first year of employment. This can be accomplished by having monthly "brown bag lunches" where new/novice faculty and their more seasoned colleagues discuss teaching innovations, challenges, and successes. Baker (2008) designed a faculty development program that fit into the organization's committee structure. New/novice faculty were assigned to one committee, the "faculty orientation committee," that met monthly to discuss the key components addressed earlier in this chapter (i.e., mission, vision, core values and faculty role expectations and responsibilities), as well as mentorship.

Another faculty development strategy implemented at the author's college of nursing was to adapt a faculty roles and responsibilities doctoral course into an online continuing education course. Modules with reading assignments and discussion questions were created and assigned continuing education units (CEUs). New faculty were expected to complete the module requirements and discussion questions on a monthly basis and submit responses for CEUs.

Research that Will Inform Successful Transitioning to the Faculty Role

Research in the area of clinicians transitioning to the nurse educator role is very limited. Possible research questions that might be considered include:

- What strategies support the successful transition of clinicians to the faculty role?
- What transitional patterns/phases are encountered by new/novice faculty?
- What differences exist in the transitioning of full-time versus part-time faculty appointments?
- What are faculty orientation program "best practices"?

Conclusion

Transitioning from the role of clinician to the role of faculty member is challenging, but it also can be one of the most rewarding experiences one undertakes. The sense of fulfillment that a nurse educator receives when preparing future nurses to provide safe, quality patient care is indescribable. While clinical teaching requires a strong clinical knowledge base and clinical competence, both of which a clinician brings to the position, it also requires skills such as assessing student learning needs, designing meaningful learning activities, and evaluating students' clinical performance based on stated student outcomes. Individuals who pursue this path must realize that it requires commitment and a sense of determination to learn the faculty role and responsibilities related to clinical and classroom teaching, research and service. Nursing education research is needed to provide evidence to support successful transition in order to retain these vital clinicians-turned-academic-educators.

References

AACN (American Association of Colleges of Nursing). (2008). *Nursing faculty shortage fact sheet.* Retrieved from http://www.aacn.nche.edu/Media/FactSheets/NursingShortage.htm

Baker, S. (2008, September). *New faculty orientation program: A strategy to retain nurse educators.* Paper presented at the National League for Nursing Educational Summit, San Antonio, TX.

Bartel, J. (2007). Preparing nursing faculty for baccalaureate-level and graduate-level nursing programs: Role preparation for the academy. *Journal of Nursing Education, 46*(4), 154-157.

Billings, D., & Kowalski, K. (2008). Managing your career as a nurse educator: Considering an academic appointment. *Journal of Continuing Education in Nursing, 39*(9), 392-393.

CCNE (Commission on Collegiate Nursing Education). (2008). *CCNE standards for accreditation of baccalaureate and graduate degree nursing programs.* Retrieved from http://www.aacn.nche. edu/accreditation/.

Culleiton, A., & Shellenbarger, T. (2007). Transition of a bedside clinician to a nurse educator. *MedSurg Nursing, 16*(4), 253-257.

Durham-Taylor, J., Lynn, C., Moore, P., McDaniel, S., & Walker, J. (2008). What goes around comes around: Improving faculty retention through more effective mentoring. *Journal of Professional Nursing, 24*(6), 337.

Gibson, S. (2009). Enhancing intergenerational communication in the classroom: Recommendations for successful teacher-student relationships. *Nursing Education Perspectives, 30*(1), 37-39.

Grossman, S. (2007). *Mentoring in nursing: A dynamic and collaborative process.* New York: Springer Publishing.

Halstead, J. (2007). *Nurse educator competencies: Creating an evidence-based practice for nurse educators.* New York: National League for Nursing.

Hand, M. (2008). Formalized new faculty orientation programs: Necessity or luxury? *Nurse Educator, 33*(2), 63-66.

Ignatavicius, D. (2009). *Best practices for improving student success and retention.* Paper presented at the meeting of the Alabama Council of Administrators of Professional Nursing Education Programs, Montgomery, AL.

NCSBN (National Council of State Boards of Nursing). (2008). Nursing faculty qualifications and roles. Retrieved from https://www.ncsbn.org/Final_08_Faculty_Qual_Report.pdf

NLN (National League for Nursing). (2002). The preparation of nurse educators [Position Statement]. Retrieved from http://www.nln.org/aboutnln/PositionStatements/prepartion 051 802.pdf

NLN (National League for Nursing). (2005a). Nursing faculty shortage fact sheet. Retrieved January 30, 2009, from http://www.nln.org/governmentaffairs/pdf/NurseFacultyShortage.pdf

NLN (National League for Nurisng). (2005b). *Core competencies of nurse educators with task statements.* Retrieved from http://www.nln.org/facultydevelopment/pdf/corecompetencies.pdf

NLN (National League for Nursing). (2006). *Mentoring of nurse faculty* [Position Statement]. Retrieved from http://www.nln.org/aboutnln/PositionStatements/mentoring_3_21_06.pdf

NLNAC (National League for Nursing Accrediting Commission). (2008). *NLNAC accreditation manual: Assuring quality for the future of nursing education* (2008 ed.). Retrieved from http://www.nlnac.org/manuals/Manual2008.htm

Penn, B., Wilson, L., & Rosseter, R. (2008). Transitioning from nursing practice to a teaching role. *The Online Journal of Issues in Nursing, 13*(3), 1-17.

Portner, H. (1998). *Mentoring new teachers.* Thousand Oaks, CA: Corwin Press.

Siler, B., & Kleiner, C. (2001). Novice faculty: Encountering expectations in academia. *Journal of Nursing Education, 40*(9), 397-398.

Smith, J., & Zsohar, H. (2007). Essentials of neophyte mentorship in relation to the faculty shortage. *Journal of Nursing Education, 46*(4), 184-186.

US Department of Education (DOE). (2008). *Family educational rights and privacy act (FERPA).* Retrieved from http://www.ed.gov/print/policy/gen/guid/fpco/ferpa/index.html

CLINICAL NURSING EDUCATION

Chapter 9

DEMONSTRATING EXPERTISE IN CLINICAL EDUCATION: ESSENTIAL FACULTY COMPETENCIES

Judith A. Halstead, DNS, RN, ANEF

For many nursing faculty, teaching students in the clinical setting is a significant part of their role. Immersed in the clinical setting with students, nursing faculty have a unique opportunity to role model clinical decision-making, nursing skills, interprofessional communication, patient-nurse interactions, and professional values for students, thereby helping shape the future practice of these emerging professionals. As important as the clinical educator role is, the competencies that are needed to successfully implement this role are seldom addressed in a comprehensive manner in evidence-based literature. Often it is assumed that an expert nurse clinician will be able to effortlessly and automatically translate that expertise into the academic role without needing any specialized pedagogical knowledge base. This is a false assumption that can ultimately lead to frustration and dissatisfaction on the part of the faculty and squandered learning opportunities for students.

Clinical nursing education is a complex enterprise, one that is too often left to the least academically prepared individuals. While there are many highly competent practicing nurses who hold undergraduate nursing degrees, there are few nurses prepared at the undergraduate level and not that many more with master's preparation who also have the depth of theoretical understanding of educational principles needed to successfully teach diverse learners how to practice in complex and chaotic health care systems. The role of the nurse educator is an advanced practice role, best assumed by nurses who have been prepared at the graduate level to be nurse educators. The purpose of this chapter is to demonstrate the complexity of the clinical nurse educator role by describing the competencies required to successfully implement that role, and discussing how clinicians can acquire and maintain these competencies to become more capable of teaching students in the clinical setting.

Faculty Competencies Specific To Clinical Education

In 2005, the National League for Nursing published Core Competencies of Nurse Educators (NLN, 2005a). While no one core competency singularly addresses clinical education, threaded throughout the eight core competencies are statements that describe attributes (knowledge, skills, and attitudes) that are essential to developing expertise in the clinical educator role. The core competencies that are most closely aligned with expertise in clinical education are the following: 1) facilitate learning; 2) facilitate learner development and socialization; 3) use assessment and evaluation strategies; 4) participate in curriculum design and program outcomes; 5) function as a change agent and leader; and 6) engage in scholarship.

Attributes found within these core competencies that contribute to developing clinical teaching expertise have been categorized into six themes for the purposes of the discussion here. Those categories are as follows:

1. developing personal attributes and interpersonal skills with students, peers and clinical personnel;

2. developing evidence-based teaching strategies for facilitating clinical teaching;

3. assessing and evaluating students' clinical performance;

4. designing curricula and evaluating program outcomes;

5. maintaining clinical competence as an academic clinical educator; and

6. developing interdisciplinary and collaborative partnerships.

By intentionally seeking out experiences that foster development of competency in each of these thematic areas, individuals will acquire the knowledge, skills and attitudes associated with expertise in clinical education.

How does a nurse educator most effectively develop and maintain expertise in clinical teaching? What strategies are most likely to facilitate a scholarly approach to the role of the clinical educator? What type of organizational support is necessary to foster the development of faculty expertise in clinical education? How can educational environments be created within nursing programs that demonstrate a valuing of faculty who are expert clinical teachers, similar to the value placed on nursing faculty who are expert researchers? Questions such as these will provide the context for a discussion of each of the themes noted above.

Developing Personal Attributes and Interpersonal Skills with Students, Peers and Clinical Personnel

Being able to develop and use personal attributes to facilitate student learning is a key competency that directly impacts the effectiveness of clinical faculty. A review of research on clinical teaching indicated that one of the areas consistently associated with educator expertise in clinical teaching is the interpersonal skills and intrapersonal attributes of the educator her/himself (Halstead, 2007). Findings from such research indicates that students often view the clinical educator's personal characteristics as more important than their clinical competence, and that the attitudes of faculty can influence whether or not students perceive them to be effective in their role as a clinical educator (Halstead, 2007; Tang, Chou, & Chiang, 2005). Clearly it is not enough for clinical educators to be clinically competent in order to facilitate learning; they must also be able to demonstrate the ability to develop professional relationships with students that convey a sense of respect and genuine interest in the individual learner, as well as an enthusiasm for teaching, learning and nursing process that inspires students (NLN, 2005a). Interestingly enough, most of the nursing literature is focused on student-faculty interactions at the undergraduate level, with very little discussion about the nature of graduate student-faculty relationships in the clinical environment.

As one example of the effect of professional relationships in the teaching-learning process, Cook (2005) stated that the presence of "inviting" teacher behaviors lessened the state of anxiety that students felt during their clinical learning experiences. She reported research findings that suggested "inviting" behaviors accounted for 41 percent of the variance in students' state of anxiety in clinical learning experiences. "Inviting" behaviors is a concept derived from invitational education theory (Novak & Purkey, 2001), which holds the belief that (a) individuals are invited by educators into the teaching-learning process to realize their potential, and (b) behaviors of teachers can be either intentionally or unintentionally inviting or disinviting. The goal for educators is to be intentionally inviting with students, consistently and deliberately conveying positive thoughts and attitudes in their interactions with students. Core values associated with inviting behaviors include respect, trust, intentionality, care and optimism (Cook; Novak & Purkey). Cook recommended that all clinical faculty intentionally practice "inviting" behaviors in their interactions with students.

Using a research- and theory-based foundation, such as the one just described to influence and guide the approach one uses to create and enhance student-faculty interactions, is one means by which a clinical educator can demonstrate a scholarly approach to developing expertise in the role. Far too often in the nursing profession we have left it to clinical educators to "find their own way" in establishing relationships with learners, resulting in much uncertainty regarding how to most effectively interact with students in clinical settings. Grounding one's interactions theoretically, actively reviewing evidence-based practices shared in the literature, and seeking role models all can help clinical educators develop effective, learner-centered relationships with students. As an organizational strategy, schools of nursing can implement faculty development programs that focus on the concept of developing mutually respectful and reciprocal student-faculty interactions in clinical learning experiences, instead of authoritarian, hierarchically based relationships. With many schools of nursing reporting that a significant amount of clinical education is delivered by part-time faculty and new faculty, such programming becomes even more important to provide opportunities for novice clinical faculty to be partnered with more experienced clinical faculty who can serve as expert role models.

It is not enough that clinical educators develop collegial working relationships with students, however. There is also a need for clinical educators to develop these same relationships with preceptors and other clinical agency personnel. As clinical educators gain expertise in their role, they must gain the ability to establish and nurture partnerships that will meet the needs of both partners while creating a learning environment that fosters student goal attainment. To maximize learning experiences for students, clinical educators must be able to effectively interact with agency staff so that the expertise of staff can be meaningfully integrated into the learning experiences. This means that clinical educators must invest the time and energy to develop meaningful relationships with individual agency staff, respect the potential of their contributions to the learning process, and create opportunities where the clinical decision-making and priority-setting skills of staff nurses can be specifically highlighted and used as models of practice for students.

Individual partnerships with clinical agency personnel often take on the shape of preceptor/faculty partnerships, where preceptors are used to working one-on-one with individual students to facilitate their clinical experiences. Preceptors have most often been used in advanced practice graduate programs, but they are increasingly being utilized in prelicensure programs. The effectiveness and success of preceptor partnerships at any level of education is frequently associated with how well faculty collaborate with preceptors to clarify and clearly establish the roles and responsibilities of all parties — students, faculty, and preceptors.

Partnerships with clinical colleagues are essential if clinical educators are to create optimum learning experiences for students. In order to further develop evidence-based "best practices" in the use of collaborative relationships with individual clinical agency personnel and clinical preceptor educational models, more research is needed in both pre-licensure and graduate education (Halstead, 2007).

Developing Evidence-Based Teaching Strategies for Facilitating Clinical Teaching

Individuals who are expert clinical educators strive to develop and incorporate evidence-based teaching strategies into their practice as educators. While such evidence is growing for cognitive and classroom teaching and learning, it is sorely lacking for clinical teaching and learning. As a result, many clinical nursing educators continue to teach students in ways that reflect how they were taught in their own educational programs, instead of basing their practices upon educational theories and evidence-based strategies. The Institute of Medicine (2001) attributed the historic failure to change clinical education to four primary factors: 1) lack of funding to investigate clinical teaching methodologies; 2) little regard in the disciplines for teaching; 3) the need for faculty development; and 4) the inherent difficulty in documenting cause/effect-type relationships because of the complexity of the clinical environment and the complexity of learning.

Demonstrating competency in facilitating learning in the clinical setting requires nurse educators implement a variety of teaching strategies, ground those teaching strategies in a theoretical foundation, and engage in self-reflection about ways in which teaching practices can be improved. Clinical educators are particularly called upon to develop and implement teaching-learning strategies that will model critical and reflective thinking for students and create learning experiences that foster the development of students' clinical reasoning skills. In the technology-driven environments in which health care is now practiced, it is also essential that clinical educators be able to effectively use information technology and demonstrate electronic communication skills to support student learning in patient care situations (NLN, 2005a).

It is not enough that clinical educators design and implement strategies that foster the cognitive and psychomotor development of students. Clinical educators are also professional role models for students and are responsible for creating learning environments that socialize students into the profession. Therefore, they must also facilitate learning experiences that foster affective domain learning and encourage students' abilities to engage in self-reflection on their developing professional values and skills. It is important for clinical educators to understand that teaching and learning are influenced by cultural, gender and experiential factors that students bring with them to the teaching-learning process (NLN, 2005a), and these must be respected and capitalized on.

As mentioned previously, it is likely that many clinical educators teach the way they themselves were taught. The Institute of Medicine (2003) has stated that teaching in the health professions continues to be guided by educators' personal beliefs and dominated by tradition instead of scholarly inquiry. To grow in competence and develop expertise in clinical teaching strategies, nurse educators must embrace the scholarship of teaching and bring a spirit of inquiry, creativity and reflective practice to the clinical teaching process, and be open to critique and evaluation.

There are a number of strategies that can help the clinical educator develop expertise in facilitating student learning in the clinical setting. Basing clinical teaching strategies upon research helps educators develop best practices that can be reproduced and replicated by others, further adding to the evidence base that supports the strategies. Identifying an issue and posing a question is the first step an educator can take when beginning to examine teaching practices. Once a question has been posed, the educator can review the literature to seek out potential research-based interventions that can be pilot-tested in his or her own practice. Participating in a team research effort with other clinical educators is one way to facilitate such efforts, making the process more manageable and generating enthusiasm and collegiality as the questions are formulated and addressed.

As possible teaching strategies are designed for implementation, the educator should proactively plan how to evaluate them. Deciding how to evaluate the effect of a new teaching strategy prior to implementing it ensures that the outcomes of the teaching interventions will be measured in a systematic fashion. Taking the step to obtain institutional review board approval also ensures that the outcome data can be publicly disseminated to others, thus adding to the knowledge base on clinical teaching and allowing others to replicate the teaching strategies.

Clinical teaching provides the educator with many opportunities to be innovative and creative in the teaching strategies that are chosen for use in the clinical environment. Consistently using a process of scholarly inquiry helps clinical educators gain expertise in their role and infuse their teaching with evidence-based practices.

Assessing and Evaluating Students' Clinical Performance

Another competency that is essential to the success of the clinical educator is being able to assess and evaluate the clinical performance of students, which has historically been a challenge for educators. The subjective nature of the evaluation process and the lack of standardized, valid and reliable evaluation tools have contributed to the challenge, as has the unpredictable and complex environment within which much of the evaluation of student outcomes occurs. There is very little evidence-based literature about the subject of clinical evaluation, and much of what has been written, again, addresses prelicensure education, with little attention being paid to graduate nursing education (Halstead, 2007). However, certain educator competencies in assessing and evaluating student outcomes have emerged from the literature and can be applied to clinical teaching.

Evaluating students' clinical performance requires that educators be skilled in evaluating the cognitive, psychomotor and affective domains of learning. Evaluation strategies that are appropriate and sensitive to measuring learning in each domain must be utilized, and the educator must develop skill in designing and using a variety of tools (NLN, 2005a). Clinical performance can be assessed and evaluated through direct observations, performance in simulated exercises, interactions with standardized patients, return demonstrations, participation in role play exercises, contributions to reflective exercises, and written or oral presentations of case studies. The use of clinical concept maps and journaling has also been reported to be useful evaluation tools (Halstead, 2007). Given the varied nature of evaluation strategies, clinical educators can benefit from formal academic preparation in evaluation and measurement strategies as one means to begin to develop the knowledge and skills required to evaluate clinical learning outcomes.

In addition to having knowledge of a variety of evaluation strategies, it is also important that the educator consider how feedback is provided to students about their performance. The educator should place an emphasis on providing timely and constructive feedback to students (Chickering & Gamson, 1987; NLN, 2005a) so that students can benefit from the feedback and modify their performance as appropriate. As discussed in a previous section, the interpersonal competencies of the clinical educator and how feedback is delivered to students are critical factors in how students perceive the effectiveness of their teachers. Finally, legal and ethical aspects of evaluating students must also be understood and adhered to by educators to ensure that confidentiality of the evaluation process is maintained and due process afforded to all students.

Designing Curricula and Evaluating Program Outcomes

Demonstrating expertise in clinical education requires faculty to be skilled and actively involved in designing curricula that are reflective of contemporary trends in health care and nursing, as well as designing program evaluation plans that serve to document student achievement of program outcomes (NLN, 2005a). Curricula must be dynamic and capable of responding quickly to our changing environments, and the clinical learning experiences that faculty design and integrate throughout the curriculum for students must be relevant. To be effective clinical educators, faculty must be cognizant of trends affecting health care and nursing practice and act to revise the curriculum as necessary to ensure effective and contemporary learning experiences for students.

Being knowledgeable of professional standards is one means by which a clinical educator can remain current about concepts that must be integrated into the curriculum. As an example of professional standards, the American Association of Colleges of Nursing's (AACN) recently updated *Essentials for Baccalaureate Education for Professional Nursing Practice* (AACN, 2008) delineates the areas of knowledge required for contemporary nursing practice at this entry level. Concepts such as informatics, clinical reasoning, patient safety and patient-centered care, quality improvement, genetics, cultural sensitivity, evidence-based practice and interprofessional teams are identified as being essential for baccalaureate education (AACN, 2008), all of which have implications for clinical learning experiences. Further, examples of professional standards that could have significance for the clinical educator would include the American Nurses Association's *Code of Ethics (2001)*, *Nursing's Social Policy Statement (2003)* and *Scope and Standards of Nursing Practice (2004)*. Graduate nursing education has similar statements of professional standards and curriculum content, such as the AACN *Essentials of Master's Education for Advanced Practice Nursing (1996)* and the National Organization of Nurse Practitioner Faculties' *Domains and Core Competencies of Nurse Practitioner Practice (2006)*, that guide clinical experiences for advanced practice nurses. Specialty areas of nursing practice have also developed sets of standards to guide practice. Since professional standards such as these cited here frequently serve as the framework for developing and measuring program outcomes, as well as designing clinical experiences, clinical educators must be fully aware of them.

While it is important for faculty to respond to health care trends and reform efforts with appropriate curriculum revisions, the National League for Nursing (NLN) also sounded a cautionary note in its 2005 position statement on *Transforming Nursing Education* that faculty must "base their curriculum decisions, teaching practices and evaluation methods on current research findings" (p. 5) and not on the potentially politically driven mandates of special interest groups (NLN, 2005b).

Since the research on curriculum design is limited, one may wonder how faculty proceed with making curriculum decisions that are evidence based and research driven. How do they decide upon program outcomes that are based in evidence that suggests such outcomes will lead to qualified graduates? How do clinical educators apply these curricular decisions in the clinical setting and implement learning experiences that are, themselves, evidence based?

One strategy for ensuring a scholarly approach to curriculum design and establishment of relevant program outcomes is to base curricular decisions upon data that comes from environmental scans. In other words, data related to health care trends, geographically specific diseases and illness prevention, societal trends, interprofessional team collaboration, student needs, and external stakeholder needs all can be most valuable. For example, if external stakeholders have expressed a need for graduates to better understand how to implement evidence-based practices in acute care settings, conduct a review of the literature regarding the effect of evidence-based practice on patient outcomes in acute illness and identify concepts related to evidence-based practice and the measurement of outcomes. Then faculty can use this information to design program outcomes, curriculum threads, learning activities, clinical learning experiences, and evaluation strategies. This is especially true when the information is combined with and substantiated by data acquired from other sources, such as graduates of the program. The decision of how this information can then be applied in the clinical setting is a process that can best be led by a clinical educator with expertise in clinical practice and curriculum design.

Obviously, to design a curriculum using such an approach requires the investment of organizational resources to support faculty efforts. Providing faculty development opportunities to acquire expertise in curriculum design is an important first strategy, specifically including clinical educators in such development opportunities is essential to ensure that curriculum revisions actually extend into the clinical environment. Another strategy that also communicates organizational support and valuing of the scholarship of teaching is to provide release time or funding to support faculty efforts in data collection and curriculum revision, especially when extensive program redesign is being contemplated. Unfortunately, a more common approach is to expect faculty to undertake curriculum redesign "on top" of their regular teaching, service, and scholarly efforts — such an approach does not allow faculty to achieve and maintain their competence in curriculum design, and ultimately undermines faculty efforts.

Another challenge that must be addressed organizationally is how best to connect part-time clinical educators to the overall curriculum so they can clearly understand how the courses they teach fit into the overall scheme. It is important that all faculty bring a sense of intentionality to their role as clinical educators, so their teaching efforts remain congruent with the curriculum. Since this intentionality is harder to achieve with clinical educators who are associated with the program only on a part-time basis, full-time faculty and schools must institute programs that will bridge this gap. With large portions of the clinical instruction in many nursing programs being delivered by part-time faculty, this is a critical issue that all nursing programs must address. The expert clinical educator is in a position to play a valuable role in these efforts, and such efforts should be rewarded by the institution.

Maintaining Clinical Competence

To remain credible and effective in the clinical educator role and serve as role models for students, faculty must seek opportunities that will enable them to maintain a knowledge base related to their professional practice as a nurse (NLN, 2005a). Students observe how faculty conduct themselves in the clinical setting and are aware of when their clinical faculty are not comfortable with clinical skills and equipment. Yet, it can be difficult to remain clinically competent in nursing practice when primarily employed in an academic setting. The additional responsibilities associated with the teaching, research and service aspects of the faculty role can create role overload for full-time faculty who teach clinically and are expected to demonstrate and maintain clinical competence.

Little and Milliken (2007) addressed what they labeled the "balance" between expectations to be an educator and a clinician, asking if it was even a reasonable or sustainable goal to expect educators to be able to achieve a balance between the two sets of expectations. It is very challenging to remain current with one's practice skills in today's complex health care environment when one does not practice in that environment on a regular basis, so how realistic is it to expect full-time faculty to remain current in their practice? This is especially true in acute care settings. Little and Milliken asserted that the word "competence" is a more apt description of what should be expected of academic faculty in terms of clinical skills, instead of the word "expertise." In addition, these authors raised the question of how the clinical competence of faculty is being evaluated in our academic nursing programs and if these evaluation data are being used to ensure appropriate clinical placement of faculty when clinical teaching assignments are made.

It is an individual responsibility of faculty to maintain the clinical competence required for their role as clinical educators. However, educational institutions also have a responsibility to create organizational environments that support faculty in maintaining this competence and can employ a number of strategies to help make achieving the "balance" between academic responsibilities and practice responsibilities more feasible. For example, structuring teaching assignments so that faculty can schedule one practice day/week as part of their workload assignment allows the faculty to integrate the practice day into the overall portfolio of academic responsibilities. Joint appointments can also be arranged in which academic clinical faculty time is formally shared with a clinical agency; such arrangements need to be carefully structured, however, so that there is a complementary nature between the appointments, and the faculty are not overextended when each institution ends up expecting a full-time commitment. Other forms of collaborative arrangements between the practice and education settings can be established that provide opportunities for faculty to remain connected to the clinical setting. Promotion and tenure criteria can be written to explicitly address the value of clinical practice to the academic environment and reward faculty for demonstrating scholarship related to clinical practice. As the nature of our health care environments continue to become more complex, the discussion of how to best maintain the clinical competence of faculty, and what are realistic expectations regarding faculty clinical competence, will remain an important one within the profession, likely leading to new collaborative practice models between academia and practice.

Developing Interdisciplinary and Collaborative Partnerships

With the shortage of nursing faculty reaching proportions not previously seen in our profession, it has become increasingly important for nursing faculty to be able to establish and maintain collaborative partnerships with community and clinical agency stakeholders as one means by which to extend program capacity. This is especially true for clinical educators who rely heavily upon such partnerships to deliver quality learning experiences for students in clinical settings. In addition, the emphasis within health care on the value of interdisciplinary teamwork in achieving positive patient care outcomes has created a mandate for nursing programs of all levels to explore means by which interdisciplinary learning can become more integrated throughout the program. Therefore, demonstrating expertise in clinical education requires the educator to (a) create and maintain partnerships with external stakeholders that support the educational goals of the nursing program, and (b) engage in interdisciplinary educational efforts to address health care needs at regional, national and international levels (NLN, 2005a).

The value and advantages associated with education-practice partnerships that mutually meet the needs of both partners and often demonstrate the outcomes of augmenting faculty effort and allowing nursing programs to expand student enrollment capacity have been addressed (AACN, 2002). Participating in such partnerships can serve to revitalize the practice of staff nurses, benefit the institutions by promoting synergy between practice and academe, expose students to clinical experts in the practice setting, and decrease the nursing program's reliance on part-time clinical instructors (Kowalski et al., 2007). The clinical educator is a key stakeholder in such arrangements and must possess the interpersonal, collaborative and negotiating skills needed to successfully broker and sustain such arrangements.

Conclusion

In summary, this chapter has presented the competencies that nurse educators must possess in order to demonstrate expertise in the role of clinical educator. Clinical education is a multifaceted, complex process that requires educators to be clinically competent and capable of bringing a sense of innovation, creativity and scholarly inquiry to the role while in the practice setting. It is essential that we continue to embrace an evidence-based approach to the redesign of the clinical education models that we currently utilize within the curricula of our nursing programs. This includes applying an evidence-based approach to reexamining the competencies in which faculty need to develop expertise so that they can effectively teach in these new models of clinical education. As some examples of areas that would benefit from further study, research questions about faculty expertise in clinical education include the following:

1. What evaluation competencies must clinical faculty demonstrate to most effectively evaluate learner outcomes in the clinical learning environment?

2. How can clinical faculty most effectively form partnerships with clinical agency staff to create innovative and scholarly clinical learning environments for students?

3. What institutional supports are most effective at facilitating the development of faculty in the role of the expert clinical educator?

Clinical educators have a unique opportunity to shape the nursing practice of students, and they are in a position to serve as change agents in leading clinical education redesign. The role of the clinical nurse educator is an advanced practice role, requiring the educator to be competent in practice issues as well as educational issues. Given the complexity of the role, it is best assumed by those who have graduate level preparation, and it is a role that should be valued and rewarded within our academic institutions.

References

American Association of Colleges of Nursing. (1996). *Essentials of master's education for advanced practice nursing.* Washington, DC: Author.

American Association of Colleges of Nursing. (2002). *Using strategic partnerships to expand nursing education programs.* Washington, DC: Author.

American Association of Colleges of Nursing. (2008). *Essentials for baccalaureate education for professional nursing practice.* Washington, DC: Author.

American Nurses Association. (2001). *Code of ethics.* Washington, DC: Author.

American Nurses Association. (2003). *Nursing's social policy statement.* Washington, DC: Author.

American Nurses Association. (2004). *Scope and standards of nursing practice.* Washington, DC: Author.

Chickering, A., & Gamson, Z. (1987). Seven principles for good practice in undergraduate education. [Special insert]. *Wingspread Journal, 9*(2).

Cook, L. (2005). Inviting teaching behaviors of clinical faculty and nursing students' anxiety. *Journal of Nursing Education, 44*(4), 156-161.

Halstead, J. A. (Ed.). (2007). *Nurse educator competencies: Creating an evidence-based practice for nurse educators.* New York: National League for Nursing.

Institute of Medicine. (2001). *Crossing the quality chasm: A new health system for the 21st century.* Washington, DC: National Academies Press.

Institute of Medicine. (2003). *Health professions education: A bridge to quality.* Washington, DC: National Academies Press.

Kowalski, K., Horner, M., Carroll, K., Center, D., Foss, K., Jarrett, S., et al. (2007). Nursing clinical faculty revisited: The benefits of developing staff nurses as clinical scholars. *Journal of Continuing Education in Nursing, 38*(2), 69-75.

Little, M., & Milliken, P. J. (2007). Practicing what we preach: Balancing teaching and clinical practice competencies. *International Journal of Nursing Education Scholarship, 4*(1), Article 6, 1-14.

National League for Nursing. (2005a). *Core competencies of nurse educators.* New York: Author.

National League for Nursing. (2005b). [Position statement]. *Transforming nursing education.* New York: Author.

National Organization of Nurse Practitioner Faculties. (2006). *Domains and competencies of nurse practitioner practice.* Washington, DC: Author.

Novak, J. M., & Purkey, W. W. (2001). *Invitational education.* Bloomington, IN: Phi Delta Kappa Educational Foundation.

Tang, F., Chou, S., & Chiang, H. (2005). Students' perceptions of effective and ineffective clinical instructors. *Journal of Nursing Education, 44*(4), 187-192.

Chapter 10

SIMULATION: INTEGRAL TO CLINICAL EDUCATION

Angela M. McNelis, PhD, RN
Pamela R. Jeffries, DNS, RN, FAAN, ANEF
Desiree Hensel, PhD, RNC
Mindi Anderson, PhD, RN, CPNP-PC

Prelicensure education strives to produce nurses who can perform essential nursing skills, think critically, and communicate effectively (AACN, 2008). As a practice-based discipline, clinical education in nursing has traditionally served as the venue where students learn to apply theoretical knowledge and gain the essential knowledge, skills, and attitudes required to practice in complex health care systems (AACN, 1999, 2008). Decreasing clinical sites and increasingly complex patients challenge clinical nurse educators to develop the most effective ways to prepare students for future practice (Billings & Halstead, 1998; Jeffries, 2005). Failure to provide sufficient quality learning experiences may leave students lacking the competence and confidence to provide safe care when entering the work force (Olson, 2009). Furthermore, failure to gain a strong professional self-concept by the completion of prelicensure education has been associated with lower rates of job retention at the end first year of practice (Cowin & Hengstberger-Sims, 2006). Simulation has been proposed as one solution to ensure that students receive quality clinical learning experiences.

Nursing is just beginning to fully appreciate what the field of aviation has known for years, namely, that key elements from practice can be simulated for the purpose of education (Hovancsek, 2007). Not only are airline pilots trained initially using flight simulators, their ongoing training for emergencies, including engine failures, also are done through simulation (Prince, 2009). Such training was credited as one of the reasons all 155 lives were saved on the U.S. Airways flight 1549 forced to land in the Hudson River after a double-engine failure. So what can nursing learn from the airline industry? One basic conclusion is that simulation has value in preparing individuals for practice roles in which high-stakes decisions often need to be made.

Nursing simulation is defined as an event or situation made to closely resemble clinical practice (Jeffries, 2005). Simulations vary in format and complexity and include case studies, role-playing, interactive computer programs, and mannequins, which can range from low-fidelity task trainers to high-fidelity patient simulators (Hovancsek, 2007). Reported outcomes from using simulation include enhanced knowledge, skill performance, therapeutic communication, critical thinking, self-confidence, self-efficacy and learner satisfaction, suggesting this educational strategy has the potential to positively affect student's cognitive, psychomotor, and affective domains (Jeffries, 2005; Laschinger et al., 2008; Leigh, 2008; Sleeper & Thompson, 2008). This chapter discusses the opportunities for using simulation as a component of preparation for clinical practice, types of simulations, quality design features, and challenges surrounding the use of simulation in nursing education.

How Does Simulation Prepare a Student for Clinical Practice?

Similar to the emergency training used in aviation, simulation may help bridge the theory-practice gap for high-risk and/or rare situations that students would not likely experience. For instance, Schoening, Sittner, and Todd (2006) created a two-part, high-risk obstetrical simulation for the care of a preterm labor patient. Sixty baccalaureate (BSN) students participated in the study that showed that confidence, skills, integration of concepts, teamwork, and quick response to emergencies all improved after the simulation experience. Disaster response is another practice area where few students would have the opportunity to gain hands-on experience outside of simulation. To reinforce lecture content, Doran and Mulhall (2007) created a simulation related to caring for a patient suspected of being exposed to smallpox or anthrax. The authors reported students met the simulation objectives by correctly identifying the exposure, utilizing appropriate barrier and isolation measures, and administering necessary vaccines. Students reported the simulation was an effective learning strategy that improved their confidence to care for such clients.

Developing Knowledge, Skills, and Attitudes

Beyond preparing for unusual aspects of practice, simulations are typically designed to teach and evaluate the basic knowledge, skills, and attitudes needed for everyday clinical practice. Used early in a curriculum, simulations help prepare students for their first clinical experiences. In one study, students who practiced on the human patient simulator (HPS) were better at following patient identification procedures and assessing vital signs than the control group (Radhakrishnan, Roche, & Cunningham, 2007). In another study, when the patient simulator was used to teach basic head-to-toe assessment skills to novice BSN students, 61 percent of the students felt improved confidence with physical assessment skills (Bremner, Aduddell, Bennett, & VanGeest, 2006). This learning experience was also reported to decrease the stress associated with the first day of clinical in 42 percent of the students.

Simulations can teach more than psychomotor skills. They can be used to teach and evaluate higher-level critical thinking, communication, and teamwork skills (Jeffries, 2005; Lasater, 2007; Rhodes & Curran, 2005; Schoening et al., 2006). In one randomized controlled study, students who completed a traditional problem-solving task after an educational intervention felt their educational strategy had less problem-solving features than the students who engaged in high-fidelity simulation after the same intervention (Jeffries & Rizzolo, 2006). In another randomized controlled study, researchers found that students who participated in an intensive care simulation scenario, in addition to traditional lecture, scored significantly higher on the posttest *Objective Structured Clinical Examination* (OSCE), than the control group (Alinier, Hunt, Gordon, & Harwood, 2006). While these studies used simulation as a supplement to other learning strategies, Brannan, White, and Bezanson (2008) used simulation as a lecture replacement. In this study, students whose only method of learning to care for a patient with a myocardial infarction (MI) was a simulation scored higher on a posttest related to care of an MI patient than students whose only method of learning this material was a traditional lecture.

Perhaps the greatest potential for simulation lies in influencing the affective domain. Studies suggest that simulations are particularly effective in improving self-confidence. Lasater (2007) posits that confidence is necessary for the development of clinical judgment in nurses. In one multisite simulation study, students viewed a video on postoperative care, followed by randomization to a paper and pencil task group, a static mannequin simulation group, or a high-fidelity simulation group (Jeffries & Rizzolo, 2006). Two of the simulation groups assigned students to four different roles: nurse one, nurse two, family member, or observer. The paper and pencil groups were not assigned roles, but worked together to complete a task. Following the simulation experience, the simulation groups reported significantly more self-confidence in caring for the postoperative patient than did the paper and pencil groups. Furthermore, this self-confidence did not vary by the assigned simulation role.

The self-confidence factor of self-efficacy (i.e., the belief one can successfully master a task. is thought to predict behavior — students with high self-efficacy scores are expected to readily undertake difficult tasks (Bandura, 1977). Goldenberg, Andrusyszyn, and Iwasiw (2005) found role-playing simulations increased self-efficacy for health teaching in third year BSN students, and Leigh (2008) found increases in self-efficacy in 65 BSN students after they participated in simulation. While these findings are useful, neither study examined the link between self-efficacy and actual clinical behavior, thereby identifying this relationship as an area in need of research.

Translation to Practice

Perhaps the biggest question surrounding simulation is, "How does learning through simulation transfer to practice?" While basic nursing skills have long been taught using mannequins, it is unclear how well higher-level skills translate to practice. In a study of students involved in a simulation of care of a patient with a chronic obstructive pulmonary disorder, Feingold, Calaluce, and Kallen (2004) found 100 percent of the faculty felt skills performed in the simulation would transfer to the clinical setting, but only half of the students agreed. While 69 percent of the students felt the simulation was a valuable learning experience and 86 percent felt it was realistic, less than half of the students believed the teaching strategy increased confidence. The researchers felt differences between faculty and student perceptions of transferability reflected students' inability to see the big picture; however, it is highly possible that instructors perceived the value of simulation as higher due to a desire to find alternate learning experiences in a climate of declining clinical opportunities. One systematic review of 23 studies found the use of simulation in health care education provided high learner satisfaction and was useful in teaching higher levels skills. However, the gains in knowledge and skills appeared to be short term and decreased over time (Laschinger et al., 2008).

The research is beginning to show how simulation can improve patient outcomes. For instance, a reduction in newborn birth injuries was seen in one study after implementing simulated shoulder dystocia management training to the maternal-newborn health care team (Draycott et al., 2008). While this study did not include student nurses, it does highlight the translation to practice potential of simulation. Longitudinal studies examining the sustained effects of this learning modality need to be conducted and include nursing students, novice nurses, and new skill acquisition. Moreover, more studies need to investigate differences in knowledge, skills, and attitudes between traditional clinical learning and simulated experiences.

TYPES OF SIMULATIONS USED IN CLINICAL PRACTICE

Simulation has been used in nursing for as long as many nurses can remember. Over the years, simulation has become more sophisticated and complex as additional human functions and tasks are able to be mimicked (Kneebone, Scott, Darzi, & Horrocks, 2004). It is increasingly becoming an important part of nursing education (Nehring, 2008), and agencies such as the National Quality Forum (n.d.), have endorsed training with simulation as a means to decrease patient harm. With many nursing schools now using simulation, the question has arisen as to in what context and how much simulation can serve as or be substituted for clinical practice. In order to address this question, one must consider different types of simulation, issues specific to nursing education, benefits of using simulation, and considerations for using simulation as clinical practice.

One definition of simulation is ". . . a technique, not a technology, to replace or amplify real experiences with guided experiences, often immersive in nature, that evoke or replicate substantial aspects of the real world in a fully interactive fashion" (Gaba, 2004a, p. i2). This definition implies that simulation can replace or augment clinical practice; however, to be used in this way, it must replicate real life. A simulated learning experience is defined as one that mimics the real world and enables the learner to incorporate psychomotor skills, decision-making processes and critical thinking in managing the situation (Decker, Sportsman, Puetz, & Billings, 2008). The ability to do this may depend on the type of simulation — low-fidelity, moderate-/high-fidelity, virtual reality, standardized patients, haptic systems, student role-playing, patient-focused, and screen-based computer.

Low-Fidelity Simulation

Fidelity in simulation is defined as how close something is replicated (Gaba, 2004b) or how realistic it is (Hovancsek, 2007). Partial task trainers are often called low-fidelity simulation (Broussard, 2008) and are recommended for learning, improving upon, or evaluating competency of a particular skill (Decker et al., 2008). Partial task trainers are defined as "models or mannequins used to learn, practice, and gain competency in simple techniques and procedures" (Decker et al., 2008, p. 75). Therefore, with partial task trainers, only a portion of something is replicated (Cooper & Taqueti, 2004; Decker et al., 2008; Gaba, 2004a). Examples include intravenous arms/hands, blood pressure arms, and auscultation chests. Static mannequins also fall into the low-fidelity category (Jeffries & Rogers, 2007) as well as case studies (National League for Nursing [NLN], n.d.). In nursing education, low-fidelity simulation, particularly partial task trainers and static mannequins, is often used for the novice student in a Foundations/Fundamentals or Assessment course. It could also be used for beginning graduate acute care nurse practitioner students, as they learn new skills such as performing a lumbar puncture.

Moderate-Fidelity and High-Fidelity Simulators

High-fidelity simulators (mannequins) are generally defined as those that are computerized and "breathe," with the chest rising and falling (Jeffries & Rogers, 2007). These types of patient simulators are realistic and provide an opportunity for students to practice complex skills in a safe environment (Nehring, Lashley, & Ellis, 2002). Patients of both genders can be portrayed as well as almost any disease process or age. In addition, high-fidelity simulators provide for both pharmacologic and physiologic interventions (Nehring et al., 2002). In contrast, moderate-fidelity simulators often have heart and breath sounds, but do not simulate actual breathing with chest rise and fall (Jeffries & Rogers, 2007). Both high and moderate-fidelity simulators are often called full-scale simulation, as these mannequins have a full body, not just selected parts (e.g., arm, thorax), and respond physiologically to interventions (Decker et al., 2008).

Virtual Reality

Another type of simulation is virtual reality, which combines a computerized environment with other stimuli that activate the senses, including tactile, sound, and visual, which are provided through partial trainers to increase realism (Decker et al., 2008). This type of simulation often falls into the high-fidelity category (NLN, n.d.) and is used for skill attainment and evaluation (Decker et al., 2008).

Standardized Patients

According to Gliva-McConvey (n.d.), a standardized patient (SP) is "...a person trained to portray a patient scenario, or an actual patient using their own history and physical exam findings, for the instruction, assessment, or practice of communication and/or examining skills of a health care provider. In the health and medical sciences, SPs are used to provide a safe and supportive environment conducive for learning or for standardized assessment." SPs may also be hired to play a role in the simulation learning experience and may include actors, volunteers, or other individuals (Decker et al., 2008). An SP, therefore, may play the actual patient (e.g., for physical assessment practice or competency evaluation), or may play an "extra" role in the simulation learning experience (e.g., the distraught wife of the "patient"). A great advantage to using SPs is that communication skills can be developed and validated (Decker et al., 2008), along with psychomotor and decision-making skills. This type of simulation is often categorized as high-fidelity (NLN, n.d.).

Haptic Systems

A haptic system is "a simulator that combines real-world and virtual reality exercises into the environments" (Decker et al., 2008, p. 75) and that gives participants a sense of touch, such as a surgical instrument haptic device used for practicing surgery (The Free Dictionary, 2009). This type of simulation is often used for skill development and evaluation (Decker et al.).

Student Role-Playing. Role-playing is another form of simulation that can be used to teach nursing skills. It can be utilized as a substitute for or augmentation of other types of simulation technology (Comer, 2005). For example, students can "act out" playing the nurse and patient in different care situations that include recognition of certain patient conditions and implementation of nursing interventions. Students have reported that this type of simulation helps reinforce information learned in lecture (Comer). Role-playing is often considered a low-fidelity simulation (NLN, n.d.).

Patient-Focused Simulation

Patient-focused simulation is defined as combining an inanimate object, such as a task trainer or virtual reality device, with an SP in a simulated scenario (Kneebone, Nestel, Vincent, & Darzi, 2007). For example, an SP wears an IV arm in a simulated learning experience where the student has to start the IV while still communicating to the patient. The SP then gives feedback to the student (Kneebone et al., 2007).

Screen-Based Computer Simulation

Screen-based computer simulations are defined as "programs to train and assess clinical knowledge and decision making..." (Ziv, Wolpe, Small, & Glick, 2003, p. 784). This two-dimensional form of simulation (Jeffries, 2005) is often used for specific skills development and evaluation as well as integration of skills into scenarios where students must use critical thinking (Decker et al., 2008).

Issues in Clinical Nursing Education

Nursing education and student clinical placements today are plagued with multiple issues, including scarcity of clinical sites, higher patient acuity in the hospital setting, inability of assuring that students care for a variety of patients, insufficient use of student clinical time, and lack of student experience with critical events (Jeffries, 2005; Morton, 1997; Rhodes & Curran, 2005; Tanner, 2006). For example, in high-risk situations, such as a code, patient safety takes precedence and student learners may be unable to participate (Decker et al., 2008). This can leave students at a disadvantage when they graduate, as they may have no experience managing critical events. Infrequent critical events make it challenging to meet required clinical objectives (Haskvitz & Koop, 2004).

Additional issues include limited time in clinical areas and shortened hospital stays (Rhodes & Curran, 2005). Rural areas often have problems finding clinical sites, especially for specialty populations such as pediatrics. Many hospitals limit what students can do, not allowing them, for example, to give medications or document care in the patient's record, even though skills such as these are a performance expectation upon graduation and schools of nursing are under increasing pressure from employers to produce competent nurses upon graduation (Jeffries, 2005; Morton, 1997).

Another issue with clinical placement is that many students do not get experience caring for patients outside the acute setting (Tanner, Gubrud-Howe, & Shores, 2008). Finally, the shortage of qualified faculty and the push to increase the number of graduates have many educators and institutions looking for ways to accommodate more students with fewer faculty (Board of Nurse Examiners for the State of Texas, 2006).

Benefits of Using Simulation in Clinical Education

Literature abounds describing the benefits of using simulation, much of which has been about the use of high-fidelity simulators. The simulation process allows students to critically think, use their clinical judgment, and obtain knowledge (Rhodes & Curran, 2005), and all domains of learning, including cognitive, affective, and psychomotor, can be addressed (Morton, 1997; Nehring et al., 2002) through simulated experiences. Simulation provides for both skill acquisition and management of care (Hawkins, Todd, & Manz, 2008), and it allows faculty to control the complexity of the situation with which the student is faced (Jeffries, 2005), something that cannot be done in an actual clinical setting. Moreover, faculty can control the amount of information given to the students and the response the "patient" has to various interventions. Faculty can give cues during a simulation to help students make appropriate decisions (Jeffries, 2005), which may be difficult to do in real life at the patient's bedside. Opportunities or patient conditions that may be hard to find in clinical may also be simulated (Morton, 1997) and presented to students with less variability than would be seen in the actual clinical setting (Scherer, Bruce, Graves, & Erdley, 2003). Simulation also can be used for all levels of learners (Gaba, 2004a) and, therefore, incorporated throughout the curriculum.

In addition to these benefits, simulation allows for collaborative learning (Jeffries, 2005) and can be used to achieve multidisciplinary team training goals. Such an experience gives members of a health care team an opportunity to learn diverse roles as well as develop an appreciation of what each member can contribute (Childress, Jeffries, & Dixon, 2007; Jeffries, McNelis, & Wheeler, 2008). During the simulated learning experience, communication among team members can be taught (Jeffries, et al., 2008) so that individuals are not forced to "figure it out" after graduation.

A critical advantage to using simulations is that students are able to make mistakes, such as giving the wrong dose of a medication, and see the consequences (Broussard, 2008; Kneebone et al., 2004). Simulation, therefore, has been described as "risk free" (Comer, 2005; Decker et al., 2008; Morton, 1997). Scenarios can be repeated (Henneman & Cunningham, 2005; Kneebone et al., 2004; Nehring et al., 2002), and students are able to get immediate feedback in the post-simulation debriefing from instructors and peers who observed the scenario (Kneebone et al., 2007; Rhodes & Curran, 2005). Use of video playback after a simulation learning experience allows students to observe and then evaluate their own performance, leading to self-reflection (Graling & Rusynko, 2004; Rhodes & Curran). None of these advantages are possible in a real-life clinical encounter.

Finally, both formative and summative evaluation can occur with the use of patient simulators (Nehring et al., 2002). When simulations are used as a teaching-learning activity, the idea is to improve student performance. Formative evaluation focuses on giving student feedback that will facilitate self-reflection on and ultimate growth in their knowledge, skills, and critical thinking relative to the simulation. When simulations are used in a summative fashion to assign grades or make progression decisions in a course or program, learners receive feedback about "…attainment of learning objectives and/or final competency goals" at the conclusion of the teaching-learning activity (Jeffries et al., 2008, p. 472).

Considerations for Using Simulation as Clinical Practice

The question nursing educators may ask is this: If there are so many benefits to using simulation, and if simulation can replicate the "real-life" environment, why should it not be used as clinical practice? Perhaps the best response to this question lies in the lack of evidence-based research on where best to incorporate simulated learning experiences, how best to develop and use scenarios, what technology or approach is most effective, and so on. For example, should simulation be done as part of lecture, as part of clinical laboratory (lab) experience, or as part of clinical? Or should it be incorporated in all of these areas? Some have described using simulation as lab experience (Morton, 1997) or as a lab course (Scherer et al., 2003), while others have incorporated it into lecture, such as using a high-fidelity infant simulator to demonstrate newborn examination (Anderson, 2007). Still others have described using simulation, particularly high-fidelity simulators, as clinical or clinical hours (Bantz, Dancer, Hodson-Carlton, & Van Hove; 2007; Bearnson & Wiker, 2005; Linder & Pulsipher, 2008; Nehring & Lashley, 2004; Schoening et al., 2006).

Are schools of nursing using simulation as clinical practice? In an international survey done by Nehring and Lashley (2004), schools of nursing and simulation centers associated with schools of nursing were surveyed to determine the use of human patient or high-fidelity simulators. Respondents included 34 schools of nursing as well as six simulation centers. Most respondents (approximately 58 percent) of the almost 88 percent who responded to the question reported using simulation as part of clinical, whereas 43 percent reported either never of rarely using the simulator for clinical time. The amount of hours or specific placement of simulations was not reported.

Another consideration for using simulation as clinical is how it connects to actual clinical practice. Kneebone et al. (2004) caution that "to realize its full potential as a learning aid, simulation must be used alongside clinical practice and linked closely with it" (p. 1095). Tanner (2006) agrees that simulation must complement experiences in clinical practice. Therefore, nurse educators must make sure simulation and clinical practice build upon one another. Development of quality simulations is paramount and faculty would be well advised to consider collaborating with practicing nurses to create real-life scenarios (Murray, Grant, Howarth, & Leigh, 2008).

Examples of Simulation in Clinical Education

There are only a few examples in the literature discussing using simulation specifically as clinical; however, it is clearly being used in this capacity by many schools of nursing (Nehring & Lashley, 2004). Schoening et al. (2006) described a simulated clinical experience where 60 BSN students took part in an obstetrics simulation using a high-fidelity simulator in the last two weeks of their clinical rotation. Results showed that students felt they met the simulation objectives and they had overall positive perceptions. Students' qualitative data from reflective journals showed that students liked the hands-on learning, felt their skills increased, were more confident, were able to critically think, thought the experience had value and was realistic, and they liked the teamwork and communication skills. This simulation was used in place of clinical hours in the hospital setting.

Literature describing the use of simulation as an entire clinical day was limited. Bantz et al. (2007) described a 6-hour clinical day where students participated in eight different stations — including moderate- and high-fidelity simulators, task trainers, and games — related to labor and delivery, postpartum, and newborn care. Students felt that the simulation helped them connect a concept learned in the classroom to clinical practice and provided them with the practical skills to perform well in future clinical settings. Students also reported increased confidence and they gained skills that would help them in the clinical setting.

Linder and Pulsipher (2008) described a 6-hour pediatric simulation used prior to the hospital rotation. Patient simulators were used to teach physical assessment and resuscitation of pediatric patients, as well as prioritization of nursing interventions. Students participated in case studies and an electronic medical record exercise. Anecdotal feedback from students was that the simulation was realistic, and students felt more confident about being prepared for clinical. In addition, students felt less anxious about clinical, and thought the simulation helped them with prioritization of interventions.

A study by Bearnson and Wiker (2005) examined benefits and limitations of utilizing a high-fidelity patient simulator or "mannequin" as a substitution for one clinical day for junior level nursing students. Students participated in three different postoperative patient scenarios and completed post-experience questionnaires. Results showed that students perceived their knowledge about medication side effects, ability to administer medications in a safe manner, confidence about medication administration, and understanding of patient differences in responses was increased. Interestingly, many students felt that the simulation should augment clinical, not replace a day.

Although there are few examples of simulation being used as actual clinical, empirically, it makes sense that simulation could be used in this capacity. However, how much clinical can be simulated as well as whether simulation is better than or equal to clinical has yet to be determined with research.

Considerations for Setting Up a Quality Scenario

Quality simulations have objectives that are appropriate to the desired learning goals and for the level of the learner, thus they must be set up with careful consideration of what students need to learn. To ensure quality simulations, a small group of researchers funded by the National League for Nursing developed *The Nursing Education Simulation Framework* (see Figure 10-1) that included five design characteristics for a simulation to ensure high quality (Jeffries, 2007). Inclusion of these design features makes certain that all important components needed in a simulation are present. The five simulation design characteristics are briefly described and the importance of each is discussed.

Objectives/Information

The objectives of the simulation need to be considered so that the targeted activities meet the needs of the course. A simulation can target just one or many areas of practice. For example, one 20-minute scenario may focus on enhancing communication skills, safe medication delivery, and care of a newborn. Literature suggests between three and five learning objectives for a simulation are adequate to help direct and provide a quality learning experience for students (Jeffries, 2007).

In addition to objectives, providing students with a preview of basic information about the simulation is an integral component of the learning experience. Enough information should be given so that students can anticipate what is expected and how much time they have to achieve the objectives of the activity, without divulging the content of the scenario. Providing students with pre-simulation information such as worksheets, web-based modules, or simple reading assignments to review prior to the scenario also enhances the quality of the simulation experience (Jeffries, 2007).

Fidelity (Realism)

Clinical simulations need to be clinically accurate, valid, real, and process-based (Cioffi, 2001). Authenticity is essential in making the learning experience more relevant to the real world (Hotchkins, Biddle, & Fallacaro, 2002; Jones, Cason, & Mancini, 2002; Peterson & Bechtel, 2000). Developing a completely realistic simulation is impossible; however, every effort should be made to create the best scenario to promote student learning. It is important to remember that there is more to the simulation than the high-fidelity patient simulator. Beaubien and Baker (2004) describe three dimensions of fidelity: equipment, environment, and psychology, and they posit the latter is the most important for team training. Quality scenarios mandate that consideration be given to what learners are thinking and feeling during the simulation

Figure 10 – 1
The Simulation Framework

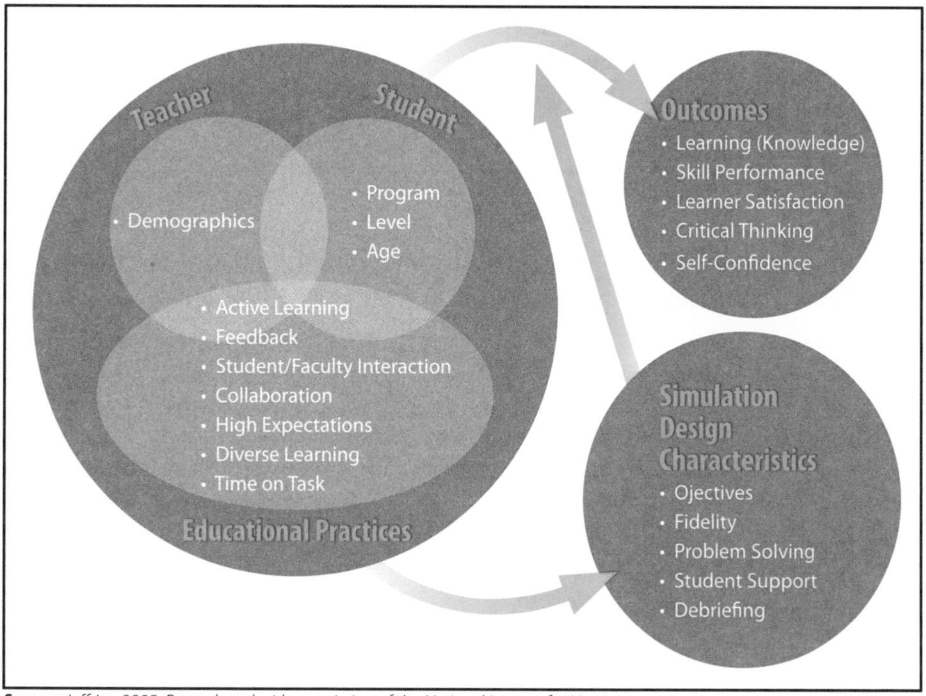

Source: Jeffries, 2005 Reproduced with permission of the National League for Nursing.

experience. The simple addition of props to make the patient and environment more realistic helps accomplish this goal.

Complexity

The third design characteristic to consider when developing a quality simulation is complexity or problem-solving. This feature requires decision-making around a real-life clinical situation. Providing opportunities for decisions during simulations creates a safe, nonthreatening environment in which learners can make decisions and see the consequences, and it assists educators in assessing students' critical thinking and problem-solving skills (Jeffries, 2007).

Cueing

Cueing, also referred to as student support, is a design characteristic discussed as important in the literature, but little evidence supporting this feature is published. Support can come in the form of providing cues or hints during the simulation to direct student participants, and it also occurs during debriefing sessions when facilitating student learning and achievement of course outcomes.

Debriefing

The final design feature that characterizes quality scenarios is debriefing, the process in which a facilitator promotes the learner's development of insight using semistructured cue questions once the simulation scenario is completed (Decker, 2007). During debriefing, the real or simulated event is explained, analyzed and synthesized by the participants, and information is shared regarding how they are feeling (psychologically) and ways to improve performance in similar and future situations.

Despite the progress made in the development and testing of simulations, as well as the evidence showing improved learning outcomes when using simulations, challenges to using simulation in nursing education remain pervasive, particularly in relation to the question of whether simulated learning experiences can be substituted for actual clinical learning experiences.

Challenges to the Acceptance of Simulation as a Partial Substitute for Clinical Learning Experiences

As the number of simulation centers increases and actual clinical sites become more difficult to access, educators are developing, implementing, and immersing students in clinical simulations in safe, nonthreatening environments. Nurse educators also are constantly engaged in an exploration to find the most effective strategies to facilitate learning. In light of the increased demand for nursing graduates to be better prepared for real-world practice and to have the knowledge and skill sets essential for the 21st century practice (Landeen & Jeffries, 2008), clinical simulations are increasingly being incorporated into the curricula. However, challenges to accepting simulation as a substitute for real clinical practice time remain.

Faculty Need to Learn How to Effectively Use Simulation Pedagogy

As new clinical models are being called for and the use and incorporation of simulations in nursing curricula are increasing, schools of nursing are purchasing simulation equipment and faculty are expected to embrace the new technology and incorporate it into their teaching. Unfortunately, many faculty are not prepared for this type of teaching. Without proper preparation regarding how to incorporate simulations into the curriculum, faculty often have to experiment with the simulators in a trial-and-error manner, wasting time and often becoming frustrated. Until recently, there were very few faculty development materials to help faculty design, implement, and evaluate simulations in clinical nursing education, but in June 2008, the National League for Nursing launched a website called the Simulation Innovation Resource Center (SIRC) (http://sirc.nln.org) to serve as a repository of information, guidance, and resources for nurse educators. The nine web-based courses, developed by simulation experts across the country and included on the SIRC website, have been developed to promote faculty development in using simulation. In addition, conferences and seminars across the country are focused on faculty development in simulation. The UK Simulation in Nursing and the International Nursing Simulation/Learning Resource Centers Conferences both focus on this emerging pedagogy.

Using Simulation Requires Changing from a Teacher-Centered to a Student-Centered Approach

If simulation is to be accepted as a partial substitute for clinical experiences, faculty must change their perspective from a teacher-centered one to a student-centered one (Jeffries 2007). In a student-centered approach to using simulation, students are at the center of the simulation and the instructor observes students caring for a clinical, simulated patient, often from behind a one-way mirror or in a control room. This teaching structure promotes a sense of autonomy in students, expects them to be self-directed, and challenges students to think critically, solve problems independently, and make decisions on their own. Teachers accustomed to the traditional teacher-centered approach, often find it difficult to place students at the center and let them make mistakes. Such a shift is essential, however, to take full advantage of this pedagogy and allow students to be totally emerged in the simulation experience.

The Faculty Role in Using Simulation Pedagogy Must Be Defined

Faculty need to fully understand what simulation is and what it is not, and they must view it as a strategy that holds promise in providing students complex, "real-life" clinical experiences in a safe, nonthreatening environment (Billings, 2007). Part of the hesitation with faculty to attempt this innovative pedagogy and to substitute simulations for a certain percent of clinical practice is the lack of defined expectations regarding roles. Faculty need to ask what role they play when developing and integrating simulations into the classroom, or when using them to enhance or substitute for clinical experiences, as the expectations can be quite varied (Henneman, Cunningham,

Roche, & Cumin, 2007; Jeffries, 2008; Medley & Horne, 2005). For example, some educators are expected to do everything in a simulation, including setting it up, running the simulator, assessing student behaviors/actions, cueing or providing helpful hints to the students, and conducting the debriefing session. Requiring that a single individual take on all these responsibilities creates great concern for many educators, and they wonder how they can do it all and do it well (Kardong-Edgren, Starkweather, & Ward, 2008). Thus, the role of the educator, as well as that of laboratory assistants, needs to be clearly defined to ensure that faculty are available to serve as the coach and facilitator of student learning.

Regulatory and Accreditation Body Mandates and Standards Must Be Met

Regulatory bodies are beginning to show an interest in clinical simulation; however, there are currently no preset national or international standards or standardization on how much clinical practice time can be substituted with clinical simulations. For example, in the United States, many states, including Florida and California, have set mandates on the percentage of clinical hours that can be obtained through simulations (Nehring, 2008). While the positions and regulations set by these bodies on clinical hours and the use of simulation vary by country (and by state and province), all accrediting bodies consider clinical experience as one aspect of their reviews. In the reviews of the regulatory bodies, the need for evidence-based outcomes is crucial before decisions are made. Until more clear standards are set for clinical practice allowing simulations to be substituted for clinical time, this area will continue to be a challenge in nursing education.

Space, Resources, and Simulation Center Availability Must Be Appropriate

Location, space availability, equipment, and resources all need to be considered when substituting clinical time with simulations, particularly if quality simulations are to be designed and implemented in place of clinical hours. Financial resources must be sufficient to not only purchase simulator equipment and supplies, but also for faculty development (Jeffries, 2008).

Depending on the simulation delivery model selected, resources will be needed for technical support and/or laboratory staff to run the simulator, as well as for set-up and take-down for each simulation experience (Jones & Hegge, 2008).

Evidence Regarding Effectiveness of Simulation as a Substitute for Clinical Learning Experiences Must Be Built

There has been exponential growth in clinical simulation laboratories worldwide, with many descriptive articles appearing in the literature over the past five years. Yet the research into the effectiveness of clinical simulation for nursing remains in its infancy (Landeen & Jeffries, 2008). The future calls for more rigorous testing of hypotheses and practices related to using simulation. We must be able to answer questions such as the following: What can we not simulate? What can we not teach our students using this pedagogy? How much simulation time can we substitute for actual clinical experiences? What types of simulations are most effective in teaching nursing students to think critically and solve problems? All these questions and more lack evidence at this time and must be answered to promote quality student learning outcomes.

Summary/Conclusions

Nursing is a practice profession and, as such, "medical training must at some point use live patients to hone the skills of health professionals" (Ziv et al., 2003, p. 783). However, simulation offers an environment where students can work on improving their skills, observe others providing care, and sharpen clinical decision-making without placing patients at risk. Patient safety must be a priority along with provision of the best care and treatment possible. Use of simulation certainly protects patients and may be a more effective tool for teaching students nursing practice. Nurse educators, however, are challenged to find "... the right mix of traditional learning, simulation-based learning, and actual patient care experience ..." (Gaba, 2004a, p. i6).

The use of clinical simulations as a substitute for clinical practice reflects the direction of nursing education. Different types of simulated experiences are being used in today's classroom, laboratory, and/or clinical teaching to promote more realism in the practice environment, enhance learning outcomes, and promote safe patient care environments in clinical practice. To keep up with our changing society and the technological advances in nursing practice, educators have to be creative in developing new, innovative models of teaching, including the use of clinical simulations, and they need to conduct research that will help us find the best way to incorporate these new methods into the teaching-learning process.

Leighton (2008) describes a future where 25 percent of nursing clinical practice hours will be completed in the simulation lab. However, more research is needed to support and direct the use of simulation in nursing education (Nehring, 2008) and using simulation as clinical practice. Future research is first needed to test the differences between simulation and traditional clinical teaching on learning outcomes. Based on these findings, further research will be needed to determine when, where, how, and what type of simulation can be substituted for traditional clinical hours, as well as whether simulation translates to clinical practice (Murray et al., 2008). Additional questions that must be answered to provide evidence-based support for this pedagogical approach include:

- Are there differences in learning outcomes between students completing simulation rotations and students completing traditional clinical rotations?

- Are there differences between the types of simulation on learning outcomes? Should only a certain type of simulation experience, such as those using high-fidelity simulators or standardized patients, count as clinical hours?

- Should the type of simulation dictate where it is incorporated (e.g., case studies in the classroom and task trainers in the lab)?

- What are the best practices for using simulation as clinical, attending to each design element of a quality?

- How much simulation time can we substitute for clinical practice time for optimal student learning and outcomes?

- What are the most important educator behaviors and skills needed to implement quality simulations in nursing education?

- Should simulation hours be counted the same as clinical hours? Are the outcomes of one hour of simulation the same as one hour of clinical? Because simulation experiences may be more concentrated, with less down time and more opportunity for repetitive practice than traditional clinical experiences, should one hour of simulation experience count as more than one hour of clinical experience?

- How does incorporating simulations as a substitute for clinical impact the transition to clinical practice for the new nursing graduate?

References

AACN (American Association of Colleges of Nursing). (1999). *The essential clinical resources for nursing's academic mission.* Retrieved February 8, 2009, from http://www.aacn.nche.edu/Education/pdf/ClinicalEssentials99.pdf

AACN (American Association of Colleges of Nursing). (2008). In *The essentials of baccalaureate education for professional nursing practice.* Retrieved February 8, 2009, from http://www.aacn.nche.edu/Education/pdf/BaccEssentials08.pdf

Alinier, G., Hunt, B., Gordon, R., & Harwood, C. (2006). Effectiveness of intermediate-fidelity simulation training technology in undergraduate nursing education. *Journal of Advanced Nursing, 54*(3), 359-369.

Anderson, M. (2007). *Effect of integrated high-fidelity simulation in knowledge, perceived self-efficacy and satisfaction of nurse practitioner students in newborn assessment.* Unpublished dissertation, Texas Woman's University, Denton.

Bandura, A. (1977). *Social learning theory.* Englewood Cliffs, NJ: Prentice-Hall.

Bantz, D., Dancer, M. M., Hodson-Carlton, K., & Van Hove, S. (2007). A daylong clinical laboratory: From gaming to high-fidelity simulators. *Nurse Educator, 32*(6), 274-277.

Bearnson, C., & Wiker, K. M. (2005). Human patient simulators: A new face in baccalaureate nursing education at Brigham Young University. *Journal of Nursing Education, 44*(9), 421-425.

Beaubien, J. M., & Baker, D. P. (2004). The use of simulation for training teamwork skills in health care: How low can you go? *Quality and Safety in Health Care, 13*(Suppl. 1), i51-i56.

Billings, D. M. (2007). Foreword. In P. R. Jeffries (Ed.), *Simulation in nursing education: From conceptualization to evaluation* (pp. ix). New York: National League for Nursing.

Billings, D. M., & Halstead, J. A. (Eds.). (1998). *Teaching in nursing: A guide for faculty.* Philadelphia: Saunders.

Board of Nurse Examiners for the State of Texas. (2006). *Strategic plan for fiscal years 2007-11.* Retrieved January 1, 2009, from http://www.bon.state.tx.us/about/pdfs/strat06.pdf

Brannan, J. D., White, A., & Bezanson, J. L. (2008). Simulator effects on cognitive skills and confidence levels. *Journal of Nursing Education, 47*(11), 495-500.

Bremner, M. N., Aduddell, K., Bennett, D. N., & VanGeest, J. B. (2006). The use of human patient simulators: Best practices with novice nursing students. *Nurse Educator, 31*(4), 170-174.

Broussard, L. (2008). Simulation-based learning: How simulators help nurses improve clinical skills and preserve patient safety. *Nursing for Woman's Health, 12*(6), 521-524.

Childress, R. M., Jeffries, P. R., & Dixon, C. F. (2007). Using collaboration to enhance the effectiveness of simulated learning in nursing education. In P. R. Jeffries (Ed.), *Simulation in nursing education: From conceptualization to evaluation* (pp. 123-135). New York: National League for Nursing.

Cioffi, J. (2001). Clinical simulations: Development and validation. *Nurse Education Today, 21,* 477-486.

Comer, S. K. (2005). Patient care simulations: Role playing to enhance clinical understanding. *Nursing Education Perspectives, 26*(6), 357-361.

Cooper, J. B., & Taqueti, V. R. (2004). A brief history of the development of mannequin simulators for clinical education and training. *Quality &Safety in Health Care, 13*(Suppl. 1), i11-i18.

Cowin, L. S., & Hengstberger-Sims, C. (2006). New graduate nurse self-concept and retention: A longitudinal survey. *International Journal of Nursing Studies, 43*(1), 59-70.

Decker, S., Sportsman, S., Puetz, L., & Billings, L. (2008). The evolution of simulation and its contribution to competency. *The Journal of Continuing Education in Nursing, 39*(2), 74-80.

Doran, A. J., & Mulhall, M. (2007). Bioterrorism in the simulation laboratory: Preparing students for the unexpected. *Journal of Nursing Education, 46*(6), 292.

Draycott, T. J., Crofts, J. F., Ash, J. P., Wilson, L. V., Yard, E., Sibanda, T., et al. (2008). Improving neonatal outcomes through practical shoulder dystocia training. *Obstetrics and Gynecology, 112*(1), 14-20.

Feingold, C. E., Calaluce, M., & Kallen, M. A. (2004). Computerized patient model and simulated clinical experiences: Evaluation with baccalaureate nursing students. *Journal of Nursing Education, 43*(4), 156-163.

Gaba, D. M. (2004a). The future vision of simulation in health care. *Quality & Safety in Health Care, 13*(Suppl. 1), i2-i10.

Gaba, D. M. (2004b). A brief history of mannequin-based simulation and application. In W. F. Dunn (Ed.), *Simulators in critical care and beyond* (pp. 7-14). Des Plaines, IL: Society of Critical Care Medicine.

Gliva-McConvey, G. (n.d.). *Definition of an SP.* Retrieved January 31, 2009, from http://www.aspeducators.org/sp_info.htm

Goldenberg, D., Andrusyszyn, M. A., & Iwasiw, C. (2005). The effects of classroom simulation on nursing students' self-efficacy related to health teaching. *Journal of Nursing Education, 44*(7), 310-314.

Graling, P., & Rusynko, B. (2004). Kicking it up a notch — Successful teaching techniques. *AORN Journal, 80*(3), 459-68, 471-475.

Haskvitz, L. M., & Koop, E. C. (2004). Students struggling in clinical? A new role for the patient simulator. *Journal of Nursing Education, 43*(4), 181-184.

Hawkins, K., Todd, M., & Manz, J. (2008). A unique simulation teaching method. *Journal of Nursing Education, 47*(11), 524-527.

Henneman, E. A., & Cunningham, H. (2005). Using clinical simulation to teach patient safety in an acute/critical care nursing course. *Nurse Educator, 30*(4), 172-177.

Henneman, E., Cunningham, H., Roche, J. P., & Cumin, M. E. (2007). Human patient simulation: Teaching students to enhance provide safe care. *Nurse Educator, 32*(5), 212-217.

Hotchkins, M., Biddle, C., & Fallacaro, M. (2002). Assessing the authenticity of the human simulation experience in anesthesiology. *AANA Journal, 70*, 470-473.

Hovancsek, M. T. (2007). Using simulation in nursing education. In P. R. Jeffries (Ed.), *Simulation in nursing education: From conceptualization to evaluation* (pp. 1-9). New York: National League for Nursing.

Jeffries, P. R. (2005). A framework for designing, implementing, and evaluating simulations used as teaching strategies in nursing. *Nursing Education Perspectives, 26*(2), 96-103.

Jeffries, P. R. (2007). *Simulation in nursing education: From conceptualization to evaluation.* New York: National League for Nursing.

Jeffries, P. R. (2008). Getting in S.T.E.P. with simulations: Simulations take educator preparation. *Nursing Education Perspectives, 29*(2), 70-73.

Jeffries, P. R., McNelis, A. M., & Wheeler, C.A. (2008). Simulation as a vehicle for enhancing collaborative practice models. *Critical Care Nursing Clinics of North America, 20*(4), 471-480.

Jeffries, P. R., & Rizzolo, M. A. (2006). *Designing and implementing models for the innovative use of simulation to teach nursing care of ill adults and children: A national, multi-site, multi-method study.* Retrieved February 8, 2009, from http://www.nln.org/research/LaerdalY2End.pdf

Jeffries, P. R., & Rogers, K. J. (2007). Theoretical framework for simulation design. In P. R. Jeffries (Ed.), *Simulation in nursing education: From conceptualization to evaluation* (pp. 21-33). New York: National League for Nursing.

Jones, T., Cason, C., & Mancini, M. (2002). Evaluating nurse competency: Evidence of validity for a skills re-credentialing program. *Journal of Professional Nursing, 18*(1), 22-28.

Jones, A., & Hegge, M. (2008). Simulation and faculty time investment. *Clinical Simulation in Nursing, 4*, e5-e9.

Kardong-Edgren, S., Starkweather, A., & Ward, L. (2008). The integration of simulation into clinical foundations of nursing students' therapeutic communication skills course: Student and faculty perspectives. *International Journal of Nursing Education Scholarship, 5*(1), 1-16.

Kneebone, R. L., Nestel, D., Vincent, C., & Darzi, A. (2007). Complexity, risk and simulation in learning procedural skills. *Medical Education, 41*(8), 808-814.

Kneebone, R. L., Scott, W., Darzi, A., & Horrocks, M. (2004). Simulation and clinical practice: Strengthening the relationship. *Medical Education, 38*(10), 1095-1102.

Landeen, J., & Jeffries, P. R. (2008). Simulation. *Journal of Nursing Education, 47*(11), 487- 488.

Lasater, K. (2007). High-fidelity simulation and the development of clinical judgment skills: Student's experiences. *Journal of Nursing Education, 46*(6), 269-275.

Laschinger, S., Medves, J., Pulling, C., McGraw, R., Waytuck, B., Harrison, M., et al. (2008). Effectiveness of simulation on health profession students' knowledge, skills, confidence, and satisfaction. *International Journal of Evidence-Based Healthcare, 6*, 278-302.

Leigh, G. T. (2008). Examining the relationships between participation in simulation and the levels of self-efficacy reported by nursing students. *Dissertations Abstracts International, 68*(11), DAIB. (UMI No. 3288617)

Leighton, K. (2008). Simulation for the future: Message from the president-elect. *Clinical Simulation in Nursing, 4*, e35-e36.

Linder, M. S., & Pulsipher, N. (2008, October). Implementation of simulated learning experiences for baccalaureate pediatric nursing students. *Clinical Simulation in Nursing, 4*, e41-e47.

Medley, C. F., & Horne, C. (2005). Using simulation technology for undergraduate nursing education. *Educational Innovations, 44*(1), 31-34.

Morton, P. G. (1997). Using a critical care simulation laboratory to teach students. *Critical Care Nurse, 17*(6), 66-69.

Murray, C., Grant, M. J., Howarth, M. L., & Leigh, J. (2008). The use of simulation as a teaching and learning approach to support practice learning. *Nursing Education in Practice, 8*, 5-8.

National League for Nursing. (n.d.) Simulation Innovation Resource Center. Retrieved February 9, 2009, from http://sirc.nln.org

National Quality Forum. (n.d.). Safe practices for better healthcare: 2009 update. Retrieved February 16, 2009, from http://qualityforum.org/projects/ongoing/safe-practices/

Nehring, W. M. (2008). U.S. boards of nursing and the use of high-fidelity patient simulators in nursing education. *Journal of Professional Nursing, 24*(2), 109-117.

Nehring, W. M., & Lashley, F. R. (2004). Current use and opinions regarding human patient simulators in nursing education. *Nursing Education Perspectives, 25*(5), 244-248.

Nehring, W. M., Lashley, F. R., & Ellis, W. E. (2002). Critical incident nursing management using human patient simulators. *Nursing Education Perspectives, 23*(3), 128-132.

Olson. M. E. (2009). The "Millennials": First year of practice. *Nursing Outlook, 57*, 10-17.

Peterson, M., & Bechtel, G. (2000). Combining the arts: An applied critical thinking approach in the skills laboratory. *Nursing Connections, 13*(2), 43-49.

Prince, A. (Executive Producer). (2009, January 19). *Water landing part of pilot training.* [Radio broadcast]. Washington, DC: National Public Radio. Retrieved February 1, 2009, from http://www.npr.org/templates/story/story.php?storyId=99480314

Radhakrishnan, K., Roche, J. & Cunningham, H. (2007). Measuring clinical practice parameters with human patient simulators: A pilot study. *International Journal of Nursing Education Scholarship, 4*(1), Article 8.

Rhodes, M. L., & Curran, C. (2005). Use of the human patient simulator to teach clinical judgment skills in a baccalaureate nursing program. *Computers, Informatics, Nursing, 23*(5), 256-262.

Scherer, Y. K., Bruce, S. A., Graves, B. T., & Erdley, W. S. (2003). Acute care nurse practitioner education: Enhancing performance through the use of clinical simulation. *AACN Clinical Issues, 14*(3), 331-341.

Schoening, A. M., Sittner, B. J., & Todd, M. J. (2006). Simulated clinical experience: Nursing students' perceptions and the educators' role. *Nurse Educator, 31*(6), 253-258.

Sleeper, J. A., & Thompson, C. (2008). The use of hi fidelity simulation to enhance nursing students' therapeutic communication skills. *International Journal of Nursing Education Scholarship, 5*(1), Article 42.

Tanner, C. A. (2006). The next transformation: Clinical education. *Journal of Nursing Education, 45*(4), 99-100.

Tanner, C. A., Gubrud-Howe, P., & Shores, L. (2008). The Oregon Consortium for Nursing Education: A response to the nursing shortage. *Policy, Politics, & Nursing Practice, 9*(3), 203-209.

The Free Dictionary. (2009). Haptic interface. Retrieved February 15, 2009, from http://medical-dictionary.thefreedictionary.com/haptic+interface

Ziv, A., Wolpe, P. R., Small, S. D., & Glick, S. (2003). Simulation-based medical education: An ethical imperative. *Academic Medicine, 78*(8), 783-788.

INTERDISCIPLINARY CLINICAL EDUCATION

Rita D'Aoust, PhD, RN, ACNP, ANP, CNE
Camille Martina, PhD
Andrew Wall, PhD
Denham Ward, MD, PhD

Clinical education simply has not kept pace with or been responsive enough to shifting patient demographics and desires, changing health system expectations, evolving practice requirements and staffing arrangements, new information, a focus on improving quality, or new technologies…Once in practice, health professionals are asked to work in interdisciplinary teams, often to support those with chronic conditions, yet they are not educated together or trained in team-based skills.

Greiner & Knebel, 2003, pp.1-2

Increasingly, the practice of health care is one that requires those trained in different health disciplines to work together to improve patient safety and health outcomes and to curtail increasing health care delivery costs (Steinert, 2005). The value and benefits of health care professionals working together in the planning and delivery of care is evident; however, in practice, concerns associated with communication, accountability, organizational limitations, power, leadership, and professional prestige have created barriers and impediments for meaningful collaboration. In a recent report by the Institute of Medicine (Greiner & Knebel, 2003), health care professions education is being called upon to develop professionals who are more highly skilled at collaboration across traditional disciplinary boundaries as a means to advance quality health care. In particular, interprofessional education, or the learning together of two or more health professions, has been seen as an educational tool in the process of creating a mechanism of learning that models the desired collaboration of health care delivery (Oandasan & Reeves, 2005a; Oandasan & Reeves, 2005b).

Interprofessional educational experiences for nursing students brings to light both the opportunities and the challenges of interprofessional health care education and practice, generally. The opportunities point toward the potential of students from different health professions learning with and from each other in ways that this collaborative learning expands, deepens and reinforces learning. However, the challenges of interprofessional education rest in the traditional nature of health professions education, which has primarily been discipline specific, focused on the contributions and roles of that discipline only, and attendant only to intradisciplinary learning. In other words, nurses learn nursing only with other nursing students, physicians learn medicine only with other medical students, and so on. In this chapter, the opportunities and challenges of interprofessional education are examined. We argue that interprofessional health education is a process that must first take on the task of transforming current teaching and learning practices of health professions educators in order to create an environment that supports collaborative learning and practice for students.

The Evolution of Health Professions Education

Health professions education has been intertwined with the evolution of higher education in the United States. Just as higher education has grown from modest beginnings at Harvard in 1636, where a few faculty and students gathered to study a limited and prescribed curriculum, the education of health professions also has evolved from a limited curriculum to the highly organized, regulated and specialized educational processes of today (Cohen, 1998; Ludmerer, 1999).

The development of professional practice in nursing, medicine, pharmacy and dentistry, as well as in many other health fields, reflect the increase of health-related knowledge, increased integration of technology in practice, growing ethical dilemmas and other factors. The expanded roles of health care professionals in today's society, and the learning experiences needed to prepare individuals for such complex roles, demand in-depth study in one's profession or discipline to develop minimum competency. It is this specialized knowledge and practice that has been a hallmark of a profession (Rudolph, 1990) and that depth of learning in one's field is not easily abandoned.

The development of a profession and the unique educational path to preparation of its members also have been hallmarks that separated the health professions by their discrete educational practices (Ludmerer, 1999). Health professional education, similar to higher education generally, is organized in a vertical manner or in what has been termed "organizational silos" (Keeling, Underhile, & Wall, 2007). This "siloed" organization of health professions education has promoted highly specialized knowledge and competition for prestige and resources, rather than mutual respect, understanding, and collaboration. For example, nursing education programs are accountable to professional accreditation in nursing. Nursing faculty are promoted by their professional nursing peers, and the nursing program is likely to have perceived itself to be in competition with other schools (or silos) for both resources and prestige. The challenges of interprofessional education, therefore, are rooted in a history that has valued separation, rather than integration, of educational practice (Hall & Weaver, 2001).

The challenge to the "siloed" nature of education resonates with Max Weber's discussion that bureaucratic specialization of tasks ultimately places individuals into black boxes of isolation (Weber, Mills, & Gerth, 1948). Specialized knowledge and practice have the most value not when they isolate, but when they operate in concert with professionals who possess other complementary skills, as occurs with the artistry of a symphony. A symphony contains skilled musicians, each of whom has spent intensive time mastering his respective instrument, but who has also trained with a group to develop the ability to play in an ensemble. Such learning allows each musician to exhibit his/her uniqueness and strength while complementing the talents of the other players to create beautiful music. Interprofessional health education requires that discipline-specific silos be transformed in ways that allow professionals to work in concert to deliver better patient care, with greater safety and with greater efficiency.

Although it is evident that a teamwork approach is essential among all health care providers (Institute of Medicine, 2001), the clinical education of two key providers, physicians and nurses, deserves special attention, since each remains largely independent of the other, yet their clinical practices are closely intertwined. A brief historical overview of the clinical education of physicians and nurses helps place into context both the possibilities and challenges of interdisciplinary clinical learning.

Clinical Education of Physicians, Nurses, and Other Health Professionals

Although the roles of physician and nurse have been played since antiquity, the education of these two partners in health care have had somewhat different roads to today's professional education. But modern educational practices and the routes to professionalism for both started in the mid to late 19th century.

Florence Nightingale's *Notes on Hospitals and Notes on Nursing: What It Is and What It Is Not* established nursing as a profession and placed nursing education firmly within the hospital's sphere. In this time period, preparation for the medical doctor (MD) degree consisted solely of two four-month terms of didactic lectures, often in proprietary medical schools, and clinical education was not included in the educational program itself. Instead, students were left to arrange their own apprenticeship experiences with a practicing physician or in a city hospital.

The more fortunate students were able to complete their clinical training in established medical clinical education programs in France or Germany, since there were few well-trained physicians in this country to guide their learning (Ludmerer, 1985).

By the end of the 19th century, medical educators were acknowledging the inadequate core requirements and the limited access to quality clinical education, and the profession began to call for physician education to include a four-year college undergraduate degree (bachelor of arts (BA)/bachelor of science (BS)), followed by an additional four years of medical school. Such programs were taking shape at Johns Hopkins University, the University of Michigan and Harvard University, among others. The new four-year medical program consisted of two years of basic sciences and two years of clinical experience. Postgraduate clinical training, while initially only a year of internship prior to general practice, soon evolved into longer, more specialized clinical training experiences. The seminal *Flexner Report* in 1909 completed the transition to the *modern* physician education model clearly still recognizable in today's medical schools (Cooke, Irby, Sullivan, & Ludmerer, 2006).

During this same time period, official nursing training programs were established in the leading hospitals using Nightingale's model. Thus, while medical education was pushed into the university and the level of scientific instruction increased, nursing education, while becoming more scientifically rigorous, remained in the workplace. State licensure for both nurses and physicians started in the first years of the 20th century and, at the same time, nurse specialization in anesthesia and midwifery began. In 1923, the *Goldmark Report*, the nursing equivalent of the *Flexner Report*, advocated for collegiate nursing programs, and Yale started the first university nursing program with a curriculum based on an educational plan rather than on hospital service needs. By 1938, Duke was offering the baccalaureate degree in nursing. But nursing education remained primarily hospital based and the entry into the profession was marked by professional registration (at the state level) rather than an academic degree. It was not until well into the last half of the 20th century that nursing education became academically based, but controversy remained as to whether an associate degree or a bachelor's degree should be the professional entry level academic degree.

There are several concurrent themes in the education of physicians and nurses today: balance of practical clinical and academic instruction; competency-based clinical evaluation; and a focus on patient safety as highlighted by the Institute of Medicine reports (Institute of Medicine, 2000; 2001). The medical school experience, while still leaning heavily toward the classroom-based, basic science education in the first two years, now commonly includes some early clinical experiences. The introduction to the performance of a complete patient history and physical examination often begins in tandem with the study of physiology and anatomy, traditionally the first two subjects in medical school. Additional direct patient contact, frequently in a primary care physician's office, is scheduled together with the other basic science classes. Yet the greater part of clinical medical education does not start until the third year of medical school in most instances. While the bachelor's degree nursing curriculum permits more academic education, the associate degree by necessity focuses on practical clinical instruction. The need for more advanced practice nurses, in a variety of specialties, will push nursing education to both the master's and doctoral levels. An important issue is the number of nursing professors for instruction at these levels within the university.

A competency-based education is a current educational theme that is shared across the education of all health care professionals (Greiner & Knebel, 2003). While the competencies for the different health care specialties are different, there are opportunities for values to be shared, particularly in the areas of patient-centered care and safety. However, the adoption of a competency-based education is not without controversy (Albanese, Mejicano, Mullan, Kokotailo, & Gruppen, 2008; Epstein & Hundert, 2002; Govaerts, 2008), reflecting the tension between a practical clinical training and an education in the scientific foundations of the profession. However, if the competencies are crafted correctly, they should encompass the essential characteristics of a health care professional and not diminish the role in any way (Batalden, Leach, Swing, Dreyfus, & Dreyfus, 2002). In contrast, if the competencies are poorly crafted, they can become little more than a simple checklist for students to complete.

These examples of the history of nursing and physician education are shared in many respects by the other health care professions. Any profession requires a solid grounding in its scientific foundations, but at the same time requires that graduates have the skills needed to practice the profession. The IOM report (Greiner & Knebel, 2003) provides further information on the education of other health care professionals. While similar problems have been faced across the different health care specialties, there has been little sharing of solutions.

Interprofessional Practise and Interprofessional Education

Traditionally, professional nursing has focused on health maintenance, restoration and prevention while medicine has focused on disease, diagnosis and treatment. But the changes in health care in the 21st century, with more treatment of chronic disease, an aging population, scientific advances in the understanding of the genetic basis of disease, combined with some of the political realities of providing affordable health care to everyone, have blurred the distinctions in the professions and demand that new paradigms of education be developed. It is somewhat paradoxical that while these forces have increased specialization, the patients require more collaboration in their care (O'Neill & Pew Health Professions Education, 1998). No single discipline or health care professional can independently meet the complex needs of patients today.

Evidence now suggests that better collaboration among health care professionals in the design and delivery of care results in improved patient health outcomes, increased patient and provider satisfaction, and decreased health care costs (Baggs & Schmitt, 1997; Baggs et al., 1997; Baggs et al., 1999; Baggs, Ryan, Phelps, Richeson, & Johnson, 1992; Larson, 1999). However, health professions educators have been slow to respond to the need to prepare a collaboration-ready workforce (Schmitt, 2008) that can effectively manage the realities, expectations and regulations in the clinical practice environment. It is not far-fetched to think that while all health care professionals wish to maintain their own area of expertise, they can readily appreciate the knowledge and unique contributions that each brings to patient care (AACN, 1996). Interprofessional education (IPE) offers a venue to create an authentic collaborative-ready workforce.

Moving Toward Interprofessional Education

Interprofessional care and education in the United States has occurred largely in relation to the planning and delivery of comprehensive care for special populations such as the elderly; addressing issues of access to care for rural and poor populations; examining system issues that affect patient safety, quality and cost; and solving workforce shortages or maldistribution of primary care providers (Schmitt, 2008). In the United States, formal interprofessional education (IPE) emerged in the 1960s, when new models of care were designed to address workforce shortages, nurse practitioners became more prominent in primary adult and pediatric care, and the training of "allied" health professionals increased (Schmitt).

In the 1970s, the IOM created the first committee to study IPE as a means of preparing for team practice. The recommendations of this committee addressed three major issues. The first issue resided at the administrative level of schools and academic health centers whose obligation was to promote interdisciplinary education and advance the core competency of teamwork skills. The second recommendation was to explicitly value interdisciplinary learning experiences within the clinical setting as a way to implement interdisciplinary education. The third recommendation recognized the need for governmental and professional support of interdisciplinary education for health care delivery teams. Twenty years later, in the midst of managed care initiatives of the 1990s to control the rapidly rising costs of care, influential health professions education reports continue to call for educational reform and the expansion of IPE. That call continues into the 21st century.

The Institute of Medicine (Greiner & Knebel, 2003) suggested that accrediting agencies, licensing bodies and certification boards must be engaged if real change in curricula is expected. Recent reports also focus on the lack of synchrony between health professions education and the realities of health care practice, and recommend that "all health professionals should be educated to deliver patient-centered care as members of an interdisciplinary team, emphasizing evidence-based practice, quality improvement approaches, and informatics" (Shaver, 2005, p. 57).

Basic Elements and Models of Interprofessional Education

Interprofessional education is achieved by learning and working together. Therefore, it is the knowledge that we acquire about, from and with each other. The skills for working together, supported by opportunities to practice what it means to work together on behalf of those who receive our care — contribute to changing preexisting, usually stereotypical, attitudes toward each other (Schmitt, 2008). The knowledge base in IPE that is core to the professions is both process and relationship centered. Components of IPE include knowledge of our own role, as well as the role of other team members. We also need to consider education preparation, such as course work and clinical training, as well as the principles of communication and teamwork, which include conflict resolution, system level influences, and interprofessional improvement approaches (Schmitt). Furthermore, we need to ensure competence in interprofessional teamwork through educational preparation that is consistent with the knowledge, skills, and attitudes of teamwork. This demands a pedagogy of IPE that draws on fundamental principles and strategies for explicit preparation, such as leveling, timing and sequencing of IPE training.

Lastly, we need to combine didactic and clinical learning that is both academic and work-based, and incorporates teaching and learning strategies (Schmitt).

There are three models of IPE that are common: (1) the lecture experience, which involves sharing of courses and modules; (2) clinical education, which includes learning experiences in and through interdisciplinary care delivery; and (3) project-based experiences, which can incorporate elements of the lecture and clinical models (Fealy, 2005; Zwarenstein et al., 1999). These models point to when, where and how interactions between professionals occur in interdisciplinary professional education.

When Should Interprofessional Education Occur?

One of the challenges of IPE is that the evidence related to effective timing of interdisciplinary education is inconclusive (Reeves et al., 2009). In a literature review conducted by Wheeler, Powelson, and Kim (2007), the authors report that there is inconclusive evidence as to the most effective timing of interdisciplinary education. Several reports support education at the undergraduate level, whereas others supported education at the professional/graduate level. The argument for preprofessional interdisciplinary education suggests that early exposure to IPE facilitates the appreciation of the roles and differences among the disciplines. On the other hand, those reports that favor professional exposure to interdisciplinary education contend that it is essential for the professional to first be confident in his/her own discipline. The authors argue that the most effective time to foster interdisciplinary collaboration is while individuals are just learning their roles so that interdisciplinary collaboration becomes a natural part of their practice.

While many nursing programs report a need to revise curriculum to incorporate IPE, both the cost and preexisting overburdened curricula often impede curricular change to provide IPE. This is compounded by access to health professional students due to differences in the number of nursing schools and students relative to the number of medical and other health professional schools and students. Although most health professional schools and programs have not included IPE, professionals from all disciplines are expected to work together in the practice setting (Greiner & Knebel, 2003; Schmitt, 2008). Historically, nursing and medical students have been educated in separate settings where the traditional system of hierarchy and individual, discipline-specific responsibility and decisions are emphasized (Greiner & Knebel, 2003; Ludmerer, 1999; Wheeler, Powelson, & Kim, 2007).

Where Should Interprofessional Education Occur?

Interprofessional education occurs both in the academic environment and in the clinical practice setting. A key issue is whether the learning is interprofessional or parallel multidisciplinary learning by professionals. Multidisciplinary learning occurs when different professions learn alongside one another but not interactively. In comparison, interprofessional learning is a deliberate process where students engage in learning with, from, and about each other (Harvan, Royeen, & Jensen, 2009; Ovretweit, 1996). Interdisciplinary learning calls upon students to jointly examine common issues such as access to health care, health promotion goals, managing chronic illness, or health care financing. Such examinations highlight each profession's perspective on the issue, how those perspectives can be combined, and how the unique contributions of each professional can be tapped to resolve the issues. In this approach two or more professional groups learn with and about each other to achieve a common purpose by synthesizing and complementing one another's professional skills and perspectives (Harden, 1998). Clinical education, which is the core of health professionals' education, has long been considered an ideal method for interprofessional learning and the development of collaborative approaches. While the purpose of clinical education is generally held to be the development of students' clinical competence, it is now being viewed as an important site for interprofessional learning. The effectiveness of clinical education in preparing students for interdisciplinary collaboration, however, depends on the existence of several key elements — the role and quality of clinical faculty (D'Eon, 2005), the effective use of preceptors, and clinical practice environments that are supportive and that value all professionals. While many authors articulate the importance of such elements, little evidence exists that can inform faculty and preceptors in how to implement their roles and create positive learning environments that support interprofessional education.

Service learning or community placements are also an important venue for interprofessional learning. These supervised placements can be voluntarily undertaken in addition to the clinical requirements for a professional degree. In locating learners within working community centers and organizations, the placements offer participants the opportunity to learn collaboratively both with professionals from other disciplines and with clients, within a structured, supervised learning environment (Seifer, 1998).

How Should Interprofessional Education Occur?

To be effective, interprofessional education must involve a variety of educational approaches, techniques and strategies to achieve collaborative competencies proposed by Barr (Barr, 1996, 1998; Barr, Koppel, Reeves, Hammick, & Freeth, 2005; Oandasan & Reeves, 2005a). These competencies include:

1. describe one's roles and responsibilities to other health professions;

2. recognize and observe the constraints of one's own professional role, responsibilities, and competencies while being able to perceive the needs of patients in a wider framework that involves other professions;

3. recognize and value the roles, responsibilities, and competence of other professions in relation to one's own professional role;

4. work with other professions to effect change and resolve conflict in the provision of patient care;

5. work collaboratively with other professions to assess, plan, provide and review care for patients;

6. tolerate differences, misunderstandings and limitations in other professions;

7. facilitate interprofessional patient care meetings, such as team meetings and patient case conferences;

8. engage in interdependent relationships with other professions.

Key dimensions of learning interprofessional clinical education include the design of courses and clinical experiences/rotations, development and use of assessment/evaluation methods, institutional policies that support IPE, and participation by health professions programs. Course and clinical rotations should be designed with explicit rather than implicit concepts that support the collaborative competencies discussed earlier. Are concepts that support course and clinical designed from one discipline's perspective with participation by other disciplines or as a shared perspective? Clinical rotations should be designed so that placements support planned interaction and integration of other health professions students. Are students exposed to and interact with faculty from other disciplines in a purposeful manner? The design and use of standardized assessments/evaluations is an important component of IPE clinical education. Assessments range from no IPE/collaborative assessment to a common IPE assessment that is conducted within a single discipline to a common assessment that is used among all learners. The participation of a health professions program in clinical IPE varies based on availability of a professional program as well as intra - and interagency support. However, the participation in some level of IPE is essential; this participation can vary from providing collaborative on-site care to case conferences or project/service learning. While the literature reports the design of course and clinical IPE, the literature is sparse in discussing the faculty development and incentives for IPE. Institutional policies that support and reward faculty participation in IPE is critical. Faculty often participate due to interest; however, release time for collaboration on an IPE/teaching team is essential to ensure well developed course and clinical experiences. Furthermore, participation in IPE is a form of scholarship that should be included in promotion and tenure decisions for faculty.

Presently, the use of learning strategies such as problem-based learning, experiential learning, active learning, and reflective practice all appear to support learning in general (Billings & Halstead, 2005; Young & Paterson, 2007), as well as interprofessional learning. What distinguishes the use of these strategies for IPE lies within the design of the educational experience that allows collaborative learning and competency development (Freeth, Hammick, Reeves, Koppel, & Barr, 2005). Schmitt (2008) identifies pedagogical approaches for IPE that include educational principles and strategies that focus on the leveling, timing, and sequencing of IPE as well as combining didactic and experiential learning that is both education and work-based. Educational methods include learning about each other's professions, such as reviewing the evolution of different professions, and examining stereotypes. Experiential strategies include having students learn with each other and interview persons from other professions; shadowing other professions, and completing clinical learning under the supervision of another professional. Integration skills of teamwork and collaborative endeavors can be facilitated by educational strategies such as reading about basic principles of teamwork, observing role models in practice, learning quality improvement approaches to team meetings, care delivery, patient outcomes (e.g., TeamSTEPPS), and teamwork exercises to learn about communication distortions, cooperation, assertion, hand-off communication, coordination of care, and responding under pressure. Second Life families can be created that are jointly cared for by students across the professions. The culmination of IPE learning is student engagement in real life activities to deliver health care through student-run clinics or action-based research that focuses on community needs assessment and health improvement projects such as those supported by grant funding for Community Based Quality Improvement Education or Achieving Competence Today.

Changes in technology and educational methods have also affected learning and teaching approaches, and have led to more learner-driven approaches (Billings & Halstead, 2005; Young & Paterson, 2007). Examples of these are evident in the increased use of computer-based learning (e.g., Second Life families, use of wikis, blogs, and discussion boards for collaborative assignments across institutions and geographic settings), simulation learning (see previous chapter), and problem-based learning (PBL) (Hughes & Lucas, 1997; Jeffries, McNelis, & Wheeler, 2008).

Problem-based learning cases are structured around practical problems that are presented to students. Students take an active role, working within small groups. They take responsibility for seeking out the information that they perceive as relevant to the case and later share this in the group to achieve a more adequate understanding. It is usual for the group to apply some aspect of this information to the case study, such as developing an assessment and appropriate intervention. Each case enables students to learn about several aspects of the discipline under study, assisting the development of an integrated web of personal knowledge. Collaborative cases can include such topics as pain management, end-of-life issues, medication errors, coordination of care, miscommunication, and others. The collaborative PBL process is often regarded by faculty, students and staff as encouraging the development of interpersonal skills, working in teams and respect for each other's roles. This respect is a core component of collaboration and team skills necessary for professional practice (Hughes & Lucas, 1997; Reynolds, 2003).

Another professional practice team building approach is the use of patient simulation, which can be thought of as the re-creation of an event that is as close to reality as possible. A patient simulator is used to establish realism in simulated scenarios and includes both noncomputerized and computerized types. Non-computer-based simulators have been used in nursing education for many years. Recently, sophisticated computer-based, high-fidelity human patient simulators have been used in health professionals education. Human patient simulators offer a high degree of realism, particularly when integrated into simulated scenarios, because of their advanced and responsive computerized physiological functions. Students and other learners integrate a full range of knowledge, attitudes and skills to respond effectively. In addition, they are able to observe the outcomes of their clinical decisions and actions as well as a videotape of their performance. Thus, the use of high fidelity patient simulators with clinical scenarios can provide the dynamic realism of the practice setting, using, for example, cardiac arrest or other emergency situation, but in an environment where errors or omissions do not jeopardize a real patient. Furthermore, there is growing research evidence of the transferability of competencies learned through simulation to the practice setting (Rosen et al., 2008).

Creating an Interprofessional Health Education Agenda

Interprofessional health education asks health professions educators to reconceptualize their practice. It is not simply students who must change how they understand health care. It is educators who must alter the models of teaching and learning through which students learn. One of the lessons that can be taken from the field of education is that teachers tend to teach as they were taught. The process of IPE demands that health professions educators teach in a way that is counter to dominant models of learning in professional silos. IPE is an interdependent model of collaborative learning in which students learn with and from each other, not just about each other. Building a practice of IPE can be created at any number of different time points, in both education and clinical settings, and taking advantage of different educational practices. But, developing a model of IPE as a means to effective collaborative teaming in health care delivery requires first developing a means for interdisciplinary teaming between faculty located in discrete departments, and likely schools, within higher education institutions. It is necessary to train the trainers (faculty) first, rather than assume faculty inherently versed in IPE.

The process of faculty teaming to foster meaningful interprofessional education opportunities requires time, listening, collaborative learning and reconsideration of existing discipline-based reward structures. The authors of this chapter had recent experience with interprofessional education that suggests that building the partnership between instructors is a necessary platform for forming meaningful educational environments where learning from and about each others' professions is valued, facilitated and enhanced. An authentic process of interprofessional teaming to create interprofessional learning requires reflecting upon process and outcome, taking the best from our own discipline and learning from our partners. The challenge is that too often the stresses of our disciplinary or professional demands cause us to resort to the models of teaching and learning that are comfortable, tried and true, and do not strain the organizational dynamics. The opportunity that IPE presents is to develop models of learning that mimic the kind of care that patients need; take advantage of the strengths of many different health care professions; and is learned collaboratively, thus building toward a stronger health care environment.

Research on IPE Outcomes

There is little research that meets the stringent Cochrane criteria for systematic review of research studies. However, a Joint Evaluation Team (JET) for Interprofessional Education in the United Kingdom conducted a systematic meta-analysis of worldwide reviews of IPE outcomes with the establishment of widened yet rigorous criteria using the same search strategies and definitions of IPE as the Cochrane review (Hammick, 2000). Instead of asking whether IPE changes practice and benefits patients, as asked by the Cochrane review, the JET or "Parallel Review" asked what kind of IPE, under what circumstances, produces what kind of outcomes. Thus, a wider range of research methodologies using both qualitative and quantitative methods were included that inform the process and form of IPE.

The JET review used a typology proposed by Barr (1996), which identified the following typology for IPE outcomes: 1) learner reactions, 2) changes or modification of learners' attitudes or perceptions, 3) acquisition of knowledge and skills, 4) change in learner behavior, 5) change in organizational practice, and 6) benefits to patients. This typology serves as a framework to guide the classification and design of IPE and evaluate outcomes. Learner reactions center on the student's satisfaction and view of their learning experience. The second level moves from an individual student to changes in reciprocal attitudes/perceptions between student groups and move toward patients and their condition, care, and treatment. The third typology considers the acquisition of problem-solving knowledge, attitudes or skills linked to the collaborative learning experience. The fourth level, change in behavior, covers the transfer from learning environment to workplace as a result of modifications or applications of newly acquired knowledge or skills in practice, whereas the fifth classification focuses more on organizational practice. The sixth, and perhaps most important, is the benefit to patients as a direct result of the IPE.

Systematic reviews conducted report that the majority of research centers on the first three levels (Cooper, Carlisle, Gibbs, & Watkins, 2001; Reeves et al., 2009). These reviews report that the largest effect was on learner knowledge, attitudes, skills, and understanding of professional roles and teamwork. The smallest effects were reported for transfer of learner into experiential practice and learning environment. However, this finding reflects methodological shortcomings associated with reporting practices and research design issues such as length of follow-up measures. In short, there is little evidence that demonstrates either the effectiveness or ineffectiveness of IPE.

Future research that meets methodological criteria of systematic reviews is needed. Funding for IPE should include the costs of rigorous evaluation. Studies reported in the literature need to be transparent and adequately described in order to allow inclusion for a systematic review. The typology used by the JET review should serve as a framework for future research, with attention given to transfer of knowledge, attitudes, and skills from the academic setting to the practice setting and subsequent effect on patients and organizations.

In summary, research and educational approaches to interprofessional educational experiences for nursing and other health professions students brings to light both the opportunities and the challenges that exist in health care education and practice. Interprofessional practice that exists in today's health care environment drives the need for IPE and is broader than patient safety and quality issues. Clinical education provides experiential learning opportunties for nursing and other health professional students to learn about and with each other in order to provide and coordinate care.

References

Albanese, M.A., Mejicano, G., Mullan, P., Kokotailo, P., & Gruppen, L. (2008). Defining characteristics of educational competencies. *Medical Education, 42*, 248-255.

American Association of Colleges of Nursing [AACN]. (1996). Position statement: Interdisciplinary education and practice. *Journal of Professional Nursing, 12*(2), 119-123.

Baggs, J. G., & Schmitt, M. H. (1997). Nurses' and resident physicians' perceptions of the process of collaboration in an MICU. *Research in Nursing and Health, 20*(1), 71-80.

Baggs, J. G., Ryan, S., Phelps, C., Richeson, J., & Johnson, J. (1992). The association of interdisciplinary collaboration and patient outcomes in a medical intensive care unit. *Heart & Lung, 21*(1), 18-24.

Baggs, J. G., Schmitt, M. H., Mushlin, A. I., Eldredge, D. H., Oakes, D., & Hutson, A. D. (1997). Nurse-physician collaboration and satisfaction with the decision-making process in three critical care units. *American Journal of Critical Care, 6*(5), 393-399.

Baggs, J. G., Schmitt, M. H., Mushlin, A. I., Mitchell, P. H., Eldredge, D. H., Oakes, D., et al. (1999). The association between nurse-physician collaboration and patient outcomes in three intensive care units. *Critical Care Medicine, 27*, 1991-1998.

Barr H. (1996). Ends and means in interprofessional education: Towards a typology. *Education for Health, 9*(3), 341-352.

Barr, H. (1998). Competent to collaborate: Towards a competency-based model for interprofessional education. *Journal of Interprofessional Care, 12*, 181-187.

Barr, H., Koppel, I., Reeves, S., Hammick, M., & Freeth, D. (2005). *Effective interprofessional education: Argument, assumption and evidence*. London: Blackwell.

Batalden, P., Leach, D., Swing, S., Dreyfus, H., & Dreyfus, S. (2002). General competencies and accreditation in graduate medical education. *Health Affairs* (Millwood.), *21*, 103-111.

Billings, D. M., & Halstead, J. A. (2005). *Teaching in nursing: A guide for faculty* (2nd ed.). Philadelphia: Evolve Elsevier.

Cohen, A. M. (1998). *The shaping of American higher education: Emergence and growth of the contemporary system*. San Francisco: Wiley & Sons.

Cooke, M., Irby, D. M., Sullivan, W., & Ludmerer, K. M. (2006). American medical education 100 years after the Flexner report. *New England Journal of Medicine, 355*, 1339-1344.

Cooper, H., Carlisle, C., Gibbs, T., & Watkins, C. (2001). Developing an evidence base for interdisciplinary learning: A systematic review. *Journal of Advanced Nursing, 35*(2), 228-237.

D'Eon, M. (2005). A blueprint for interprofessional learning. *Journal of Interprofessional Care, 19*(Suppl. 1), 49-59.

Epstein, R. M., & Hundert, E. M. (2002). Defining and assessing professional competence. *Journal of the American Medical Association, 287*, 226-235.

Fealy, G. M. (2005). Sharing the experience: Interdisciplinary education and interprofessional learning. *Nursing Education in Practice, 5*, 317-319.

Freeth, D., Hammick, M., Reeves, S., Koppel, I., & Barr, H. (2005). *Effective interprofessional education: Development, delivery, and evaluation*. London: Blackwell.

Govaerts, M. J. B. (2008). Educational competencies or education for professional competence? *Medical Education, 42*, 234-236.

Greiner, A., & Knebel, E. (Eds.). (2003). *Health professions education: A bridge to quality*. Washington, DC: National Academies Press.

Hall, P., & Weaver, L. (2001). Interdisciplinary education and teamwork: A long and winding road. *Medical Education, 35*, 867-875.

Hammick, M. (2000). *Interprofessional education: evidence from the past to guide the future, Medical Teacher, 22*(5), 461-467.

Harden, R. M. (1998). AMEE Guide No. 12. Multiprofessional education: Part 1 — Effective multiprofessional education: A three-dimensional perspective. *Medical Teacher, 20*(5), 402-408.

Harvan, R. A., Royeen, C. B., & Jensen, G. M. (2009). Grounding interprofessional education and practice in theory. In C. B. Royeen, G. M. Jensen, & R. A. Harvan (Eds.), *Leadership in interprofessional health education* (pp. 45-62). Sudbury, MA: Jones and Bartlett.

Hughes, L., & Lucas, J. (1997). An evaluation of problem-based learning in the multiprofessional education curriculum for the health professions. *Journal of Interprofessional Care, 11*(1), 77- 88.

Institute of Medicine. (2000). *To err is human: Building a safer health system*. Washington, DC: National Academies Press.

Institute of Medicine. (2001). *Crossing the quality chasm: A new health system for the 21st century*. Washington, DC: National Academies Press.

Jeffries, P. R., McNelis, A. M., & Wheeler, C. A. (2008). Simulation as a vehicle for enhancing collaborative practice models. *Critical Care Nursing Clinics of North America, 20*(4), 471-480.

Keeling, R., Underhile, R., & Wall, A. (2007). Horizontal and vertical structures: The dynamics of organization in higher education. *Liberal Education, 93*(4), 22-31.

Larson, E. (1999). The impact of physician-nurse interaction on patient care. *Holistic Nursing Practice, 13*(2), 38-46.

Ludmerer, K. M. (1985). *Learning to heal: The development of American medical education*. Baltimore: Johns Hopkins University Press.

Ludmerer, K. M. (1999). *Time to heal. American medical education from the turn of the century to the era of managed care*. New York: Oxford University Press.

O'Neill, E. H., & Pew Health Professions Education. (1998). *Re-creating health professional practice for a new century*. The fourth report of the PEW Health Professions Commission. San Francisco: Pew Health Professions Commission

Oandasan, I., & Reeves, S. (2005a). Key elements for interprofessional education. Part 1: The learner, the educator and the learning context. *Journal of Interprofessional Care, 19*(Suppl. 1), 21-38.

Oandasan, I., & Reeves, S. (2005b). Key elements of interprofessional education. Part 2: Factors, processes and outcomes. *Journal of Interprofessional Care, 19*(Suppl. 1), 39-48.

Ovretweit, J. (1996). Five ways to describe a multidisciplinary team. *Journal of Interprofessional Care, 10*(2), 163-172.

Reeves, S., Zwarenstein, M., Goldman, J., Barr, H., Freeth, D., Hammick, M., et al. (2009). [Review]. Interprofessional education: Effects on professional practice and health care outcomes. *Cochrane Library.* Retrieved January 26, 2009, from http://www.thecochranelibrary.com

Reynolds, F. (2003). Initial experiences of interprofessional problem-based learning: A comparison of male and female students' views. *Journal of Interprofessional Care, 17*(1), 35-44.

Rosen, M., Salas, E., Wu, T., Silvestri, S., Lazzara, E., Lyons, R., et al. (2008). Promoting teamwork: An event-based approach to simulation-based teamwork training for emergency medicine residents. *Academic Emergency Medicine, 15*(11), 1190-1198.

Rudolph, F. (1990). *The American college & university: A history.* Athens, GA: University of Georgia Press.

Schmitt, M. (2008, November). *Interprofessional education: Finding our way forward 35 years after the first Institute of Medicine report.* Paper presented at the meeting of the American Association of Medical Colleges, San Antonio, TX.

Seifer, S. D. (1998). Service-learning: Community-campus partnerships for health professions education. *Academic Medicine, 73*(3), 273-277.

Shaver, J. L. (2005). Interdisciplinary education and practice: Moving from reformation to transformation. *Nursing Outlook, 53*, 57-58.

Steinert, Y. (2005). Learning together to teach together: Interprofessional education and faculty development. *Journal of Interprofessional Care, 19*(1), 60-75.

U.S. Department of Health and Human Services. Office of Disease Prevention and Health Promotion. (2000). *Healthy People 2010.* Retrieved January 26, 2009, from http://www.health.gov/healthypeople/

Weber, M., Mills, C. W. (Ed.), & Gerth, H. H. (Trans.). (1948). *From Max Weber: Essays in sociology.* New York: Routledge.

Wheeler, B. K., Powelson, S., & Kim, J. (2007). Interdisciplinary clinical education: Implementing a gerontological home visiting program. *Nurse Educator, 32*(3), 136-140.

Young, L. E., & Paterson, B. L. (2007). *Teaching nursing: Developing a student-centered learning environment.* Philadelphia: Lippincott, Williams, & Wilkins.

Zwarenstein, M., Atkins, J., Barr, H., Hammick, M., Koppel, I., & Reeves, S. (1999). A systematic review of interprofessional education. *Journal of Interprofessional Care, 13*(4), 417-424.

CLINICAL NURSING EDUCATION

CLINICAL EDUCATION AND REGULATION

Nancy Spector, PhD, RN

While planning for course innovation,
Our mantra for nurse education
Is, "Please be aware
That face-to-face care
Is vital for nurses' formation."

Introduction

Because U.S. states, territories, and the District of Columbia approve nursing programs, it is important for educators to understand the regulatory perspective on clinical education in nursing prelicensure programs. This chapter will explore in detail the regulatory perspective on clinical education and why boards of nursing take the position that nursing programs need to provide supervised clinical experiences for their students. Some of the myths about regulatory barriers are dispelled, and some of the differences among boards of nursing are discussed. Current issues, such as the regulatory perspective on the use of simulation in prelicensure programs and the use of exit exams, also are explored. Lastly, the importance of collaboration between education, practice, and regulation is integrated throughout the chapter.

Background of Regulation in Nursing Education

In 1903, North Carolina enacted the first registration law for nursing, followed by New York, New Jersey, and Virginia (Dorsey & Schowalter, 2008). Soon thereafter, boards of nursing began to regulate nursing. The mission of all 60 boards of nursing in the United States[1] is to protect the public. Boards of nursing accomplish this through four major domains: (1) approving and enforcing educational standards, (2) licensing on the basis of psychometrically and legally defensible testing, (3) monitoring and decision making related to practice issues, and (4) using the disciplinary process to remove from practice those nurses who fail to maintain standards (Hudspeth, 2008).

By 1906, inspectors of schools or hospitals with nurse training programs began making program visits for regulatory approval. As boards of nursing developed, they began approving nursing education programs as part of their mission to protect the public. Currently 58 of the 60 boards of nursing approve nursing education in their jurisdiction. Furthermore, in the other two states (Mississippi and New York), approval is done through the Board of Higher Education by nurses who hold an earned doctorate. A more detailed history of the regulation of nursing education programs in the United States, and the processes used when approving programs, can be found elsewhere (NCSBN, 2004b; Spector, in press).

Approval of nursing programs ensures that nursing is practiced by minimally competent licensed nurses within an authorized scope of practice. With the Institute of Medicine's (IOM) report on medical errors (Kohn, Corrigan & Donaldson, 1999), followed by other IOM and national reports on safety in health care, national attention has been directed to patient safety issues. While nurse leaders assert that there is a direct relationship between safe patient care and the quality of nursing programs (ICN, 1997), nurse researchers need to conduct studies that document this relationship between nursing education and patient outcomes.

It is also important for educators to remember that the licensure examinations, the NCLEX-RN® and NCLEX-PN®, are not designed as stand-alone assessments of the ability to practice nursing. Passage of the licensing examination is predicated on the nurse graduate successfully

---

[1] The boards of nursing reside in the 50 states; four states have a registered nurse board and a practical nursing board; one state has an APRN board, the District of Columbia and four territories each have a board.

completing a board-approved nursing education program. Therefore, while regulators have the responsibility for approving nursing programs, educators have the responsibility for deciding whether the student should graduate, thereby affirming that the student is safe, clinically competent, and eligible to take the NCLEX®. This decision by faculty members should not be taken lightly.

Another regulatory principle that is important to nurse educators is that nurse licensure is for general nursing practice. In other words, nurses who graduate from prelicensure programs are not licensed for specialties, such as obstetrics or medical-surgical nursing. Thus, when boards of nursing review nursing programs, many of them look for learning experiences across the lifespan. Educators sometimes argue that students should be able to specialize in a field of their choice, especially during these times when clinical experiences are hard to find. However, because licensure covers a broad practice, such an option is not feasible for regulation. Educators, therefore, need to explore creative clinical experiences, such as using day care centers, physician or nurse practitioner offices, or schools for pediatrics experiences. There are some excellent innovative clinical models available (Gubrud-Howe & Schoessler, 2008).

How Regulation of Nursing Education Varies Across the Jurisdictions

Educators often complain about the inconsistency in nursing regulation of education programs across the United States. There is no doubt that this inconsistency exists, and it is particularly the case for practical nursing programs. Processes of approval vary across the country, so that educators, particularly administrators, often find it difficult when they move from one state to another and take a new position. In the fall issue of NCSBN's *Leader to Leader*, Hobbs (2007) discusses the implications of these inconsistencies when educators move to other states and offers some tips to effectively manage the differences (see Box 12-1). For example, one state might require 500 hours of clinical experience and limit the faculty-student ratio in the clinical setting to 1:10, while another state may have no minimal requirements for clinical hours but allow only a 1:8 ratio in clinical; still another might have no requirements for either of those situations.

Other differences are that at least one board (Louisiana-RN) regulates nursing students in that jurisdiction. In most states, practicing nursing as a student who is enrolled in an approved nursing program is an "exempted" or "excepted" practice in the practice act (see the discussion below under Myth #3). However, in the Louisiana-RN board, while students are not licensed, they are under the jurisdiction of the board and can be disciplined for violating their provisions.

Other states require that the board of nursing be notified in writing of any change in faculty and program administrator positions (Hobbs, 2007). A comparison of nursing education requirements across the boards of nursing can be found in the National Council of State Boards of Nursing's[2] (NCSBN) Member Board Profiles (NCSBN, 2007). This document can be valuable

---

2 The National Council of State Boards of Nursing (NCSBN) is a national organization, composed of the boards of nursing, and its mission is to provide leadership to advance regulatory excellence for public protection.

Box 12 – 1
Regulatory Tips When Educators Move (Hobbs, 2007)

For All Faculty

- Once contracts are finalized, initiate licensure by endorsements. This can take months in some states; others might be able to provide a temporary work permit.

- Read new jurisdiction s nurse practice act and education administrative rules (often available on the Web). Most have curricular requirements, such as student-faculty ratios.

- Is there oversight of RN to BSN programs or MSN programs?

- Texas requires a jurisprudence exam (assessment of knowledge of the nurse practice act and administrative rules) for all nurses who it endorses; see http://www.bon.state.tx.us/olv/je.html. Other states may follow.

- Board may have an orientation course for faculty.

- Some states require that the board be notified of any faculty changes.

For Administrators

- Contact the education consultant at the board of nursing for developing a line of communication.

- Attend dean and director meetings as the board of nursing may be represented.

- Find out required faculty qualifications for that jurisdiction.

- Find out when annual reports are due and how site visits are conducted. A template for approval processes is available on NCSBN s website (NCSBN, 2004b).

- Know what your jurisdiction s requirements are for the NCLEX® pass rates.

for educators to analyze similarities and differences among how boards regulate nursing education. If the educator would like to suggest rule[3] changes to the board, this document could provide convincing evidence by showing what the other boards are doing.

Because of these differences, it is incumbent upon each faculty member to read the nurse practice act[4] and administrative education rules of the state(s) in which she/he is teaching to fully understand the requirements of each jurisdiction. Many states now have their current rules posted on their website (Hobbs, 2007). Some boards of nursing have started orientation programs for new administrators to highlight the educational rules, and, in many jurisdictions, deans and directors invite a representative from the board of nursing to their regular meetings to discuss any regulatory issues related to nursing education. This is an excellent way to improve communication between educators and regulators. Furthermore, nursing program administrators are encouraged to contact the board of nursing's education consultant, or the person who is assigned to program approval in that state, if there are any questions about the approval requirements.

---

3 Rules and regulations are consistent with The Nurse Practice Act. The rules cannot go beyond the law, and once enacted, they have the force of the law. Some states refer to these as the regulations (Spector, in press).

4 Statutes that authorize the board of nursing to promulgate rules that are necessary for the implementation of The Nurse Practice Act (Spector, in press).

NCSBN is often asked why all these inconsistencies exist, and stakeholders ask our organization to "mandate" more consistency. However, it is not that simple. Licensure and the state-based regulatory system in the United States are founded in the 10th Amendment of the US Constitution, thus falling under "individual state jurisdiction with its inevitable variations and uniqueness" (Poe, 2008, p. 268). Therefore, each jurisdiction has its own laws and administrative rules, and these laws/rules differ across jurisdictions. In an attempt to provide some regulatory guidelines and consistency to boards of nursing as they promulgate rules and revise their Nurse Practice Acts, NCSBN, through committees of its membership, maintains a model Nurse Practice Act and model administrative rules (NCSBN, 2004a). The model Act and rules are a living document that is regularly reviewed by experts in nursing regulation. However, NCSBN can only provide recommendations to the boards of nursing; it cannot mandate legislative language because of our state-based regulatory system. In addition, NCSBN has provided its members with Evidence-Based Nursing Education for Regulation (EBNER) (NCSBN, 2006a), which is evidence upon which the Boards can base their administrative rules. This document will be discussed in more detail later.

Regulatory Position on Clinical Experiences: The Evidence

These are exciting times in nursing education. There has been a call for transforming how we teach clinical education (Benner, Sutphen, Leonard-Kahn & Day, 2008; Greiner & Knebel, 2003; Gubrud-Howe & Schoessler, 2008; NLN, 2003). At the same time there a major focus on evidence-based nursing education (Oermann, 2007), and journals are seeing more nursing education research being submitted (Tanner, Bellack & Harker, 2009). Regulation welcomes innovation in nursing education and evidence upon which to base their rules for nursing curricula and teaching strategies.

However, one point that regulation is quite firm on is that all prelicensure students should have sufficient supervised clinical experiences with actual patients, at the scope of practice to which the students are aspiring, to meet the program's outcomes. Nursing is a practice discipline, so actual contact with patients is an essential component of prelicensure nursing education. All other health professions require supervised clinical experiences, and nursing should be no exception. Yet, from time to time, programs have presented boards of nursing with curricula that incorporate minimal or no clinical experiences. Therefore, the following discussion will provide rationale for why nursing regulation has taken this position.

At NCSBN's 2004 annual meeting, the membership presented the organization with a resolution asking NCSBN to develop a position statement that provides boards with guidance on evaluating clinical experiences in both traditional and alternative nursing education programs (NCSBN, 2005). An NCSBN committee was established to look at this question, and its members spent a year investigating the evidence as to whether supervised clinical experiences, at the aspired level of licensure, were an essential component of a nursing education program. To accomplish this goal, the committee members took several steps. They reviewed the available literature and research, surveyed boards of nursing, surveyed education organizations, consulted with renowned simulation experts, participated in simulated scenarios at a simulation center, and sought input from practice.

Box 12 – 2
Recommendations from NCSBN 's Position Paper on Clinical Experiences in Prelicensure Nursing Programs (NCSBN, 2005)

Prelicensure nursing educational experiences should be across the lifespan.

Prelicensure nursing education programs shall include clinical experiences with actual patients; they might also include innovative teaching strategies that complement clinical experiences for entry into practice competency.

Prelicensure clinical education should be supervised by qualified faculty who provide feedback and facilitate reflection.

Faculty members retain the responsibility to demonstrate that programs have clinical experiences with actual patients that are sufficient to meet program outcomes.

Additional research needs to be conducted on prelicensure nursing education and the development of clinical competency.

The committee findings and recommendations were presented in a position paper at NCSBN's 2005 annual meeting, and the membership nearly unanimously adopted the statement (NCSBN, 2005). This position paper calls for supervised clinical experiences, at the level of licensure that the graduates are seeking, to be an essential component of prelicensure education. The specific recommendations of this paper are highlighted in Box 12-2.

While NCSBN's position paper on clinical experiences was released in 2005, the American Organization of Nurse Executives (AONE) released a similar position statement in 2004 (AONE, 2004). See Box 12-3 for that position statement.

Furthermore, both national nursing accreditation organizations (i.e., CCNE and NLNAC) provide expert opinions that prelicensure nursing students should have supervised clinical experiences in their standards and criteria. Standard 4.8 from the 2008 National League for Nursing Accrediting Commission (NLNAC) Standards and Criteria (NLNAC, 2008) addresses

Box 12 – 3
AONE Position Statement on Prelicensure Clinical Experiences (AONE, 2004)

AONE firmly believes that solutions to the nursing shortage require innovation and creative approaches to education, practice and the delivery of systems of care. We strongly support efforts to address the shortage that align with the guiding principles that have been developed by the AONE Board to describe the future work of the nurse. Such initiatives are critical to our ability to secure a competent, professional workforce that can deliver safe, quality care to populations in our communities.

AONE also believes that the education programs for the nurses of the future will require a balance of didactic content and supervised clinical instruction.

Although innovative approaches may be developed, it is the position of AONE that all prelicensure nursing education programs must contain structured and supervised clinical instruction and that the clinical instruction must be provided by appropriately prepared registered nurses.

clinical education, and Standard 4.8.1 specifically states that "Student clinical experiences reflect current best practices and nationally established patient health and safety goals." Similarly, the Commission on Collegiate Nursing Education (CCNE) uses the *2008 Essentials of Baccalaureate Education for Professional Nursing Practice* (AACN, 2008) as a guiding document when accrediting baccalaureate programs. Throughout this document, the essentiality of supervised clinical experiences in baccalaureate programs is highlighted, as evidenced by the following example (p. 4): "Learning opportunities, including direct clinical experiences, must be sufficient in breadth and depth to ensure the baccalaureate graduate attains these practice focused outcomes and integrates the delineated knowledge and skills into the graduate's professional nursing practice."

Boards of nursing, however, are vested in basing their administrative rules on research findings, as well as consensus statements of experts, and, as NCSBN's recommendation number five stated, there is the need for additional research on this subject. For that reason, NCSBN conducted a study to identify evidence-based elements of nursing education. In this study, a sample of 410 education programs provided information on the characteristics of their programs. Then a sample of 7,497 graduates from those programs was obtained and graduates were matched to the program from which they graduated; at least five graduates had to graduate from a particular program in order for that program to be included. The two outcomes measures explored were the new nurses' self-reports of (a) adequacy of preparation and (b) difficulty with client care assignments. Whereas these were only self-reports, the last outcome measure is closely related to actual patient outcomes. If nurses are having difficulty with their current workplace assignments, it is likely that will affect patient outcomes. Content validity and reliability (Cronbach's alpha scores ranged from 0.87 to 0.91) were established on the research tools; separate tools were used for new graduates and nursing programs. Multiple regression, when the data were continuous, and logistic regression, when the data were dichotomous, analyses were used to link the curriculum elements and outcomes. Significant results are summarized in Table 12-1.

NCSBN's National Study of Elements of Nursing Education was a beginning effort toward describing the evidence-based elements of nursing education. The findings on clinical education provide evidence that clinical education is important to student learning outcomes and the ability to practice. For example, the finding on faculty members being available to assist with clinical skills during clinical experiences found that those graduates were 1.4 times more likely to report having no difficulty with their current assignment.

One limitation of this study is that it relies on student reports of being prepared or of having difficulty with assignments. Future studies might look at actual patient outcomes. There are no studies that link nursing education to actual patient outcomes, and that would be a next step.

After reviewing the results of the National Survey of Elements of Nursing Education, NCSBN conducted a systematic review of nursing education outcomes (NCSBN, 2006c), which found 25 studies that met the study criteria. The studies were categorized as to strength of study design. Five studies in this review provided evidence that clinical experiences improve students' abilities to think critically when caring for patients, though no study investigated numbers of clinical hours that are necessary for quality education. Since clinical experiences are so variable

Table 12 – 1
Summary of Significant Results from NCSBN's Elements of Nursing Education Study
(NCSBN, 2006b)

Graduates were more likely to report they were adequately prepared (multiple regression analysis) when their nursing program:
- Had a higher percentage of faculty who taught both didactic and clinical courses (β=0.34).
- Taught use of information technology (β=0.42) and evidence-based practice (β=0.44).
- Integrated pathophysiology β =0.33) and critical thinking (β=0.34) throughout the curriculum.
- Taught content related to specific client populations (such as medical surgical β=0.20), care of clients with psychiatric disorders β=0.24), and women's health β=0.41) as separate courses.

Graduates were more likely (multiple regression analysis) to report they were adequately prepared when their faculty were able to:
- Demonstrate clinical skills (β=1.15)
- Assist with classroom projects (β=0.84
- Provide current information in the classroom (β=1.15)
- Assist with clinical skills (β=0.67)
- Require students to demonstrate skills (β=0.51)
- Answer questions during clinical (β=0.73)
- Answer questions about content (β=0.33)

- Availability of faculty to assist with clinical skills is also predictive of difficulty with current care assignments (Odds Ratio OR)=1.44

Relationship between perceived adequacy of education preparation and difficulty with client care assignments (logistic regression analysis):
- Work effectively within the health care team (OR=2.2)
- Understand the pathophysiology underlying a client s condition (OR=1.5)
- Delegate tasks to others (OR=1.4)
- Analyze multiple types of data when making decisions (OR=1.3)
- Administer medications to groups of patients (OR=1.3)

(Gubrud-Howe & Schoessler, 2008) and since educators have many different strategies for teaching clinical education, it is not likely that specific numbers of clinical hours will ever be supported by research findings. It is the quality of clinical learning experiences that researchers should be addressing, as well as their relationship to patient outcomes.

NCSBN's National Survey of Elements of Nursing Education (NCSBN, 2006b) and the systematic review of nursing education outcomes (NCSBN, 2006c) were used to develop

Box 12 – 4
EBNER Recommendations Related to Clinical Education (NCSBN, 2006a)

Assimilation to the role of nursing
- Provide experiences for relationship-building with professionals
- Provide experiences for students to gain comfort in nursing role
- Provide experiences for students to work effectively in a team
- Provide transition programs
- Deliberate practice with actual patients
- Provide experiences for relation-building with patients
- Provide clinical experiences with actual patients
- Provide experiences for gaining confidence
- Provide opportunities for reflection

Faculty-student relationships
- Faculty teach clinical and didactic courses
- Faculty are available to demonstrate and assist with skills in clinical activities
- Faculty are available to answer questions during clinical activities
- Faculty provide current information

Teaching methodologies
- Integrate critical thinking into the curriculum
- Use critical thinking strategies
- Integrate evidence-based practice into the curriculum
- Integrate information technology into the curriculum
- Integrate pathophysiology into the curriculum
- Teach population courses separately
- Require students to demonstrate skills before performing them on patients

evidence-based nursing education for regulation (EBNER) (NCSBN, 2006a) for boards of nursing to use as evidence-based guidelines when promulgating education rules. Recommendations that directly related to clinical education are outlined in Box 12-4.

Two studies similar to NCSBN's National Survey of Elements of Nursing Education (NCSBN, 2006b) were conducted more recently. Candela and Bowles (2008) conducted a descriptive study of nurses who were registered in the state of Nevada and had graduated within the past five years. A total of 352 nurses returned the survey with 43 percent being in practice from one to three years and 57 percent practicing from three to five years. The data collection instrument, which was researcher designed, showed adequate reliability (Cronbach's alpha of 0.87). A factor analysis determined that the items were loaded onto three factors: skills for practice, professional development, and clinical performance. As with the NCSBN national study, this statewide study is limited because its outcomes measures are based on student self-reports. Some of the significant findings for clinical education included:

- Need to be better prepared to administer medications
- Need for more clinical hours in the education program
- Need for more management/leadership in the education program
- Need for better preparation in using electronic medical records
- More than half of the respondents believed that their programs prepared them to pass the NCLEX-RN®

The findings support more focused clinical experiences in areas of medication administration, management and leadership, as well as practice with electronic medical records.

The Nursing Executive Center conducted a large national study regarding new graduate nurses. The researchers surveyed 53,000 "frontline" nurse employers, and more than 5,700 responded. An online survey asked employers to rate their satisfaction (from "strongly agree" to "strongly disagree") with new graduates (defined as those with less than 12 months of practice) on 36 mutually-agreed-upon competencies that are essential to safe and competent care (Berkow, Virkstis, Stewart & Conway, 2008). The researchers also surveyed more than 400 nursing school deans/directors/department chairs for relative curricular emphasis on these competencies. Results of the study found that about 25 percent of the employers were fully satisfied with new graduate performance, while more than 25 percent were somewhat dissatisfied or worse. Indeed, new graduates met the expectations of more than 50 percent of their employers on only two competencies: utilization of information technologies and rapport with patients and families (Berkow et al.). In another publication (Advisory Board Company, 2008), the Nursing Executive Center plotted the 36 competencies by relative curriculum emphasis (as reported by the educators) and new graduate proficiency (as reported by employers). See Box 12-5 for the competencies with the least curricular emphasis and the least proficiency in practice.

The national findings by the Nursing Executive Center support the need for focused and well-planned clinical experiences. For example, there is evidence to support more emphasis of delegation in nursing clinical courses. NCSBN's studies have also found delegation and supervision of others to be a weakness reported by new graduates (NCSBN, 2006b). Further,

Box 12 – 5
New Graduate Competencies with Least Curricular Emphasis and Least Practice Proficiency (Advisory Board Company, 2008)

- Follow-up
- Initiative
- Understanding of quality improvement
- Completion of tasks within expected time frame
- Track multiple responsibilities
- Conflict resolution
- Delegation

when new nurses reported inadequate preparation to delegate, they were 1.4 times more likely to have difficulty with their patient assignments (logistic regression analysis; Odds Ratio of 1.4).

While the report of Carnegie's national study of nursing education has not been released yet, this study (Benner et al., 2008) also cites the importance of well-planned clinical experiences. In this multi-method national study, the researchers found that clinical and didactic education frequently are taught separately, and they call for an integration of classroom and clinical teaching.

Taken together, all of these studies and expert opinions provide evidence that education for nursing should include supervised experiences with actual patients. Future research should address innovative strategies and relate them to actual outcomes. While boards of nursing take the position that direct patient care is important in prelicensure programs, no board of nursing mandates how this should be done.

Myths and Realities in Regulation of Education Programs

Educators sometimes complain about regulatory barriers that don't actually exist. The following includes a discussion of some of those myths.

Myth 1: All Boards of Nursing Require Specific Numbers of Clinical Hours

At a national meeting, a nurse leader stood up and said, "All boards of nursing require specific numbers of clinical hours, and this limits innovation." This is a common misunderstanding of faculty, and could easily be dispelled had that leader gone to her/his own board's administrative rules. Table 12-2 shows how many boards of nursing require specific numbers of hours and makes clear that this practice is more frequent in practical nursing education than in RN education.

Myth 2: Boards of Nursing Limit Innovation Because of Their Prescriptiveness

Nursing regulation supports innovations in nursing education. In March 2008, for example, NCSBN hosted a roundtable with leaders from nursing education, regulation and practice. The purposes of that meeting were as follows:

- Analyze possible barriers to implementing innovations in education put in place by education, practice and regulation

- Discuss ways to maintain quality while implementing innovation

- Discuss the future vision of innovation in nursing education

Currently, an NCSBN committee has delivered a document that identifies regulatory parameters that may prevent innovation, though also acknowledging that practice, education, and the students themselves can set up barriers. The committee members developed a flyer for boards of nursing that provides recommendations for breaking down regulatory barriers and another to share with educators for encouraging innovative approaches. It is hoped that these handouts (available online) will promote innovative approaches and that the flyer for educators will stimulate dialogue between the regulators and educators about the myths and realities of implementing innovations, thus enhancing communication. The committee members also developed a model to explain the regulatory influences on innovations in nursing education;

Table 12 – 2
Number of Boards that Require Numbers of Clinical Hours (NCSBN, 2007)

Type of Program	Number Requiring Hours	Number Not Requiring Hours	Does Not Apply
PN Certificate or Diploma	17	35	7
PN Associate Degree	8	36	15
Associate Degree RN	8	46	5
Diploma RN	3	35	19
Baccalaureate RN	7	46	6

these influences include the laws/rules themselves, the board's approval processes (which can sometimes be lengthy), and communication between faculty and the board of nursing. The final report from this committee work can be found on the NCSBN website: www.ncsbn.org.

Most boards of nursing, however, do not have highly prescriptive administrative rules, and innovations are not limited at present. In fact, three boards (Texas, Minnesota, and North Carolina) have, or have had, specific laws that allow exemptions to rules for innovative projects. Sadly, none of the three boards has received many proposals. In the 15 years Minnesota has had a rule allowing exemptions for innovations in nursing education, they have received no proposals for exemptions. Similarly, North Carolina had an innovation rule from 1984 to 2005, at which time it was repealed because no one used it. Texas's law and administrative rules that allow programs to be exempted from specific rules for an innovative project is more recent, but there have been very few programs that have applied. To stimulate proposals for innovation, Texas has created a link on their website (http://www.bon.state.tx.us/nursingeducation/innovative.html) where they report on all the innovative projects in that state (whether or not the programs need an exemption for the project). Such an approach might be an exemplar for other boards of nursing, particularly since communication between regulation and education is crucial as more innovations in nursing education are developed.

Myth 3: *Clinical Students Work Under the License of Their Faculty Member*

A similar question was addressed in the Spring 2005 issue of Leader to Leader (https://www.ncsbn.org/LDR_to_LDR_March_05.pdf), and the comments here mirror the response to that question. Although nurse educators frequently talk about students practicing under their (i.e., the nursing instructor's) license, the fact is that the only person who works on a nurse's license is the person named on the license. Nurse practice acts include statutory language that specifies exemptions or exceptions to the requirement for a nursing license. Typically, practicing nursing as a student who is enrolled in an approved nursing program is one of the exempted (or excepted) practices. The nursing student is accountable for nursing actions and behaviors to patients, the instructor, the clinical facility and the nursing program. The accountability for nursing instructors is for their decisions and actions as an instructor. For example, the instructor is accountable for the selection of patients for nursing students' assignments, supporting students in preparing for the clinical experience, monitoring students' clinical performance, and, most critically, intervening as necessary to protect patients when situations are beyond the abilities of students. Instructors must identify "teaching moments" as well as assess and evaluate students' clinical performance. This broader accountability reflects the education, experience and role of the instructor, who is accountable to the patient, the student, the facility, the nursing program and the professional licensing board.

Myth 4: Boards Require Acute Care Experiences in the Specialties

As clinical sites become saturated with nursing students, NCSBN often hears complaints from educators that their board is so prescriptive that they must offer acute care obstetric, psychiatric or pediatric experiences, all of which are difficult to find. While the majority of boards do require clinical experiences to be across the lifespan, they do not specify that these be hospital-based experiences. Educators, therefore, are encouraged to be creative about where they will provide specialty experiences. For example, Lamaze classes, children's day care centers, schools, assisted living, ambulatory clinics, community centers, free clinics and homeless shelters are all places where students could have excellent learning experiences to develop assessment and communication skills across the lifespan. If educators are unsure about specific settings, they are encouraged to contact the education consultant at their board of nursing for advice.

Myth 5: Boards of Nursing Regulate Online/Distance Programs Differently from Traditional Programs

The nurse practice act and education administrative rules in each jurisdiction cite regulations for education programs. All programs must meet the same regulations, whether they are an online/distance learning program or a brick-and-mortar program. For example, if an online/distance program in state A wanted all students in a distant state to have preceptored experiences, but state A's administrative rules dictate that only 50 percent of clinical experiences can be accomplished with a preceptor, then the online/distance program would have to hire clinical faculty in the distant states in order to receive continued approval. There are not separate and different rules for online/distance programs versus traditional programs.

Myth 6: Annual Education Reports Are Put on the Shelf and Not Used

At a recent meeting with leaders from nursing education, an educator commented that the annual reports to the board of nursing, which can take a great deal of time to complete, get put on a shelf, never to be seen again. Those reports, however, should serve as very useful resources for nursing education in a state. For example, Arizona's board of nursing notes that their report is quoted by policy makers to establish the need for additional faculty and nursing education funding. For example, Arizona data have been used to:

1. Successfully support and secure $20 million in funding for additional faculty to expand nursing program capacity

2. Inform the media, and others who publish articles on policy, regarding the nursing shortage or nursing education issues

3. Respond to requests for information and data from various stakeholders, including the Governor's office, the Arizona Hospital Association, lobbyists, and the Arizona Nurses Association

4. Provide data utilized by prospective nursing programs to establish the need for a nursing program

Other states report similar uses of the annual data that educators send the board of nursing in most states. Thus, they do not simply "sit on a shelf."

Myth 7: All Boards Have Rules that Limit the Use of Simulation

The boards of nursing, like educators, are attempting to understand what place simulation has in nursing education today. In NCSBN's 2005 position paper on clinical experiences (NCSBN, 2005), boards of nursing recognized the importance of simulation in education. In fact, the committee members sought the expertise of Dr. William McGaghie, a co-author of a rigorously conducted, systematic review of simulation (Issenberg, McGaghie, Petrusa, Gordon & Scalese, 2005), to learn about the regulatory perspectives toward simulation. The committee members also participated in high-fidelity simulations at a leading simulation center in Chicago in order to learn how simulation can be best used in nursing education. Further, NCSBN has conducted a randomized controlled trial of simulation, and preliminary results were presented in a poster format at the 2007 ICN conference in Yokohama, Japan (Li, Hicks, & Bosek, 2007) and are available on NCSBN's website: https://www.ncsbn.org/169. In this study, baccalaureate students were randomized into one of three groups for a critical care course: 1) simulation only (n=19); 2) simulation and clinical experiences (n=19); 3) clinical experiences only (n=20). The outcome measures included knowledge acquisition, confidence scores, and clinical performance with standardized patients. Because of small numbers in each group, the results of this study were inconclusive, though trends favored the combination group. There are plans for replicating the study using multiple sites and including associate degree students. Finally, NCSBN has also funded several studies on simulation through their Center of Regulatory Excellence (https://www.ncsbn.org/389.htm), and our members are awaiting those results.

In summary, while boards of nursing are interested in how simulation is being used, they also are waiting to see the best evidence as to how simulation can or should be used. Therefore, there are few boards that have any rules on simulation. Nehring (2008) has written an excellent review of the use of simulation in nursing in her report of a survey on simulation that she sent to the boards of nursing. In that survey, she found that only one board limited the use of simulation by requiring a percentage of time that it could substitute for actual clinical experiences. Even in that state, simulation can be used when it is not substituting for clinical experiences. In a 2009 NCSBN survey sent to the boards of nursing, of the 48 respondents, only five boards reported limiting simulation to nonclinical course work. Most indicated they were waiting for further evidence on the use of simulation or that they review requests on a case-by-case basis. Yet, it is clear that boards do not want to see 100 percent of the clinical education coming from simulated experiences. Many educators, however, fear that their board will limit the use of simulation by requiring it be used as only a small percentage of actual experiences. Since most boards do not have specific clinical hours in the first place, this seems unlikely. Educators who want to substitute simulation for clinical experiences should contact the education consultant at their board of nursing and discuss the issue. Most boards are waiting for some more definitive answers on simulation before they write anything in their rules.

Other Regulatory Issues

Around the country, boards of nursing are seeing an entrepreneurial response to the nursing shortage. Businesspeople, with no nursing expertise or degrees, are developing nursing programs. Some of these are well done because they hire qualified nurses to plan the program and curriculum. However, other such programs suffer because non-nurses are developing the curricula for nursing programs. Programs that are not well conceived can take up tremendous board resources, thus preventing the board's work in other areas of public protection. Boards of nursing find that quality nursing programs have nursing administrators who are seasoned, well-educated nurses with the power to make decisions for the program. Quality programs also hire sufficient, qualified faculty members (i.e., those with master's or doctoral preparation) and have adequate resources to support nursing education, including the supervised clinical component. Sometimes, though, new nursing programs are loosely put together by people who have no experience in nursing education. Their sense of clinical experiences might be to send the students out to find preceptors in local hospitals. When this happens, there is no cohesiveness in the program, and students most likely will not be successful.

Boards of nursing also struggle with programs to maintain a qualified nursing faculty. At the 2008 annual meeting of NCSBN, the member boards voted to strengthen the model administrative rule language regarding faculty qualifications (NCSBN, 2008). The qualifications call for faculty to have a minimum of a master's in nursing with graduate preparation in clinical practice and in education for teaching in PN and RN programs. There was also a recommendation that the faculty team be balanced, so that faculty with other graduate degrees related to nursing (such as pharmacology and genetics) are encouraged to participate in the education of RNs. Faculty members with a baccalaureate in nursing may be used to assist in the clinical education of PN education. While this position elevates requirements for faculty appointment, the reality is they cannot be met in today's climate of the faculty shortage. Boards are collaborating with each other and with educators to learn how to successfully educate nurses during this severe faculty shortage. On the February 2009 education consultant conference call facilitated by NCSBN, the member boards discussed creative strategies during this faculty shortage — some are allowing waivers of qualifications, and one is facilitating the development of a pool of qualified educators that programs could use on a temporary basis. Since some areas of the country and certain settings (large urban medical centers) are temporarily no longer experiencing a nursing shortage, the boards suggest that this might be the time for nurses to go to graduate school to become nurse educators.

Boards of nursing are hearing from the nursing programs that clinical spaces for their students are becoming saturated. Programs will often use this as a reason to limit their clinical experiences, and it is a legitimate concern in some areas. When boards or others have recommended the use of clinical placement software, which is a web-based tool designed to match available clinical sites with the needs of the nursing programs in that state or region, oftentimes there has been a satisfactory outcome. One board of nursing's executive director said that once their state implemented clinical placement software, clinical site saturation, which had previously been a highly ranked problem, was no longer an issue. Boards also encourage the use of more creative clinical sites to meet program outcomes.

Another education issue that some boards of nursing face concerns nursing programs using standardized assessment exams, which are designed for benchmarking and remediation, to increase their percentage of students passing the NCLEX® . If these exams are used throughout the program for remediation, they can be excellent resources for enhancing student learning and the program's NCLEX® pass rates. However, when programs administer such exams at the end of a course or even at the end of the program and provide little or no structured remediation, the standardized tests are being misused. In a 2006 NCSBN survey of boards of nursing, 15 of the 42 respondents reported that exit exams have presented some problems for that board of nursing. Indeed, one state has taken a stance and developed a monitoring policy stating that exit exams should not be used as a bar for graduation when all other program requirements have been met (Spector & Alexander, 2006). Other states have written letters to programs explaining their recommendations for the use of exit exams, while others have counseled students to use the institutional grievance process. Often states have rules that require programs to outline the requirements for graduation and to implement those requirements as written. Therefore, in some states, the use of an exit exam could be a violation of the rules in that state (Spector & Alexander, 2006). When programs do have problems with NCLEX® pass rates, the board of nursing will work with the program and will provide them a reasonable time frame to make appropriate changes.

Conclusion

This chapter provides the regulatory perspective on clinical education in nursing. For more than 100 years, nurse regulators have been approving education programs, and how and why this is done has been explained. Some of the inconsistencies across boards of nursing have been described, as has the rationale for why differences exist. Further, the chapter has highlighted the U.S. regulatory position on the need for supervised clinical experiences, at the level of licensure that the student is seeking, and the evidence supporting this stand.

There are many myths about the regulation of education programs, and seven specific ones have been discussed, pointing out both the facts and the fiction. Issues the boards of nursing continue to struggle with have been presented, along with how the boards are working with each other and with educators to overcome some of these challenges.

While educators bring practice partners to the table when planning for educating the nurse of the future, they often do not think to invite the boards of nursing. Yet, educators and regulators have the same goal, which is to graduate safe and competent nurses in sufficient numbers to meet the needs of the public. When there is collaboration between education and regulation, this goal will be met.

References

AACN (American Association of Colleges of Nursing). (2008). The essentials of baccalaureate education for professional nursing practice. Retrieved from http://www.aacn.nche.edu/Education/pdf/BaccEssentials08.pdf

Advisory Board Company. (2008). *Bridging the preparation-practice gap: Volume I: Quantifying new graduate improvement needs.* Washington DC: Author.

AONE (American Organization of Nurse Executives). (2004). Position statement on pre-licensure supervised clinical instruction. Retrieved from www.aone.org/aone/advocacy/PositionStatementPre-licensureclinicalexperienceformatted.pdf

Benner, P., Sutphen, M., Leonard-Kahn, V. & Day, L. (2008). Formation and everyday ethical comportment. *American Journal of Critical Care, 17*(5), 473-476.

Berkow, S., Virkstis, K., Stewart, J. & Conway, L. (2008). Assessing new graduate nurse performance. *Journal of Nursing Administration, 38*(11), 468-474.

Candela, L., & Bowles, C. (2008). Recent RN graduate perceptions of educational preparation. *Nursing Education Perspectives, 29*(5), 266-271.

Dorsey, C. F., & Schowalter, J. M. (2008). *The first 25 years: 1978-2003.* Chicago: National Council of State Boards of Nursing.

Greiner, A. C., & Knebel, E. (Eds.). (2003). *Health professions education: A bridge to quality.* Washington DC: National Academies Press.

Gubrud-Howe, P., & Schoessler, M. (2008). From random access opportunity to a clinical education curriculum. *Journal of Nursing Education, 47*(1), 3-4.

Hobbs, M. (2007). Regulatory considerations when educators move. *Leader to Leader, Fall,* 4.

Hudspeth, R. (2008). Nurse administrators and understanding the enigma of nursing regulation. *Nursing Administration Quarterly, 32*(4), 265-6.

ICN (International Council of Nurses). (1997). *An approval system for schools of nursing: Guidelines.* Geneva, Switzerland: Author.

Issenberg, S. B., McGaghie, W. C., Petrusa, E. R., Gordon, D. L., & Scalese, R. J. (2005). Features and uses of high-fidelity medical simulations that lead to effective learning: A BEME systematic review. *Medical Teacher, 27,* 10-28.

Kohn, L. T., Corrigan, J. M., & Donaldson, M. S. (Eds.). (1999). *To err is human: Building a safer health system.* Washington DC: National Academies Press.

Li, S., Hicks, F., & Bosek, M. (June 1, 2007). *The effect of high-fidelity simulation on student's learning: Interim analysis of a randomized controlled trial.* Poster presentation at the International Council of Nursing Regulatory Conference, Yokohama, Japan. Retrieved from https://www.ncsbn.org/ICN_Poster(8_Hi-Fi_Sim).pdf

NCSBN (National Council of State Boards of Nursing. (2004a). Model Administrative Rules and Practice Act. Retrieved from https://www.ncsbn.org/1455.htm

NCSBN (National Council of State Boards of Nursing). (2004b). On the state of the art of approval/accreditation processes in boards of nursing. Retrieved from https://www.ncsbn.org/Final_11_05_Approval_White_Paper.pdf

NCSBN (National Council of State Boards of Nursing). (2005). Clinical instruction in prelicensure nursing programs. Retrieved from https://www.ncsbn.org/Final_Clinical_Instr_Pre_Nsg_programs.pdf

NCSBN (National Council of State Boards of Nursing). (2006a). *Evidence-based nursing education for regulation.* Retrieved from https://www.ncsbn.org/Final_06_EBNER_Report.pdf

NCSBN (National Council of State Boards of Nursing). (2006b). *A national survey of elements of nursing education.* Retrieved from https://www.ncsbn.org/367.htm

NCSBN (National Council of State Boards of Nursing). (2006c). *Systematic review of studies on nursing education outcomes: An evolving review.* Retrieved from https://www.ncsbn.org/Final_Sys_Review_04_06.pdf

NCSBN (National Council of State Boards of Nursing). (2007). Member board profiles. Retrieved from https://www.ncsbn.org/Member_Boad_Profiles_2007.pdf

NCSBN (2008). Nursing faculty qualifications and roles. Retrieved February 12, 2009, from https://www.ncsbn.org/Final_08_Faculty_Qual_Report.pdf

Nehring, W. (2008). US boards of nursing and the use of high-fidelity patient simulators in nursing education. *Journal of Professional Nursing, 24,* 109-117.

NLN (National League for Nursing). (2003). *Innovation in nursing education: A call to reform* [Position Statement]. Retrieved from http://www.nln.org/aboutnln/PositionStatements/innovation082203.pdf

NLNAC (National League for Nursing Accrediting Commission). (2008). *NLNAC 2008 standards and criteria.* Retrieved from http://www.nlnac.org/manuals/SC2008.htm

Oermann, M. (2007). Approaches to gathering evidence for educational practices in nursing. *Journal of Continuing Education in Nursing, 38*(6), 250-255.

Poe, L. (2008). Nursing regulation, the nurse licensure compact, and nurse administrators: Working together for patient safety. *Nursing Administration Quarterly, 32*(4), 267-272.

Spector, N., & Alexander, M. (2006). Exit exams from a regulatory perspective. *Journal of Nursing Education, 46*(8), 291-292.

Spector, N. (in press). Approval: National Council of State Boards of Nursing. In L. Caputi (Ed.). *Teaching nursing: The art and science, Volume 3* (2nd ed.). Glen Ellyn, IL: College of DuPage Press.

Tanner, C., Bellack, J. P., & Harker, J. (2009). The new wave of nursing education scholarship. *Journal of Nursing Education, 48*(1), 3-4.

13 Chapter

CLINICAL EDUCATION
AND ACCREDITATION

Linda D. Norman, DSN, RN, FAAN

Sharon J. Tanner, EdD, RN

The word accreditation brings forth mental images of a high-quality peer review process to some; but others may have a perception that accreditation is a set of rigid, prescriptive rules that limit creativity and innovation. Indeed, faculty may be confused or misunderstand the nature of accreditation standards, particularly in relation to clinical education. Informal anecdotal comments from nursing faculty indicate that there is a perception that the nursing accreditation standards include specific designation of (a) the number of clinical hours, (b) student/faculty ratios, and (c) types of clinical experiences that must be present in a nursing curriculum, none of which is true. Instead, nursing accreditation standards are based on guidelines/expectations that have been well known methods of program evaluation and that focus on assessment of the structure, process, and outcomes of a program. This chapter dispels some of the myths concerning accreditation and discusses accreditation standards as they relate to clinical education.

What is Accreditation?

It might be helpful to begin the discussion about accreditation by first defining it. Accreditation is a voluntary process whereby an educational program is recognized for meeting or exceeding standards for educational quality (National League for Nursing Accrediting Commission [NLNAC], 2008; Southern Association of Colleges and Schools [SACS], 2004). It is the responsibility of each accrediting agency to establish the standards and criteria to measure the effectiveness of the types of educational programs that are the focus of its concern. Regional accrediting agencies (such as SACS, the New England Association of Colleges and Schools, and the Northwest Commission on Colleges and Universities) set standards and monitor compliance for the school/college/university as a whole, while discipline-specific accrediting agencies (such as those that focus on nursing) have responsibility at the program level. Both regional and discipline accreditation agencies are concerned with the structure, processes and outcomes of educational programs in the areas of mission/governance, faculty, students, curriculum, resources, integrity, and program effectiveness; each, however, evaluates these areas at different levels and with differing expectations, though all are in compliance with Department of Education regulations.

Myths Regarding Accreditation

There are many misperceptions or myths about the nature and requirements of accreditation of nursing programs. The following section is devoted to the myths that are commonly expressed to the accreditation agencies.

Myth 1: Accreditation standards are developed by a small number of people with no input from faculty and clinicians.

Within nursing, accreditation standards and criteria are developed by the accrediting agency with input from members of the nursing profession (educators and clinicians) and the public. They are reviewed and revised regularly (every three to five years) to ensure continued relevance to the evaluation of the educational programs (Grummet, 2002; Tanner, 2008a). As an illustration of the amount of input received from stakeholders, more than 1,100 individuals provided comment and input to the most recent revisions proposed for the NLNAC standards and criteria (Tanner, 2008a). This broad participation in the process of standard setting ensures that criteria are reflective of the discipline's goals for itself and that they meet the needs of the health care delivery system. Thus, standards are set by essentially a large number of people and are not merely imposed on nursing programs by an elite handful of individuals. While the nursing accrediting commission is the body that makes the final determination about the standards and criteria, there is a significant amount of input from others before those standards are reviewed for approval. The Commission is made up of nursing faculty representatives from all program types accredited by the specific agency, and it includes representation of nurse clinicians and the public at large. Nursing faculty are encouraged to provide comment about proposed revision of standards during the public comment period, and they can expect that all comments received are reviewed and analyzed to determine the appropriate changes that need to be made in existing standards or new standards and criteria that need to be developed. This process was most recently used for the development of the Standards and Criteria for the Doctorate of Nursing Practice (DNP) Programs.

Myth 2: The accrediting agency prescribes the clinical curriculum for the nursing program.

Issues related to clinical education are included in several of the accreditation standards: curriculum, faculty, resources, and outcomes. The curriculum standard allows great flexibility in determining the clinical education strategies that are needed to accomplish the program objectives/outcomes, recognizing that faculty own their curriculum and are best able to determine how to prepare their students for practice. The NLNAC requires that the nursing faculty develop the nursing program curriculum around an organizing framework and demonstrate how it complies with nationally recognized standards for their program type, but it is the nursing program itself that determines the set of national standards that is appropriate for the program of study. The curriculum must be clearly articulated in course objectives, course syllabi and evaluation methods, and teaching methods, including clinical teaching, must be consistent with the curriculum design and contribute to the program outcomes. Despite these expectations, however, the accreditation agency does not specify what the learning objectives/outcomes, teaching strategies, evaluation methods, or clinical experiences must be. The goal is for the students and faculty to understand the expectations for learning and for faculty to be able to provide clear rationale and methods for how students will accomplish the learning outcomes (Grumet, 2002). Therefore, it is up to the faculty to determine the types of clinical experiences students will have, the clinical sites to be used, and the number of clinical hours to accomplish the course, level, and program objectives/outcomes.

Myth 3: The accrediting agency specifies the type and number of clinical hours in the nursing program.

The accrediting agency has the responsibility to review the curriculum to determine if the nursing program is in compliance with the state board of nursing requirements for clinical education for the program of study, but it does not set those requirements. Many states have regulations within their Nurse Practice Acts that mandate certain types of clinical experiences (such as medical surgical, pediatrics, maternal/child, psychiatric, geriatric) that must be included in the curriculum in order to be approved for licensure exams, both at the Registered Nurse

(RN) and Licensed Practical Nurse (LPN)/Licensed Vocational Nurse (LVN) levels, and some also specify this at the advanced practice level. In addition, many state boards of nursing set a maximum level of student-to-faculty ratio in the clinical area. Since a nursing program must have full approval from the State Board of Nursing prior to seeking initial accreditation and must maintain approval in order to maintain accreditation, mandates regarding clinical experiences and student-faculty ratios must be met, but those mandates are not issued by the accrediting agency. In fact, the accrediting agency expects that faculty will exercise their creativity to design and deliver a program of study that meets the board of nursing requirements as well as the accreditation standards.

The national standard that is applicable to the nursing program type may also prescribe clinical site and number of clinical hours as requirements for clinical education. For example, the American Association of Colleges of Nursing's (AACN) *Essentials of Baccalaureate Nursing* states that students must be provided an opportunity to care for "a variety of patients across the lifespan and across the continuum of care" (AACN, 2008, p. 33.). Their *Essentials for Master's Education* (AACN, 1996) provides specific courses that must be included in the master's of science in nursing (MSN) program and cites a specific number of clinical hours for the advanced practice roles of nurse practitioner (NP) and clinical nurse specialist (CNS). In addition, certifying bodies require that the NP and CNS programs have at least 500 clinical hours and often specify the types of experiences that the graduates must complete to be eligible to take the certification exam. Other organizations such as the National Organization of Nurse Practitioner Faculties (NONPF) and the American College of Nurse Midwives (ACNM) include specific types of clinical experiences that must be included in the program of study. In summary, there are many bodies that issue mandates that affect clinical education, but accrediting agencies are not among them. Although accrediting agencies like NLNAC do not impose the type and number of hours of clinical experiences, they do have the responsibility to make sure that the program meets national nursing standards and is organized in a way that ensures graduates are eligible to take licensing and certification exams.

Myth 4: The accrediting agency does not have a minimum passing standard for licensure and certification pass rates.

The NLNAC 2008 standards for nursing programs do specify a minimum level of achievement for licensure and certification pass rates. All programs for initial licensure must have a pass rate at least at the national mean and meet the state board of nursing pass rate requirement for approval status, and MSN or DNP programs must have a minimum pass rate of 80 percent on each certification exam for which its graduates are eligible. It is up to each nursing program, however, to design curricula that prepare graduates to be successful on licensure/certification exams, and it may be as creative and innovative in that design as it wishes and can justify.

Myth 5: Simulation is required in clinical education.

Use of simulation has been a part of nursing education for a number of years, from task training devices to full mannequins with appliances to teach such skills as wound care, trach care, and catheter insertion (Seropian, Brown, Gavilanes, & Driggers, 2004). With the advent of interactive human patient simulators, many nursing programs have included simulation scenarios as a part of the clinical education curriculum (Nehring & Lashley, 2004; Spector, Li, & Kenward, 2006). Unfortunately, some claim that if a school does not have a sophisticated human patient simulator, the recommendations of the accrediting site visit team will be negatively affected. The truth of the matter is that accreditation standards do not mandate the use of any specific type of equipment or experiences. Instead they focus on how students demonstrate the competencies needed to meet the program's identified learning outcomes. Many boards of nursing and other professional standards cite that simulation is an appropriate methodology to use for clinical teaching and evaluation, but it does not replace patient care experiences (AACN, 2008; Giddens, Brady, Brown, Wright, Smith & Harris, 2008; Spector, Li, & Kenward, 2006; Tanner, 2006). With the increased importance of patient safety in health care, simulations provide students with an opportunity to experience "controlled" situations where they can demonstrate their ability to manage patient care situations that are complex but rarely encountered in the clinical setting. Once again, it is left to the ingenuity of the faculty in each nursing program to determine the best way to teach didactic content and develop the competencies needed to achieve patient safety goals. Accreditation criteria indicate that student clinical experiences need to include activities that address patient health and safety goals (NLNAC, 2008), but they do not specify that such must be accomplished through the use of sophisticated, high-fidelity simulators.

Issues Related to Clinical Nursing Education and Accreditation

Accrediting bodies struggle with several issues related to clinical education. Two of the most common of those issues — nursing faculty qualifications and distance education — are addressed here.

Nursing Faculty

In this time of nursing faculty shortage, it is difficult for nursing programs to employ adequate numbers of individuals who are educationally and experientially prepared for the faculty role. While this is a real challenge for programs, accreditation standards related to faculty, particularly those who provide clinical education, cannot be relaxed. NLNAC defines faculty as "those persons who teach and evaluate students" (NLNAC, 2008, p. 100), so it is these individuals who are of greatest concern. Programs, therefore, must clearly define the roles and responsibilities of all who provide assistance with clinical education, specifically paying attention to the use of the term faculty (Tanner, 2008b), preceptors, clinical instructors, and those who assist in the skills labs or in the clinical area.

New models for clinical education are being tested and utilized in many areas, including partnerships with clinical agencies to share staff for clinical supervision activities (Bellack, 2004). As these methods are used to assist with the faculty shortage and increase enrollments, faculty need to be clearly responsible for teaching and evaluating students. Since preceptors are increasingly used in clinical teaching, care needs to be taken to clearly define their role and their relationship to faculty. Nursing programs need to explicate the clinical competencies that students are expected to accomplish during each course and the teaching strategies and clinical experiences that will be used to promote student learning.

Distance Methods in Clinical Education

An area that is sometimes difficult to assess is how faculty are involved in teaching and evaluating students in clinical courses when they are working with preceptors at a distance. As nursing education programs reach out to nontraditional students who may be working and to those who live in rural and remote areas, creative scheduling and use of instructional technology are frequently used. Accrediting agencies expect that the role of the faculty member in such sites is clear regarding (a) how they are involved in teaching and evaluating distance students, (b) how they participate in selecting and evaluating clinical sites, and (c) how criteria for site selection, student learning and the evaluation of students at distance locations is the same as those for face-to-face students. Care must be taken to ensure that the teaching strategies and evaluation methods used with all students are consistent with the program philosophy and outcomes.

Expectations for Clinical Education

Clinical education practices must be consistent with the program philosophy, outcomes, curriculum design, and goals to meet student learning needs. Clinical courses need to be focused on developing student competencies that will lead to accomplishment of the program outcomes, professional standards (such as those related to licensure or certification), and "the current best practices and national health and patient safety goals" (NLNAC, 2008 p. 78). It is important to avoid the temptation to intermingle or substitute externally driven program standards (such as the AACN *Essentials* documents or the NONPF competencies) with program outcomes. Each nursing curriculum should have terminal program outcomes/objectives that flow from the philosophy and curriculum framework. Clinical experiences and learning activities should then be designed to lead to the accomplishment of those terminal program learning outcomes, while meeting national professional standards. Course objectives, teaching methods, and evaluation strategies should then be mapped to the program learning outcomes to demonstrate how they are progressive in expectations and how they are linked to one another and to the ultimate goals. Faculty in each program need to create learning experiences that build from initial course(s) to capstone course(s), and clinical teaching strategies should be designed to assist students in meeting those increasingly complex course requirements and objectives/outcomes.

Faculty must demonstrate how they are involved in the selection of the clinical sites, the evaluation of the sites and how these findings are used to make determinations about maintaining or deleting clinical sites; and there must be sufficient patients with the type of nursing care responsibilities to meet the specific course objectives. When accreditation program evaluators visit clinical units, they typically interview clinical staff, faculty, and students to verify the adequacy of the clinical site and how students are involved in activities that help them learn to provide patient care.

Accreditation standards do not dictate the type of clinical experiences, nor do they dictate the teaching strategies that should be used. Instead they allow faculty to use their creativity and innovativeness to devise clinical experiences that best facilitate student learning. The rationale for the type of clinical experiences that are included in the curriculum, the teaching strategies utilized, the expectations for student learning and competency development, and the increasing complexity of clinical evaluation as students progress in the curriculum all are important elements, and all are reviewed during the accreditation process.

Summary

Accreditation of nursing programs is designed to provide a mechanism for peer review to assure the public that the program is in compliance with the appropriate educational standards relative to the program type and that the program is striving for continual improvement. Accreditation standards and criteria that are specific to the nature of clinical education, then, further explicate the requirements to ensure program quality. Clinical education occupies a major portion of the curricula in nursing programs and requires substantive attention to ensure that the program provides the necessary environment, faculty guidance, and delineation of the activities that will provide the opportunity for students to be able to achieve the program outcomes and be prepared for entry into nursing practice. While the accrediting bodies set that standards and criteria for nursing programs, the program has the opportunity to design the clinical education in a manner that is innovative, creative, and reflects its uniqueness. It is important to understand that the purpose and processes of accreditation are to guide the clinical education processes, but not to prescribe or limit educational strategies that will prepare excellent graduates for the health care environment.

References

American Association of Colleges of Nursing (2008). *The essentials of baccalaureate education for professional nursing practice.* Washington, DC: Author.

American Association of Colleges of Nursing (1996). *The essentials of master's education for advanced practice nursing.* Washington, DC: Author.

Bellack, J. (2004). Changing our tipping point. *Journal of Nursing Education, 43*(8), 339-340.

Giddens, J., Brady, D., Brown, P., Wright, M., Smith, D., & Harris, J. (2008). A new curriculum for a new era of nursing education. *Nursing Education Perspectives, 29*(4). 200-204.

Grumet, B. R. (2002). Demystifying accreditation: How NLNAC is making the process relevant for today's educators. *Nursing Education Perspectives, 23*(3), 114-117.

NLNAC. (2008). *National League for Nursing Accrediting Commission manual.* Atlanta, GA: Author.

Nehring, W., & Lashley, F. (2004). Current use and opinion regarding use of human patient simulators in nursing education: An international survey. *Nursing Education Perspectives, 25*(5), 244-249.

Seropian, M., Brown, K., Gavalines, M., & Driggers, B. (2004). Simulation, not just a mannekin. *Journal of Nursing Education, 43*(4), 164-169.

Southern Association of Colleges and Schools. (2004). *Handbook for reaffirmation of accreditation.* Decatur, GA: Author.

Spector, N., Li, S., & Kenward, K. (2006). Evidence-based nursing education for regulation. *JONA's Healthcare Law, Ethics, and Regulation, 8*(3), 84-86.

Tanner, C. (2006). Changing times: Faculty shortage, simulation, and accelerated program. *Journal of Nursing Education, 45*(3), 99-100.

Tanner, S. J. (2008a). About Accreditation. *Nursing Education Perspectives, 29*(1), 55.

Tanner, S. J. (2008b). About Accreditation. *Nursing Education Perspectives, 29*(5), 311.

QUALITY AND SAFETY EDUCATION IN NURSING (QSEN):

INTEGRATING RECOMMENDATIONS FROM IOM INTO CLINICAL NURSING EDUCATION

Gail Armstrong, ND, RN
Gwen Sherwood, PhD, RN, FAAN
M. Elaine Tagliareni, EdD, RN

Nursing education is undergoing a renaissance as national reports of staggering issues, including those related to health care quality, are forging new ways of thinking about clinical education for nursing students. The Quality and Safety Education for Nursing (QSEN) project, funded by the Robert Wood Johnson Foundation (http://www.qsen.org), seeks to reshape nurses' professional identity formation to internalize a commitment to quality and safety. A QSEN national expert panel defined six quality and safety competencies with the knowledge, skills, and attitudes needed to guide faculty in prelicensure nursing programs as they design curricula and learning experiences that will prepare graduates for working in cultures of quality. Consistent with recommendations made by the Institute of Medicine (IOM), these six competency areas are patient-centered care, teamwork and collaboration, evidence-based practice, quality improvement, safety, and informatics (IOM, 2003).

For nurses, most of these competencies are familiar, but they are now based on concepts that redefine new nursing practice roles (Cronenwett et al., 2007). This chapter addresses the reframing of nursing education — particularly clinical education — in relation to the quality and safety competencies in order to improve patient care outcomes.

Making the Case for Quality and Safety

In the last decade, there has been a convergence of national initiatives focusing on patient safety and quality improvement. In its 2001 landmark report, *Crossing the Quality Chasm: A New Health System for the 21st Century*, the IOM reported that problems with quality and safety within the United States health care system are "...not just a gap, but a chasm" (IOM, 2001, p. 1). To address this critical issue, the IOM called for a redesign of the health care system that, in turn, requires a redesign of health professions education. Such education, the report said, must focus on developing proficiency in five core areas:

- delivering patient-centered care;
- working as part of interdisciplinary teams;
- using evidence to guide care decisions;
- focusing on quality improvement; and
- using information technology to improve patient safety (IOM, 2003).

In its riveting summary of the prevalence of medication errors in the United States, the IOM (2006) found that medication errors are surprisingly common and harmful. The most striking finding reported, however, is that much of this harm is preventable. Specific strategies to reduce harm and cost were recommended: 1) a more active role by patients in medical care; 2) greater use of information technologies in prescribing and dispensing medications; 3) more research and evidence-based approaches to identifying variables that lead to errors; and 4) enhanced instruction in health professions education about systemwide safety and quality improvement mechanisms.

Nurses are vital to achieving the quality and safety goals set forth by the IOM (Hall, Moore, & Barnsteiner, 2008), and nurse educators play a significant role in helping remedy these national concerns and improve quality care. This revisioning of nurses' roles within the quality and safety framework (Draper, Felland, Liebhaber & Melichar, 2008) is challenging nurse educators to reconceptualize both classroom and clinical learning experiences to insure graduates have the necessary skills to practice in quality focused settings (Arnold et al., 2006; Finkelman & Kenner, 2007; Sherwood & Drenkard, 2007).

Nurse educators, therefore, are challenged to reframe the way they teach to incorporate quality and safety. Such teaching must be designed to help students, particularly those enrolled in prelicensure programs, learn that (a) safety and quality are systemwide issues; (b) interdisciplinary approaches, using sound communication principles, improve clinical decision making; (c) use of evidence and information technologies enhance practice across health care settings; and (d) patient-centered care, as the cornerstone of caregiving, provides a focus for delivery of the full range of integrated health care services. Through incorporation of new pedagogies that foster the acquisition of relevant knowledge, skills, and abilities, graduates of nursing programs will be educated to provide safe and competent nursing care for patients in a wide variety of health care settings.

Quality and Safety Education in Nursing (QSEN)

The IOM reports (1999, 2001, 2003) have ignited policy and regulatory changes to improve quality that are now influencing formal education requirements across the health professions (Kohn, Corrigan, & Donaldson, 2000; Wakefield et al., 2005). In response to the demand for change, QSEN addresses the challenge of preparing nurses with the knowledge, skills, and attitudes needed to continuously improve the quality of and ensure safety in the health care systems within which they work. The QSEN project adapted the IOM competencies by separating quality and safety as separate competencies, thus basing their work on six competencies (see Tables 14.1A-F).

- Patient-Centered Care
- Teamwork and Collaboration
- Evidence-Based Practice
- Quality Improvement
- Safety
- Informatics

Table 14-1A
QSEN Prelicensure Competencies - Patient Centered Care

Definition: Recognize the patient or designee as the source of control and full partner in providing compassionate and coordinated care based on respect for patient's preferences, values and needs.

Knowledge	Skills	Attitudes
Integrate understanding of multiple dimensions of patient-centered care: • patient/family/community preferences, values • coordination and integration of care • information, communication, and education • physical comfort and emotional support • involvement of family and friends • transition and continuity Describe how diverse cultural, ethnic and social backgrounds function as sources of patient, family and community values	Elicit patient values, preferences and expressed needs as part of clinical interview, implementation of care plan and evaluation of care Communicate patient values, preferences, and expressed needs to other members of health care team Provide patient-centered care with sensitivity and respect for the diversity of human experience	Value seeing health care situations "through patients' eyes" Respect and encourage individual expression of patient values, preferences and expressed needs Value the patient's expertise with own health and symptoms Seek learning opportunities with patients who represent all aspects of human diversity Recognize personally held attitudes about working with patients from different ethnic, cultural and social backgrounds Willingly support patient-centered care for individuals and groups whose values differ from own
Demonstrate comprehensive understanding of the concepts of pain and suffering, including physiologic models of pain and comfort	Assess presence and extent of pain and suffering Assess levels of physical and emotional comfort Elicit expectations of patient and family for relief of pain, discomfort or suffering Initiate effective treatments to relieve pain and suffering in light of patient values, preferences and expressed needs	Recognize personally held values and beliefs about the management of pain or suffering Appreciate the role of the nurse in relief of all types and sources of pain or suffering Recognize that patient expectations influence outcomes in management of pain or suffering

Reprinted from *Nursing Outlook;* 55, 122-131, (2007), with permission from Elsevier.

Table 14 – 1A (continued)
QSEN Prelicensure Competencies – Patient Centered Care

Definition: Recognize the patient or designee as the source of control and full partner in providing compassionate and coordinated care based on respect for patient's preferences, values and needs.

Knowledge	Skills	Attitudes
Examine how the safety, quality and cost-effectiveness of health care can be improved through the active involvement of patients and families Examine common barriers to active involvement of patients in their own health care processes Describe strategies to empower patients or families in all aspects of the health care process	Remove barriers to presence of families and other designated surrogates based on patient preferences Assess level of patient's decisional conflict and provide access to resources Engage patients or designated surrogates in active partnerships that promote health, safety and well-being, and self-care management	Value active partnerships with patients or designated surrogates in planning, implementation, and evaluation of care Respect patient preferences for degree of active engagement in care process Respect patient's right to access to personal health records
Explore ethical and legal implications of patient-centered care Describe the limits and boundaries of therapeutic patient-centered care	Recognize the boundaries of therapeutic relationships Facilitate informed patient consent for care	Acknowledge the tension that may exist between patient rights and the organizational responsibility for professional, ethical care Appreciate shared decision-making with empowered patients and families even when conflicts occur
Discuss principles of effective communication Describe basic principles of consensus building and conflict resolution Examine nursing roles in assuring coordination, integration and continuity of care	Assess own level of communication skill in encounters with patients and families Participate in building consensus or resolving conflict in the context of patient care Communicate care provided and needed at each transition in care	Value continuous improvement of own communication and conflict resolution skills

Reprinted from *Nursing Outlook; 55*, 122-131, (2007), with permission from Elsevier.

Table 14 – 1B
QSEN Prelicensure Competencies – Teamwork and Collaboration

Definition: Function effectively within nursing and interprofessional teams, fostering open communication, mutual respect and shared decision making to achieve quality patient care.

Knowledge	Skills	Attitudes
Describe strengths, limitations, and values in functioning as a member of a team	Demonstrate awareness of own strengths and limitations as a team member	Acknowledge own potential to contribute to effective team functioning
	Initiate plan for self-development as a team member	Appreciate importance of intra - and interprofessional collaboration
	Act with integrity, consistency, and respect for differing views	
Describe scopes of practice and roles of health care team members	Function completely within own scope of practice as a member of the health care team	Value the perspective and expertise of all health team members
Describe strategies for identifying and managing overlaps in team member roles and accountabilities	Assume role of team member or leader based on the situation	Respect the centrality of the patient/family as core members of any health care team
Recognize contributions of other individuals and groups in helping patient/family achieve health goals	Initiate requests for help when appropriate to situation	Respect the unique attributes that members bring to a team, including variations in professional orientations and accountabilities
	Clarify roles and accountabilities under conditions of potential overlap in team member functioning	
	Integrate the contributions of others who play a role in helping patient/family achieve health goals	

Table 14 – 1B (continued)
QSEN Prelicensure Competencies – Teamwork and Collaboration

Definition: Function effectively within nursing and interprofessional teams, fostering open communication, mutual respect and shared decision making to achieve quality patient care.

Knowledge	Skills	Attitudes
Analyze the differences in communication style preferences among patients and families, nurses and other members of the health team Describe impact of own communication style on others	Communicate with team members, adapting own style of communicating to needs of the team and situation Demonstrate commitment to team goals Solicit input from other team members to improve individual as well as team performance	Value teamwork and the relationships upon which it is based Value different styles of communication used by patients, families and health care providers Contribute to resolution of conflict and disagreement
Describe examples of the impact of team functioning on safety and quality of care Explain how authority gradients influence teamwork and patient safety	Follow communication practices that minimize risks associated with handoffs among providers and across transitions in care Assert own position/perspective in discussions about patient care Choose communication styles that diminish the risks associated with authority gradients among team members	Appreciate the risks associated with handoffs among providers and across transitions in care
Identify system barriers and facilitators of effective team functioning Examine strategies for improving systems to support team functioning	Participate in designing systems that support effective teamwork	Value the influence of system solutions in achieving effective team functioning

Reprinted from *Nursing Outlook*; 55, 122-131, (2007), with permission from Elsevier.

Table 14 – 1C
QSEN Prelicensure Competencies – Evidence-Based Practice (EBP)

Definition: Integrates best current evidence with clinical expertise and patient/family preferences and values for delivery of optimal health care.

Knowledge	Skills	Attitudes
Demonstrate knowledge of basic scientific methods and processes Describe EBP to include the components of research evidence, clinical expertise, and patient/family values	Participate effectively in appropriate data collection and other research activities	Appreciate strengths and weaknesses of scientific bases for practice Value the need for ethical conduct of research and quality improvement Value the concept of EBP as integral to determining best clinical practice
Differentiate clinical opinion from research and evidence summaries Describe reliable sources for locating evidence reports and clinical practice guidelines	Read original research and evidence reports related to an area of practice Locate evidence reports related to clinical practice topics and guidelines	Appreciate the importance of regularly reading relevant professional journals
Explain the role of evidence in determining best clinical practice Describe how the strength and relevance of available evidence influences the choice of interventions in provision of patient-centered care	Participate in structuring the work environment to facilitate integration of new evidence into standards of practice Question rationale for routine approaches to care that result in less than desired outcomes or adverse events	Value the need for continuous improvement in clinical practice, based on new knowledge
Discriminate between valid and invalid reasons for modifying evidence-based clinical practice, based on clinical expertise or patient/family preferences	Consult with clinical experts before deciding to deviate from evidence-based protocols	Acknowledge own limitations in knowledge and clinical expertise before determining when to deviate from evidence-based best practices

Reprinted from *Nursing Outlook;* 55, 122-131, (2007), with permission from Elsevier.

Table 14 – 1D
QSEN Prelicensure Competencies – Quality Improvement (QI)

Definition: Use data to monitor the outcomes of care processes and use improvement methods to design and test changes to continuously improve the quality and safety of health care systems.

Knowledge	Skills	Attitudes
Describe strategies for learning about the outcomes of care in the setting in which one is engaged in clinical practice	Seek information about outcomes of care for populations served in care setting Seek information about quality improvement projects in the care setting	Appreciate that continuous quality improvement is an essential part of the daily work of all health professionals
Recognize that nursing and other health professions students are parts of systems of care and care processes that affect outcomes for patients and families Give examples of the tension between professional autonomy and system functioning	Use tools (such as flowcharts, cause-effect diagrams) to make processes of care explicit Participate in a root cause analysis of a sentinel event	Value own and others' contributions to outcomes of care in local care settings
Explain the importance of variation and measurement in assessing quality of care	Use quality measures to understand performance Use tools (such as control charts and run charts) that are helpful for understanding variation Identify gaps between local and best practice	Appreciate how unwanted variation affects care Value measurement and its role in good patient care
Describe approaches for changing processes of care	Design a small test of change in daily work (using an experiential learning method such as Plan-Do-Study-Act) Practice aligning the aims, measures and changes involved in improving care Use measures to evaluate the effect of change	Value local change (in individual practice or team practice on a unit) and its role in creating joy in work Appreciate the value of what individuals and teams can to do to improve care

Reprinted from *Nursing Outlook;* 55, 122-131, (2007), with permission from Elsevier.

Table 14 – 1E
QSEN Prelicensure Competencies – Safety

Definition: Minimizes risk of harm to patients and providers through both system effectiveness and individual performance.

Knowledge	Skills	Attitudes
Examine human factors and other basic safety design principles as well as commonly used unsafe practices (such as work-arounds and dangerous abbreviations) Describe the benefits and limitations of selected safety-enhancing technologies (such as barcodes, Computer Provider Order Entry, medication pumps, and automatic alerts/alarms) Discuss effective strategies to reduce reliance on memory	Demonstrate effective use of technology and standardized practices that support safety and quality Demonstrate effective use of strategies to reduce risk of harm to self or others Use appropriate strategies to reduce reliance on memory (such as forcing functions, checklists)	Value the contributions of standardization/reliability to safety Appreciate the cognitive and physical limits of human performance
Delineate general categories of errors and hazards in care Describe factors that create a culture of safety (such as open communication strategies and organizational error reporting systems)	Communicate observations or concerns related to hazards and errors to patients, families and the health care team Use organizational error reporting systems for near miss and error reporting	Value own role in preventing errors
Describe processes used in understanding causes of error and allocation of responsibility and accountability (such as root cause analysis and failure mode effects analysis)	Participate appropriately in analyzing errors and designing system improvements Engage in root cause analysis rather than blaming when errors or near misses occur	Value vigilance and monitoring (even of own performance of care activities) by patients, families, and other members of the health care team
Discuss potential and actual impact of national patient safety resources, initiatives, and regulations	Use national patient safety resources for own professional development and to focus attention on safety in care settings	Value relationship between national safety campaigns and implementation in local practices and practice settings

Reprinted from *Nursing Outlook;* 55, 122-131, (2007), with permission from Elsevier.

Table 14 – 1F
QSEN Prelicensure Competencies – Informatics

Definition: Use information and technology to communicate, manage knowledge, mitigate error, and support decision making.

Knowledge	Skills	Attitudes
Explain why information and technology skills are essential for safe patient care	Seek education about how information is managed in care settings before providing care Apply technology and information management tools to support safe processes of care	Appreciate the necessity for all health professionals to seek lifelong, continuous learning of information technology skills
Identify essential information that must be available in a common database to support patient care Contrast benefits and limitations of different communication technologies and their impact on safety and quality	Navigate the electronic health record Document and plan patient care in an electronic health record Employ communication technologies to coordinate care for patients	Value technologies that support clinical decision-making, error prevention, and care coordination Guard confidentiality of protected health information in electronic health records
Describe examples of how technology and information management are related to the quality and safety of patient care Recognize the time, effort, and skill required for computers, databases, and other technologies to become reliable and effective tools for patient care	Respond appropriately to clinical decision-making supports and alerts Use information management tools to monitor outcomes of care processes Use high quality electronic sources of health care information	Value nurses' involvement in design, selection, implementation, and evaluation of information technologies to support patient care

Reprinted from *Nursing Outlook;* 55, 122-131, (2007), with permission from Elsevier.

Since the QSEN competencies were identified by IOM for all health care professionals, the first charge of QSEN was to explore specific dimensions of these broad competencies in nursing education. The knowledge, skills, and attitudes that define each of these competencies were identified (in Phase I) by an interdisciplinary national panel of experts, primarily to guide the development of curricula that would prepare graduates to work in and lead quality organizations. A key finding from Phase I was the critical need for faculty development to reframe familiar concepts to align with new science perspectives about human factors that have redefined quality and safety (Karsh, Holden, Alper, & Or, 2006). These new ideas need to be woven into the framework of the program and not simply identified as a unit of study in a single course. Active engagement of national nursing organizations (American Association of Colleges of Nursing (AACN), National Organization of Nurse Practitioner Faculty, National League for Nursing, American Nurses Credentialing Center, and National Council of State Boards of Nursing) has helped embed the competencies in curriculum essentials and required competencies across nursing. These professional organizations are incorporating QSEN competencies into their emerging standards for nursing education and nursing practice. For example, in the 2009 standards for baccalaureate education published by the American Association of Colleges of Nursing, the six QSEN competencies are clearly integrated throughout the document's criteria (AACN, 2009).

Survey and focus group data collected by the QSEN project faculty revealed new graduates did not feel they had learning experiences related to QSEN's Knowledge, Skills, and Attitudes (KSAs), and they doubted their faculties' expertise to teach this content (Cronenwett et al., 2007). In response to this finding, QSEN Phase II was developed to help faculty understand how they could weave quality and safety into nursing curricula.

In QSEN Phase II, innovators were invited to participate in a pilot school collaborative in which faculty teaching in all types of prelicensure nursing programs would develop and test pedagogical strategies to achieve the competencies. The 15 pilot schools in the collaborative demonstrated innovative ways to incorporate the six QSEN competencies into their curricula in simulated learning labs, clinical experiences, and didactic teaching. Existing courses were refined to reflect course-specific outcomes based on the QSEN competencies, and faculty demonstrated they could embed the competencies in existing courses. Clinical experiences were refocused to reflect the competencies, using techniques such as formation of a clinical education center (or dedicated education unit) and creation of tool kits and resources for clinical instructors. Clinical partners were engaged in the redesign and negotiated ways to include students and faculty in quality improvement activities, protocols for evidence-based practice, and safety initiatives such as root cause analysis. Descriptions of these teaching innovations (and more) are available on the QSEN website, a free repository of teaching strategies and annotated bibliographies for each competency, which can be accessed at www.qsen.org.

Necessary Shifts in Nursing Clinical Education Models

Nursing education models have changed little since the 1960s, when nursing education essentially moved out of the hospital and into college and university-based programs, where nursing was acknowledged as a distinct discipline (Northup et al., 2009). The one-to-ten clinical ratio, use of simple-to-complex as a core curricular framework, and not addressing concepts of leadership, management and community-based care until the end of the curriculum are all examples of teaching approaches that have not altered significantly. Nursing curricula maintain an early focus on the tasks of providing individualized patient care (e.g., in Fundamentals of Nursing and Medical/Surgical Nursing courses), then move to addressing nursing care of special populations (e.g., Pediatrics, Obstetrics, and Mental Health), then focus on care of communities (e.g., Public Health), and finally emphasize leadership, management and a systems approach to nursing. Within the traditional curricular framework, students' exposure to core concepts of patient safety and quality improvement has been episodic and inconsistent. In addition, this exposure has often been based on time-honored approaches that focus on nurse-patient relationships as the primary determinant of patient safety, rather than addressing systemwide prevention.

To effectively incorporate the QSEN Knowledge, Skills, and Attitudes (KSAs) into clinical education models, nurse educators must examine this traditional sequencing of clinical education, where the simple-to-complex progression means novice nursing students focus on nursing care of an individual and then increase complexity to families, communities and systems. By relegating discussion of systems to senior level course work, nursing students often perceive systems-focused content as little more than an "add-on" to the real core of nursing, namely caring for the individual patient. Nursing students experience the progression of nursing courses as discrete skill sets that are prioritized, with individual patient care as the highest priority or foundation. Thus, neophyte nurse clinicians may not consider quality and safety in systems as relevant elements to their emerging nursing practice and may experience difficulty transitioning to practice settings where such concerns are increasingly paramount. By embedding QSEN KSAs throughout nursing clinical education, new clinicians can emerge — clinicians who incorporate a systems approach to patient safety and quality improvement and consider such an approach just as foundational to their nursing practice as the procurement of vital signs. The connection of these competencies and foci across a student's clinical education progression replaces discrete, unconnected learning experiences and eliminates the "silos" that emerge as the result of many nursing curricula. The QSEN competencies integrate a clinically relevant framework across the classroom, learning lab and clinical rotation settings.

Application of QSEN KSAs to the Classroom Setting

While clinical education is the central theme of this book, students benefit when content threads across the classroom, clinical setting and learning laboratory. Incorporating evidence on safety and quality throughout the curriculum reflects the generalizability of the QSEN competencies across all health care professions and all health care settings. Incorporating QSEN KSAs across courses requires faculty to work collaboratively to track students' exposure to safety and quality content, such as the 5 Million Lives Campaign and National Patient Safety Goals. This collaboration will establish a strong foundation upon which to build in later classes, so to prevent repetition of the same content and assure increasing complexity of the competencies..

The QSEN KSAs offer an opportunity for students to complete ongoing or cumulative assignments as they progress from class to class, thereby developing an appreciation for patient safety and quality improvement concepts in all aspects of nursing practice. With the abundance of open source information available online, there are a wealth of resources available for all six of the QSEN competencies. An example of threading one QSEN competency (Safety) through a traditional seven-course sequence is provided in Table 14.2.

Lessons From Colorado

To further illustrate the integration of QSEN competencies into nursing curricula, an exemplar from the QSEN Phase II Learning Collaborative is described. While each school developed its own approach, the transformation of nursing education at the University of Colorado provides an innovative and comprehensive example of what can be done.

Faculty Development

Faculty development is an essential component to successfully thread quality and safety content throughout a nursing curriculum to ensure that faculty are working from the same knowledge base in teaching the QSEN competencies. At the University of Colorado, collaborative workshops for faculty and clinical instructors from partnering clinical agencies helped develop a unified approach across classroom and clinical settings. These workshops explored questions like "What is QSEN?" and "How does QSEN interface with our current curricular model?" and generated serious discussion of how thinking needs to change. In addition, Dr. Christine Tanner, a national leader in emerging models of clinical education, offered two workshops for faculty and clinical partners to address developing trends in clinical education.

Since ongoing workshops did not completely resolve the difficulty of "QSENizing" the curriculum, a QSEN Implementation Team was organized to develop strategies and plans for threading QSEN competencies into all courses. Another effective tool that enhanced faculty "buy-in" was a centralized document adapted from the "Where's Waldo?" children's book, called, "Where's QSEN?" A spreadsheet listing the QSEN KSAs helped faculty determine gaps and facilitated constructive dialogue among faculty about how they could better thread content across classroom and clinical courses.

These strategies have had great success, but faculty development remains an ongoing process because of the wide variation in how faculty alter and adjust their classes to best address QSEN. Faculty at the University of Colorado (and at other schools) are committed to sustaining these efforts.

Clinical Learning Strategies

At the University of Colorado, the QSEN competencies are introduced to students in their first clinical course, Fundamentals of Nursing, and skills traditionally taught in this course are discussed in the context of an appropriate QSEN competency. For example, mobility, falls, restraints and medication administration are taught in relation to safety; information about documentation is presented in the context of information technology and informatics; and communication techniques are taught as an integral part of teamwork and collaboration. As a result, the QSEN competencies reframed the content of this foundational course.

Several simulation activities were also introduced into Fundamentals of Nursing to enliven the students' widespread reading on the QSEN competencies. Case scenarios were developed that coincided with classroom QSEN readings, and students often came to class enthusiastic about the safety and quality concepts they were learning in those patient care scenarios. The

Table 14 – 2
QSEN Competency: Safety

Curriculum Level	Typical Class Name	QSEN Readings
Beginning Level	Fundamentals of Nursing	Introduction to National Patient Safety Goals (NPSG): See www.jointcommission.org for free PowerPoint presentation on NPSG and other reading materials
Beginning Level	Medical/Surgical Nursing I	The Agency for Healthcare Research and Quality Patient Safety Network: www.psenet.ahrq.gov/classics.aspx AHRQ Patient Safety Network editors have selected a set of "Classics": Review articles, empirical studies, reports, and books that have special relevance to patient safety.
Intermediate Level	Care of the Childbearing Family (OB)	The first article summarizes the system failures that led to a sentinel event with a newborn: Smetzer, J. L. (1998). Lesson from Colorado: Beyond blaming individuals. *Nursing Management, 29*(6), 49-51. This article looks at standardized measures in OB that contribute to patient safety: Mann, S., Pratt, S., Gluck, P., Nielsen, P., Risser, D., Greenberg, P., et al. (2006). Assessing quality in obstetrical care: Development of standardized measures. *Joint Commission Journal on Quality and Patient Safety, 32*(9), 497-505.
Intermediate Level	Pediatric Nursing	*Principles of Patient Safety in Pediatrics*: This document, written by the American Academy of Pediatrics, outlines pediatric safety initiatives, development of safety standards for pediatric patients, and recommendations for leadership in safety in pediatric care. http://aappolicy.aappublications.org/cgi/reprint/pediatrics; 07/6/1473.pdf
Intermediate Level	Mental Health Nursing	National Patient Safety Agency: This article discusses the investigation of serious patient safety incidents in mental health services. http://www.npsa.nhs.uk/nrls/
Advanced Level	Medical/Surgical Nursing II	*Nine Patient Safety Solutions* by the WHO Collaborating Centre for Patient Safety Solutions. The purpose of these solutions is to guide the redesign of care processes to prevent inevitable human errors from actually reaching patients. http://www.ccforpatient safety.org/patient-safety solutions
Advanced Level	Senior Practicum	*Committed to Safety: Ten Case Studies on Reducing Harm to Patients* by The Commonwealth Fund. This report presents ten case studies of health care organizations, clinical teams, and learning collaborations that have designed innovations in five areas for improving patient safety: promoting an organizational culture of safety, improving teamwork and commnication, enhancing rapid response to prevent heart attacks and other crises in the hospital, preventing health care associated infections in the intensive care unit, and preventing adverse drug events throughout the hospital. http://www.cmwf.org/Content/Publications/Fund-Reports/2006/Apr/Committed-to-Safety--Ten-Case-Studies-on-Reducing-Harm-to-Patients.aspx

explicit connection between their reading and clinical learning in the lab was shaping their emerging clinical awareness. As the students then began their Fundamentals of Nursing clinical experience in a long-term care setting, clinical instructors commented on their attention to issues of patient safety, as well as their sustained inquiry about quality improvement processes within the clinical agency.

As students progressed to higher level clinical courses, concerns surfaced during discussions between clinical faculty and clinical staff about the inconsistency of students' experiences at different clinical sites, especially around the implementation of safety and quality concepts. As a result, two nursing faculty developed and piloted a Clinical Learning Activity Resource Book that was made available to all clinical instructors for an intermediate level Medical/Surgical class at all clinical sites. Among other things, this resource book includes four clinical learning activities (Exploring Health Literacy, Nurse-Physician Communication, Alarm Safety, and Heparin Data Mining Exercise) that focus on the application of safety and quality processes in the provision of nursing care. Several of these learning activities are available as teaching strategies on the QSEN website (www.qsen.org).

As another example, the students' perioperative experience in Medical/Surgical Nursing I was presented in the context of QSEN competencies and national perioperative initiatives. Box 14.1 outlines the assignment given to students as they participate in this experience, again showing how the QSEN competencies can be incorporated into clinical learning experiences.

Evaluation of Clinical Learning Activities

Developing objective, competency-based evaluation measures for clinical learning is a continuing struggle for nursing faculty. Criterion-referenced measurements, or rubrics, are

Box 14 – 1
Perioperative Clinical Assignment

One week after the perioperative experience, the student will give a 10- to 15-minute presentation during the postconference to their clinical group on one of the six (6) QSEN competencies. Provide your instructor and peers a copy of your paper. Include an evidence-based article with your paper that supports the QSEN competency discussed. Consider the following questions in your paper:

a. What did you observe, experience, and participate in during the perioperative rotation?

b. What are your responses to what you observed, experienced, and/or participated with related to the QSEN competency, during the perioperative rotation?

c. What do you already know? What do you need to know about what you observed or experienced?

d. How did you feel about your observations?

e. What will you do now or in your future nursing practice related to your feelings, observations, and responses to the perioperative experience?

Developed by Leli Pedro, DNSc, RN C, OCN, CNE
Assistant Professor, University of Colorado at Denver School of Nursing

Used with permission of Dr. Leli Pedro

becoming more prevalent to evaluate learning in clinical education, as standardization of expected clinical behaviors into a rubric assists educators and students in measuring competence and progression in clinical learning. At the University of Colorado, updating evaluation tools using rubrics with QSEN competencies has contributed to an increase in academic rigor and relevance of these rubrics to actual practice. The QSEN KSAs have also increased consistency of performance expectations across didactic, simulated and clinical environments. These rubrics are used across several courses for clinical learning activities, thereby reinforcing the importance of these concepts in students' emerging nursing practice.

In addition, an evaluation rubric for simulated clinical learning was developed, a tool that has the potential to add value to learning in direct care clinical experiences. When the QSEN KSAs are incorporated in the simulated learning environment, they can then be carried into a clinical experience. In this real setting, evaluation rubrics assist with standardization of expected behaviors as the recurring elements of the rubrics become familiar, known, and predictable for students, and help them effectively address QSEN KSAs as they provide care.

Outcomes

At the University of Colorado, the increased collaboration of faculty across courses and across learning environments has resulted in earlier identification and intervention of at-risk students. With a more consistent approach for evaluation and feedback, patterned weaknesses are identified earlier and addressed with remediation more effectively. In addition, faculty noted how quickly the students adopted a culture of safety and quality. One professor who teaches research observed a significant difference in the students' appreciation and inquiry around evidence-based practice and research in general because of their early exposure to quality improvement and evidence-based practice. Another nursing professor noted that the students' ability to see clinical practice through a "safety and quality lens" and use quality and safety language in their growing bedside practice was noticeably apparent. And a third professor noticed a dramatic shift in nursing students' language as they raised questions about systemic responses to adverse events.

Potential Areas of Research Related to QSEN

Integration of the QSEN competencies into nursing curricula nationally represents a transformation in perspectives on how faculty approach student learning experiences. It is imperative that educators themselves apply to their own work the goals represented in the competencies in order to achieve evidence-based, best practice teaching strategies. Research into how the competencies are integrated, assessment of student learning outcomes, and placement of the competencies in the curriculum will direct evidence for best emerging educational practices. A common query for pilot schools in Phase II stemmed from faculty concerns about how to integrate the 162 KSAs that make up the six QSEN competencies into the program of learning. Which KSAs are fundamental? Which ones are more advanced and require a sound knowledge base to implement? Based on these recurring questions, faculty from a pilot school conducted a national Delphi Study to gain consensus on a developmental progression model for the 162 KSAs. This Delphi Study asked experts to identify where each of the KSAs should be introduced in a prelicensure curriculum, and where each KSA should be emphasized. The results of this study will be published in a QSEN issue of Nursing Outlook in December 2009 (Barton, Armstrong, Preheim, Gelman, & Andrus, in press). The Delphi results will assist programs across the county in a developmental implementation of the KSAs.

As nursing educators across the country work to more fully integrate QSEN competencies, many other QSEN-focused pedagogical questions will benefit from educational research. For example, many nursing programs will be looking to have QSEN competencies become an organizing framework of their curriculum. When this happens, nursing education research questions will , for example, focus on evaluating how the program of learning has achieved graduate competencies in new standards of quality and safety, as well as measuring how reframing the Fundamentals of Nursing course provides a stronger foundation in the QSEN competencies. Specific research questions related to these essential transformative changes are suggested below. These questions and others designed by nursing educators within their own colleges and universities have the potential to discover evidence for best emerging educational practices to incorporate quality and safety across all types of nursing education programs.

- Do graduates successfully meet program objectives to improve quality and safety for patients across the lifespan in a wide variety of practice environments? What effects does consistent inclusion of an electronic health record in a prelicensure nursing student's clinical education have on the graduate's documentation habits?

- In what ways do graduates in a prelicensure nursing program provide coordinated care for patients in full partnership with the patient and the patient's designee?

- What simulation activities best assist students to participate in a root cause analysis of a sentinel event?

- What educational pedagogies provide in-depth experiences for students in a wide variety of settings to minimize risk to patients through analysis of system effectiveness?

- What are the best clinical learning experiences to assist students and graduates to value their own role in preventing errors and contributing to meeting safety standards? What are the best ways to measure this attitude change?

- Which pedagogies are effective in transforming Fundamentals of Nursing to include all of the QSEN competencies?

- How might nursing educators measure prelicensure students' knowledge of safe systems and their ability to apply this knowledge to unfolding clinical scenarios?

- Which teaching strategies help prelicensure students develop habits of looking to clinical evidence when making clinical decisions?

- Many nursing programs include a cumulative senior project to implement a rapid change cycle project. How can quality improvement attitudes be best introduced and reinforced from the beginning of a prelicensure curriculum?

Conclusion

Widespread adoption of an idea is not always connected to an idea's distinctiveness; often the success of an idea is due to its timing. This connection is clear in the historic success of Florence Nightingale's work during the Crimean War. It is impossible to understand the uniqueness of Nightingale's ideas of a clean environment, putting the patient in the best condition for nature to act upon him/her, and emphasis on the basics of clear air, light, proper nutrition and sanitation. It is well known, however, that Nightingale's timing in implementing her methodical interventions for soldiers wounded in the Crimean War was vital to her success. The backdrop of the Crimean War in 1855 provided Nightingale with the meaningful context for her data in the reduction of soldier mortality rate from 42 percent to two percent (Neuhauser, 2003). Clearly, timing can be an influential factor in the success of an initiative.

A century after Nightingale's work, mounting data indicates a critical need to improve patient outcomes, and QSEN offers direction, tools and a map to do just that. Integrating QSEN competencies across nursing curricula — in the classroom, clinical lab, and clinical setting — will help students develop the necessary skills to practice in quality focused settings and appreciate how safety and quality improvement initiatives impact essential health care outcomes.

References

American Association of Colleges of Nursing. (2009). *The essentials of baccalaureate education for professional nursing practice*. Washington, DC: Author.

Arnold, L., Campbell, A., Dubree, M., Fuchs, M., Davis, N., Hertzler, B., et al. (2006). Priorities and challenges of health system chief nursing executives: Insights for nursing educators. *Journal of Professional Nursing, 22*(4), 213-220.

Barton, A., Armstrong, G., Preheim, G., Gelmon, S. B. & Andrus, L. C. (in press). A national Delphi to determine developmental progression of quality and safety competencies in nursing education. *Nursing Outlook*.

Cronenwett, L., Sherwood, G., Barnsteiner, J., Disch, J., Johnson, J., Mitchell, P., et al. (2007). Quality and safety education for nurses. *Nursing Outlook; 55*, 122-131.

Draper, D., Felland, L., Liebhaber, A., & Melichar, L. (2008). *The role of nurses in hospital quality improvement. Research Brief 3*. Washington, DC: Center for Studying Health System Change.

Finkelman, A., & Kenner, C. (2007). *Teaching IOM: Implications of the IOM reports for nursing education*. Silver Spring, MD: American Nurses Association.

Hall, L.W., Moore, S. M., & Barnsteiner, J. H. (2008). Quality and nursing: Moving from a concept to a core competency. *Urologic Nursing — Special Topic Issue on Quality, 28*(6), 417-425.

Institute of Medicine. (1999). *To err is human*. Washington, DC: Committee on Quality of Health Care in America, Institute of Medicine, National Academy Press.

Institute of Medicine. (2001). *Crossing the quality chasm: A new health system for the 21st century*. Retrieved from http://www.iom.edu/CMS/8089/5432.aspx

Institute of Medicine. (2003). *Health professions education: A bridge to quality*. Retrieved from http://www.iom.edu/CMS/3809/4634/5914.aspx

Karsh, B., Holden, R. J., Alper, S. J., & Or, C. K. L. (2006). A human factors engineering paradigm for patient safety: Designing to support the performance of the healthcare professional. *Quality and Safety in Health Care, 15*(Suppl. 1), i59-i65.

Kohn, L., Corigan, J., & Donaldson, M. (Eds). (2000). *To err is human: Building a safer health system*. Committee on Quality of Health Care in America, Institute of Medicine. Wash D.C.: The Natl Academies Press.

Neuhauser, D. (2003). Florence Nightingale gets no respect, as a statistician that is. *Quality and Safety in Health Care, 12*, 317.

Northrup, D. T., Tschanz, C. L., Olynk, V. G., Makaroff, K. L., Szabo, J. & Biasio, H. A. (2009). Nursing: Whose discipline is it anyway? In P. G. Reed & N. C. Shearer (Eds.), *Perspectives on nursing theory* (5th ed., pp. 79-89). Philadelphia: Lippincott Williams & Wilkins.

Sherwood, G., & Drenkard, K. (2007). Quality and safety curricula in nursing education: Matching practice realities. *Nursing Outlook, 55*(3), 151-155.

Wakefield, A., Attree, M., Braidman, I., Carlisle, C., Johnson, M., & Cooke, H. (2005). Patient safety: Do nursing and medical curricula address this theme? *Nurse Education Today, 25*, 333-340.

TRANSFORMING CLINICAL EDUCATION IN NURSING

Nell Ard, PhD, RN, ANEF, CNE
Theresa M. "Terry" Valiga, EdD, RN, ANEF, FAAN

Clinical education is often thought to be the most significant aspect of preparing a nurse because that is where the information, skills and insights gained through classroom and laboratory experience is applied and "comes alive." As such, clinical education is a vital aspect of the overall process of becoming a nurse, and it must be exquisitely designed and implemented. In recent years, however, a growing number of challenges — increasingly sick patients in acute care settings, shorter hospital stays, increased complexity in home care, increased emphasis on interdisciplinary collaboration, expectations related to systemwide thinking, errors in patient care, the shortage of nurse faculty, increased regulatory requirements, and so on — have made it impossible to continue "business as usual." Indeed, the way nurse educators design and implement clinical learning now requires a major transformation if we are to most effectively prepare the nurse of today and the future.

Nowhere was the need for transformation more evident than in the work of the National League for Nursing's (NLN) Task Group on Clinical Nursing Education, Blue Ribbon Panel, and Think Tank on Transforming Clinical Nursing Education. And nowhere is the need argued more strongly than in the chapters in this book.

Insights from the Work of National Groups Related to Clinical Nursing Education

NLN Task Group on Clinical Nursing Education

The NLN's Task Group on Clinical Nursing Education (TG) was established in 2006 and charged to study and clarify current thoughts and issues regarding clinical nursing education in the United States. Initially, this group identified three significant issues that would guide their discussions: the nature of clinical experiences, the evaluation of clinical/ laboratory performance, and new models of clinical learning. As the dialogue progressed, the need for a comprehensive review of the literature in nursing and related fields became clear; that work resulted in an annotated bibliography regarding clinical education that is included here as Appendix B.

The literature search introduced the task group to works by Parkes (1995) and Napthine (1996), both of whom described twelve principles of quality clinical education that had been developed by an interdisciplinary committee in Australia. Essentially the twelve principles indicated that good quality clinical education should (1) be shared by education and service, (2) be integrated with theory components, (3) have clear learning objectives, (4) have its plan readily shared with clinical staff, (5) be accepting of both educational and service policies regarding students, (6) include routine student evaluation and feedback on clinical placements, (7) should reflect the range of curriculum with a broad span of clinical areas, (8) be primarily experiential but could include observation and/or simulation, (9) have placements aimed at depth to meet learning objectives, (10) be structured to match the organization of work in the placement setting and promote continuity of care, (11) maximize students' time spent in nursing activities, and (12) have student assessments done by faculty in collaboration with clinical staff.

The TG used these works, as well as others, to guide their thinking and formulate answers to several questions that seemed crucial to understanding and then transforming clinical education in nursing. Those questions were as follows: *What* is clinical education? *Why* is it done? *Where* is it done? *When* does it occur? *Who* is involved in it?

The TG defined the **WHAT** of clinical education as follows: a holistic experience that attends to the intellectual (knowledge, critical thinking, decision-making, priority setting, transfer of knowledge and understanding from one situation to another, etc.), the physical (presence), and the passion (values, psychosocial aspects, professional involvement, etc.) components of *learning what it means to be a nurse and developing one's identity as a nurse.* It requires four "players" if it is to be called "clinical": the student, the teacher, the patient (family unit/community), and the clinical staff (or health care team).

The literature led the TG to conclude that the reason we incorporate clinical education experiences in the preparation of nurses — the **WHY** — is that they provide actual experiences that help students meet the health care needs of society. Clinical experiences are opportunities to "pull it together," particularly in a place where students can be taught to think on the spot. Clinical experiences occur to assist students in developing their identities as a nurse through their experiences with patients/families, and they provide opportunities to work collaboratively with the patient/family/community and other health care providers. Clinical education challenges students to enhance their critical thinking and problem solving skills, and they provide students with opportunities to demonstrate competence and to operationalize the intellectual, physical and passion components of practice in the context of the four players (i.e., student, patient/family, teacher, and clinical staff).

The TG then explored the **WHERE** of clinical education and concluded that it could occur in any setting that provides (a) integration of the intellectual, physical, and passion components of what it means to be a nurse and (b) involves all four players. Where students actually do their clinical learning should be determined by (1) the learning outcomes/goals that have been mutually developed by students and faculty, and (2) the ability to integrate the three components and four players. The TG firmly believed that clinical "placements" should not be determined by required "rotations" through medical specialty areas or by a specified number of hours that need to be "put in." Instead, they should be determined by the factors noted above, which allow for more flexibility and individualization, both of which are known to be good educational practices (Chickering & Gamson, 1987).

In considering the **WHEN** of clinical education, the TG concluded that it should occur throughout the student's program since it is very helpful for "hands-on" learners and many students do learn better from direct, rather than vicarious, experiences. The TG also agreed that all students should have at least one intensive, "immersion-like" experience where they can be part of a team, see patient progress (or lack of progress) over time, and function as a "real nurse." Finally, the TG agreed that all students should have some type of clinical experience early on in their program to help them make a decision about their career and "connect" them with nurses and others committed to the profession.

Finally, the question of **WHO** is essential for an experience to be called "clinical." The TG concluded that clinical education involves four "players": the student, the teacher, the patient/family, and the health care team/staff.

- The **student** needs to take an active part in the clinical experience and be fully engaged in the learning process. He/She must collaborate with faculty to identify learning outcomes and then seek out and take responsibility for obtaining those experiences. The TG believed that only the student can integrate the three components of clinical (intellectual, physical, and passion) to develop his/her identity as a nurse, and she/he must take responsibility to do so.

- The role of the **teacher** is to (a) work with the student to identify learning outcomes, (b) help arrange experiences, and (c) work with the clinical agency to provide a positive learning environment. Two important roles for the teacher are (1) to help students surface the learning as they engage in reflective exercises, and (2) to facilitate/guide/critique/evaluate the student's performance.

- According to the TG, the **patient/family** does not need to be a physiological entity; instead, the patient/family can be simulated or be a geographic community/group. The TG also believed that the patient could be a standardized patient or one available through telehealth — if the clinical experience was carefully constructed.

- The final player, according to the TG, was the **clinical staff/team**. These individuals are expected to facilitate student learning in order to help meet learning outcomes. They are not necessarily physically present at all times, but they also never "abandon" the student. If staff are used as preceptors or clinical instructors (as often happens on DEUs [dedicated education units]), they must be carefully selected and properly prepared for the role, and their expectations — to supervise student performances, oversee and help the student's day-to-day experiences, and have input to the student's evaluation — must be made clear.

Based on this work, the TG surveyed NLN members in spring 2007 regarding the extent to which they agreed with the statements made regarding the What, Why, Where, When and Who of clinical education. The results of this survey, which were published in *Nursing Education Perspectives* (Ard, Rogers, & Vinten, 2008), noted that respondents were in general agreement with all items on the survey. This finding, along with the insights and perspectives shared through open comments, indicated that nurse faculty are open to challenging the current model of nursing clinical education and considering new models for the future.

Throughout the TG's journey together, the group realized the lack of existing evidence-based research on clinical education and the need to transform the status quo of clinical education. It is clear that educators must think "outside the box" and consider dramatically new models for clinical education. Since there cannot be only one model that will meet the needs of all programs, faculty in each school of nursing are challenged to consider what models will work in their setting, based on the resources available, the learning objectives to be met, and the talents of faculty and clinical partners to help students achieve those objectives. (See Appendix C — Final Report of the NLN Task Group on Clinical Nursing Education.)

The results of the survey noted above — along with feedback from nurse educators to their presentations at three NLN Education Summits, the Headlines from the NLN article that was published (Ard et al., 2008), and the piece they contributed to an article on clinical education evaluation (Oermann, Saewert, Yarbrough, Ard, & Charasika, In press) — indicate that nurse educators are ready to think very differently about clinical education. This perspective was reinforced as members of the TG participated in the NLN's Think Tank on Transforming Clinical Education.

NLN Think Tank on Transforming Clinical Education

In April 2008, the NLN convened an invitational Think Tank to assist NLN and its members to answer the following questions:

- What does it mean to teach a practice?
- What are the most effective ways to help students learn the practice of nursing?
- What are the most effective ways to assess the clinical performance of nursing students in prelicensure programs? and
- What meaning do these questions have for teaching diverse student populations to care for diverse patient populations?

This group of leaders in nursing education, accreditation and regulation, as well as individuals from disciplines outside nursing, was co-facilitated by Dr. Pamela Ironside and Dr. Christine Tanner, two of nursing education's most innovative and scholarly members. See Table 15-1 for participants. The full final report of the exciting work of this Think Tank can be found at http://www.nln.org/facultydevelopment/pdf/think_tank.pdf and a partial report is included here as Appendix D-1. Readers are encouraged to review it as a source of creative ideas about the future of this highly significant aspect of the education of a nurse for practice.

NLN Blue Ribbon Panel on Priorities for Research in Nursing Education

Like the Task Group and the Think Tank, this group of nursing education leaders was convened to help the NLN identify the key areas in need of research in nursing education – studies that might be undertaken by the NLN itself and/or supported through the organization's research grants program. After extensive discussion on several separate occasions, members of the Blue Ribbon Panel reaffirmed that the primary area in need of research is the design and implementation of clinical education in nursing.

During their discussions, the Blue Ribbon Panel developed a model showing the three most significant areas in need of research: patient-centered teaching, new clinical education models, and system re-design. Figure 15-1 illustrates that these three areas are interrelated, though in any given study one may be in the forefront while the other two are in the background. For example, one study may focus primarily on new clinical education models, but such a study also should attend to the changes that occur simultaneously in the classroom (i.e., increased use of patient-centered teaching) and those that occur in the overall educational system (e.g., increased rewards for excellence in clinical teaching, enhanced preparation of clinical instructors, and so on).

Recommendations from this scholarly group guided the NLN's national study of nursing education that was conducted in 2008-2009. Results of this study are included here as Chapter 2, and they will be reported at the 2009 Education Summit, in issues of Nursing Education Perspectives, on the NLN website, and through other means; the reader is encouraged to watch

Table 15 – 1
NLN Think Tank on Transforming Clinical Nursing Education

CO-FACILITATORS

Pamela Ironside, PhD, RN, FAAN
Christine Tanner, PhD, RN, FAAN

PARTICIPANTS

Nell Ard, PhD, CNS, RNC, CNE
Linda Caputi, EdD, RN, CNE
Lisa Day, PhD, RN, CNS
Joanne R. Duffy, PhD, RN, FAAN
Linda Q. Everett, PhD, RN, FAAN
Judith Halstead, DNS, RN, ANEF
Thomas S. Inui, ScM, MD
Beverly Malone, PhD, RN, FAAN
Mary Schoessler, EdD, RN-BC
Nancy Spector, PhD, RN
Sharon Tanner, EdD, RN
M. Elaine Tagliareni, EdD, RN

OBSERVERS

Sandy Calhoun, MSN, RN, CPHQ
Kay Hodson Carlton, EdD, RN, FAAN
Sara Horton-Deutsch, PhD, CNS, RN
Maryjoan Ladden, PhD, RN, FAAN
Mary Lou Morales, MSN, RN
Clive Patrickson, PhD
Catherine Pearsall, PhD, FNP, RN, CNE
Maureen Peters
Diane Whitehead, EdD, RN
Patricia Young, PhD, RN

STAFF

Tamara Kear, MSN, RN, CNN
Theresa "Terry" Valiga, EdD, RN, FAAN

Figure 15 – 1
NLN Blue Ribbon Panel's Model on Clinical Education

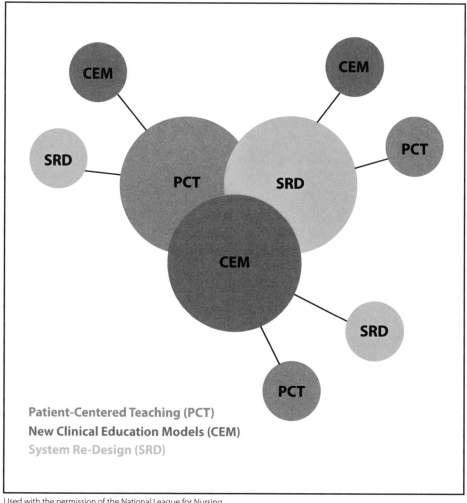

Patient-Centered Teaching (PCT)
New Clinical Education Models (CEM)
System Re-Design (SRD)

Used with the permission of the National League for Nursing.

for such reports. Think Tank members also recommended future areas in need of study, and those ideas are reflected, along with those of the authors, at the conclusion of this chapter.

Insights from Chapters Included in This Book

There is no doubt that clinical nursing education is receiving a great deal of attention today, and it is expected that this will continue far into the future. The comprehensive literature review provided in Chapter 1 acknowledges the paucity of quality, rigorous research about clinical education and encourages nurse educators to systematically explore and reflect, in a scholarly way, on new approaches to these student experiences. Selected findings from the recent national study on clinical education are reported in Chapter 2, insights from the recent Carnegie study of nursing are reported in Chapter 5, and the need for continued scholarly inquiry into clinical education is reinforced in subsequent chapters and emphasized again at the conclusion of this one.

The innovations occurring through the Oregon Consortium for Nursing Education (Chapter 3) and the evolution of dedicated education units (Chapter 4) are encouraging signs that new models for clinical education can be created and that the outcomes of such models promise to be highly positive for students, faculty, clinical staff, and patients. The use of simulation as an integral component of learning the nursing role (Chapter 10) also provides beginning evidence about the effectiveness of these new ways to think about and structure clinical learning experiences.

The authors of this book have helped readers reflect on students' perspectives of clinical learning experiences (Chapter 7) and elements of evaluating students' clinical performance (Chapter 6). In addition, the authors have assisted readers in reflecting upon aspects faculty need to consider as they plan and implement such clinical experiences (Chapter 8) and the competencies faculty need to be effective clinical educators (Chapter 9).

It is important that clinical nursing education of the future incorporate learning experiences of other health professionals, and Chapter 11 has provided a thoughtful analysis of considerations to be made as such experiences are planned. As nurse educators transform the clinical component of curricula, they must do so with clear recognition of regulatory requirements or perspectives (Chapter 12), accreditation standards and expectations (Chapter 13), and events occurring in the larger context (one example of which is examined in Chapter 14).

Conclusion

Without question, the clinical component of nursing education is critical. It is the component that is most complicated and that truly calls for integration (of cognitive learning, psychomotor skills, and values/professional standards). It is in the clinical setting where the importance of effective relationships with clinical partners — in nursing and other disciplines — is most evident. And it is in the clinical setting where students can have incredibly positive learning experiences or dreadful ones.

It is the responsibility of nurse educators to develop the competencies essential for effective teaching in this setting, to establish and nurture collegial relationships with clinical partners in order to create a positive learning environment for students, and to always keep patient safety and quality care in mind. Educators are challenged to re-think all the elements of clinical education — WHY we do it, WHAT it really is, WHERE it can occur, WHEN it should occur, and WHO needs to be involved to ensure valuable learning experiences — and be open to new approaches.

Finally, nurse educators and, in particular, our nursing education scholars are urged to reflect on the evidence that does — or that needs to — underlie the decisions we make about clinical education, and to conduct research to address the many unanswered questions about the best way to design and implement the clinical component of our curricula. The following questions are offered to stimulate such thinking:

- What percentage of clinical experiences can be done through simulation and still have students be successful in patient care and on the licensing exam?

- What happens regarding student confidence, patient care delivery, and success on the licensing exam when student do not "rotate through" all clinical settings?

- How do the roles, relationships, and responsibilities of faculty, students, and clinical partners need to change for new models of clinical education to be most effective?

- What alternative models of clinical education (e.g., immersion throughout the program vs. immersion during last-semester courses only or having all clinical experiences in the same healthcare system vs. moving from one facility to another) are most effective in enhancing student learning and confidence in the nursing role?

Through rigorous study of questions like these (and the many others proposed in other chapters) nurse educators — novice and experienced — will contribute significantly to the science of nursing education and provide a firm foundation for transforming clinical education. Such scholarship and leadership are needed, and they are needed now.

References

Ard N., Rogers K., &, Vinten, S. (2008). Summary of the survey on clinical education in nursing. *Nursing Education Perspectives, 29*(4), 238-245.

Chickering, A. W., & Gamson, Z. F. (1987). Seven principles for good practice in undergraduate education. *Wingspread Journal, 9*(2), 1-5. Retrieved from http://www.johnsonfdn.org/Publications/ConferenceReports/SevenPrinciples/SevenPrinciples_pdf.pdf

Napthine, R. (1996). Clinical education: A system under a pressure. *Australian Nursing Journal, 3*(9), 20-25.

Oermann, M. H., Yarbrough, S. S., Saewert, K. J., Ard, N., & Charasika, M. (in press). Assessment and grading practices in schools of nursing: National survey findings, part 1, and Clinical evaluation and grading practices in schools of nursing: National survey findings, part 2. *Nursing Education Perspectives.*

Parkes, R. (1995). Educating for the future. *Australian Nursing Journal, 2*(7), 22-27.

Appendix A

AUTHOR PROFILES

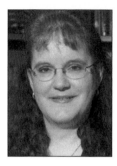

Nell Ard, PhD, RN, ANEF, CNE
Director & Professor of Nursing
Collin County Community College District (McKinney, TX)

Dr. Nell Ard has been in nursing education for twenty years and has taught at the diploma, associate, baccalaureate, and master's degree levels. She has served the NLN in several capacities: a member of the Task Group on Teaching/Learning, a member of a Task Group on Test Security, Consultant for the Centers of Excellence program, a Nominations Committee member, and as the Chair of the Task Group on Clinical Nursing Education. She is currently serving as an Ambassador, as a member of the Public Policy Committee, and as a NLNAC Site Visitor. She has presented several times at the NLN Education Summit. Dr. Ard graduated from Harding University (BSN), West Texas State University (MSN), and University of Texas Health Science Center at San Antonio (PhD in clinical nursing research). She earned NLN's Certification in Nursing Education in 2006. She has published extensively and has received numerous awards. Most recently, she authored the "Essentials of Learning" chapter in Building the Science of Nursing Education: Foundation for Evidence-Based Teaching and Learning. Dr. Ard was also recently honored by her nursing colleagues and students with the funding of a nursing scholarship named for her. Dr. Ard will be inducted into the National League for Nursing's Academy of Nursing Education in September 2009.

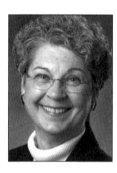

Theresa M. "Terry" Valiga, EdD, RN, ANEF, FAAN
Director of the Institute for Educational Excellence
Duke University School of Nursing (Durham, NC)

Dr. Terry Valiga received both a master's and a doctoral degree in nursing education from Teachers College, Columbia University in New York. She held faculty and administrative positions in five different universities over a 26-year period and then served as Chief Program Officer at the National League for Nursing for nine years. In July 2008, Dr. Valiga returned to academe to create and develop a variety of initiatives that advance excellence in nursing education at the Duke University School of Nursing and beyond. Throughout her career, she has collaborated with many talented students and professional colleagues to develop innovative curricula and programs, including the NLN's Centers of Excellence program, Academy of Nursing Education, Hallmarks of Excellence in Nursing Education, and Excellence in Nursing Education Model. She has received several prestigious awards for excellence in nursing education, presented on education topics at national and international conferences, published widely on issues related to nursing education, and consulted with nursing faculty groups in the United States, Canada, Japan, and China on curriculum development, program evaluation, innovations in teaching, and the faculty role. She also is an expert in the area of leadership and has co-authored a book (now in its third edition) on this complex phenomenon. Dr. Valiga will be inducted into the National League for Nursing's Academy of Nursing Education in September 2009.

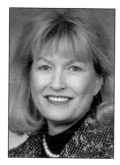

Marsha Howell Adams, DSN, RN, CNE
Professor & Director of Undergraduate Programs
The University of Alabama Capstone College of Nursing
(Tuscaloosa, AL)

Dr. Marsha Howell Adams received a BSN, MSN, and DSN-Nursing Administration from the University of Alabama School of Nursing at Birmingham and a post-master's certificate in rural case management from the University of Alabama, Capstone College of Nursing. She has extensive experience in both undergraduate and graduate education. Dr. Adams is presently serving on the NLN Board of Governors for a second term and on the Editorial Board for Nursing Education Perspectives. She also served as the chair for both the NLN Nursing Education Standards and the Excellence in Nursing Education Task Groups, where she was instrumental in the development of the NLN Hallmarks of Excellence and the Excellence in Nursing Education Model. She has been the recipient of the CCN Board of Visitors Commitment to Teaching Award, the University of Alabama National Alumni Association Outstanding Commitment to Teaching Award, the Alabama League for Nursing Lamplighter Award and the Alabama State Nurses Association Outstanding Nurse Educator/Academe Award. Dr. Adams is recognized as an NLN Certified Nurse Educator (CNE), a Nursing Academic Fellow by the American Association of Colleges of Nursing, and is certified as an on-site evaluator by the Commission on Collegiate Nursing Education. Her clinical research interests and numerous publications have focused on rural women and children and nursing education.

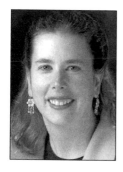

Mindi Anderson, PhD, RN, CPNP-PC
Simulation Coordinator & Assistant Professor
The University of Texas at Arlington School of Nursing

Dr. Mindi Anderson is an assistant professor and simulation coordinator at The University of Texas at Arlington School of Nursing. Her research and scholarship are focused on the most effective way to teach using simulation, multidisciplinary team training, and the use of standardized patients in nursing. She has received several research grants. Dr. Anderson is one of the course authors for Simulation Innovation Resource Center project for the National League for Nursing/Laerdal Medical. She has given multiple presentations on topics related to simulation and standardized patients.

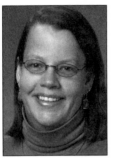

Gail Armstrong, ND, RN
Assistant Professor
University of Colorado Denver College of Nursing (Denver, CO)

Dr. Gail Armstrong is an assistant professor at the University of Colorado Denver College of Nursing. She is a Medical/Surgical nurse whose practice and teaching are focused on adult acute care nursing. Dr. Armstrong has worked in adult acute care nursing since 1995. She is the Medical/Surgical Content Coordinator for the Baccalaureate Program at the University of Colorado, and she is working with the national initiative Quality and Safety Education for Nurses (QSEN) to update prelicensure clinical courses to reflect quality and safety trends in health care delivery.

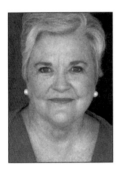

Patricia Benner, PhD, RN, FAAN
Director of National Nursing Education Research Project
Carnegie Foundation for the Advancement of Teaching (San Francisco, CA)

Dr. Patricia Benner is currently the director of a National Nursing Education Research Project under the auspices of the Carnegie Foundation for the Advancement in Teaching. This research project, which is a part of a larger project that studies the preparation for the professions (PPP), is the first national study of nursing education in 30 years. She also is the Co-Principal Director of the project entitled, Clinical Knowledge Development of Nurses in an Operational Environment, which seeks to address three research aims: (a) to articulate, describe, and interpret experiential learning regarding medical and nursing care during combat operations in order to evaluate and extend this knowledge; (b) to provide narratives of combat practice that could assist in the design and teaching of combat health care; and (c) to create a collection of narratives around practice topics or issues that are identified that can be published as a learning resource for nurses. Dr. Benner also is completing a six-year research project to develop a taxonomy of nursing error and a data collection instrument for the National Council of State Boards of Nursing entitled, Nursing Pathways to Patient Safety (TERCAP), a data collection tool that is now being implemented nationally by The Council for State Boards of Nursing.

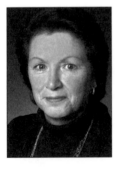

Kathleen Blust, MSN, RN-BC
Professor of Nursing
Collin County Community College District (McKinney, TX)

Ms. Kathleen Blust received her Bachelor of Science and Master of Science in nursing from the University of Phoenix. She also holds a certification in medical-surgical nursing. Her nursing experience has spanned medical-surgical, perioperative, and geriatric nursing. She currently teaches nursing at Collin College in Texas. Her primary interests in teaching include medical-surgical nursing, nursing skills, and simulation.

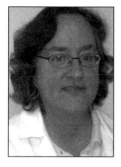

Lisa Day, PhD, RN, CSN
Clinical Nurse Specialist for Neuroscience and Critical Care
University of California San Francisco Medical Center

Dr. Lisa Day graduated from Long Beach City College in California with an Associate Degree in nursing in 1984. She has worked as a nurse in a post-anesthesia recovery room, a medical cardiac intensive care unit, and a neuroscience-critical care unit, and completed her BSN, MS and PhD (with Patricia Benner) at UCSF School of Nursing. She taught prelicensure nursing in an accelerated second degree program for eight years before recently returning to clinical practice and is now the Clinical Nurse Specialist for Neuroscience and Critical Care at UCSF Medical Center. Dr. Day has been involved as a consultant in several projects related to nursing education, including the RWJ-funded Quality and Safety Education in Nursing (QSEN; University of North Carolina, Linda Cronnenwett and Gail Sherwood); the Helene Fuld Health Trust-funded project Evaluating the Outcomes of Accelerated Nursing Education (Duke University School of Nursing, Catherine Gillis); evaluation of the Oregon Consortium for Nursing Education (OCNE), and the Carnegie Foundation for the Advancement of Teaching National Study of Nursing Education. She also participated in the 2008 National League for Nursing Think Tank on Transforming Clinical Nursing Education.

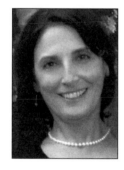

Rita Ferrari D'Aoust, PhD, ACNP, CNE
Associate Professor
University of Rochester, School of Nursing (Rochester, NY)

Dr. Rita Ferrari D'Aoust is an associate professor at the University of Rochester, in the School of Nursing. She received her PhD in 2008 from the University of Rochester in education, in the Division of Teaching and Curriculum as well as her master's and bachelor's degrees in nursing from the University of Rochester School of Nursing. Dr. D'Aoust's primary appointment is in the School of Nursing, where she has been active in developing and revising curriculum and integrating the use of technology in education and clinical practice. She has held numerous positions, assisted in integrating technology into the curriculum, and remains an active Nurse Practitioner.

Dr. D'Aoust has been active in several interdisciplinary and interprofessional education initiatives with community organizations, the University of Rochester Medical Center, and health professional students and practitioners in programs such as Community Based Quality Improvement in Education (CBQIE), Achieving Competence Today (ACT), and Health Action. She assisted in the development of a new interprofessional education program, the Master of Science Medical/Health Professionals Education that is an interdisciplinary effort across three colleges in the university: School of Medicine and Dentistry, School of Nursing and the Warner Graduate School of Education and Human Development, where she teaches one of the core courses. She has given numerous presentations and received numerous professional awards.

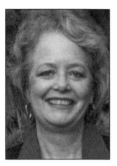

Paula Gubrud-Howe, EdD, RN
Director of Simulation
Oregon Health & Science University School of Nursing
(Portland, OR)

Dr. Paula Gubrud-Howe is the Statewide Director of Simulation at Oregon Health & Science University School of Nursing in Portland, Oregon. She is also Clinical Education Redesign Project Co-Director for the Oregon Consortium for Nursing Education (OCNE). She has been a leader in the development of OCNE from its inception and has contributed to all aspects of this innovation in nursing education. Dr. Gubrud has over 20 years of nursing education experience that spans both associate degree and baccalaureate education. Her research interests focus on use of simulation and innovative clinical education redesign. She is a founding member of the Oregon Simulation Alliance and is a frequent presenter at nursing and simulation conferences.

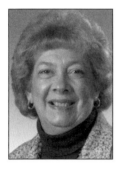

Judith A. Halstead, DNS, RN, ANEF
Executive Associate Dean for Academic Affairs
Indiana University School of Nursing (Indianapolis, IN)

Dr. Judith A. Halstead received her BSN and MSN from the University of Evansville, and her doctorate in nursing science from Indiana University. She is currently professor of nursing and executive associate dean for Academic Affairs at Indiana University School of Nursing in Indianapolis, a position she has held since 2004. Dr. Halstead has extensive experience in undergraduate and graduate nursing education. She is known for her expertise in curriculum development and online education, and is the co-editor of Teaching in Nursing: A Guide for Faculty and editor of Nurse Educator Competencies: Creating an Evidence-Based Practice for Nurse Educators. Dr. Halstead was chairperson of the NLN Task Group that developed the NLN Core Competencies for Nurse Educators. She was a 2005 recipient of the Midwest Nursing Research Society Nursing Education Research Section's Advancement of Science Award. Dr. Halstead was inducted as a fellow in the NLN Academy of Nursing Education in 2007.

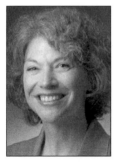

Desiree Hensel, PhD, RNC
Assistant Professor of Nursing
Indiana University School of Nursing (Bloomington, IN)

Dr. Desiree Hensel received a BSN from Indiana University, an MSN in the educator track from Ball State University, and a PhD in health and human behavior from Walden University. An NLN Health Information Technology Scholar, her research and scholarship of teaching interests include nurse self-concept development and simulations. She has been certified in high-risk neonatal nursing for over 20 years and has presented locally and nationally on the use of simulation in maternal-newborn nursing.

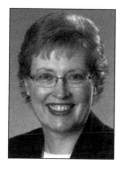

Pamela M. Ironside, PhD, RN, FAAN, ANEF
Associate Professor & Director of the Center for Nursing Education Research
Indiana University (Indianapolis, IN)

Dr. Pamela Ironside's research program includes using hermeneutic phenomenology to explicate the ways new pedagogies influence the practices of thinking in nursing classrooms and clinical courses and the ways in which nursing faculty undertake reform and innovation. She has also received funding from the National Council of State Boards of Nursing to study how multiple patient simulation experiences influence students' clinical judgment and safety competencies and, in collaboration with the Community College of Philadelphia, from the John A. Hartford Foundation to study ways to foster associate degree nursing students' knowledge, skills and abilities to care for older adults. She is a Fellow in the American Academy of Nursing and the Academy of Nursing Education. She is the recipient of the Advancing the Science of Nursing award for the Curriculum and Instruction section of the Midwest Nursing Research Society. Her work is widely published in periodicals such as Journal of Nursing Education, Journal of Advanced Nursing, Nursing Education Perspectives, Journal of Qualitative Health Research, and Advances in Nursing Science. She has presented numerous workshops on pedagogical development and using new pedagogies in classroom and clinical settings both nationally and internationally.

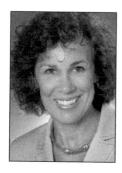

Pamela R. Jeffries, DNS, RN, FAAN, ANEF
Associate Dean of Academic Affairs
Johns Hopkins School of Nursing (Baltimore, MD)

Dr. Pamela Jeffries is associate dean for academic affairs at Johns Hopkins University School of Nursing in Baltimore, Maryland. Her research and scholarship of teaching are focused on learning outcomes, instructional design, new pedagogies, innovative teaching strategies, and incorporating the use of technology and simulated learning. She has been awarded several grants to support her research and has received several teaching awards, including the NLN Lucile Petry Leone Award for nursing education, the prestigious Elizabeth Russell Belford Award for teaching excellence given by Sigma Theta Tau International, the NLN nursing education research award, and numerous outstanding faculty awards presented by graduating nursing classes.

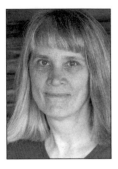

Vickie Leonard, PhD, RN, FNP
Family Nurse Practitioner, California Childcare Health Program
University of California, San Francisco

Dr. Vickie Leonard is a family nurse practitioner and Child Care Health Consultant at the California Childcare Health Program (CCHP). She is a trainer for Child Care Health Consultants in California, and does trainings and presentations for child care providers in the state on health and safety issues. She also researches and writes educational materials on health and safety for child care providers and Child Care Health Consultants. Dr. Leonard has taught in the nurse practitioner program at the University of San Francisco and has worked at both Children's Hospital Oakland and Kaiser in pediatric subspecialty clinics. She was part of the research team for the Study of Nursing Education at the Carnegie Foundation for the Advancement of Teaching. She has also consulted on a longitudinal research study of teen mothers and their infants for the past 15 years. She received her PhD from the School of Nursing, University of California, San Francisco.

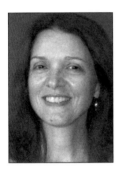

Camille Anne Martina, PhD
Research Assistant Professor
University of Rochester School of Medicine and Dentistry
(Rochester, NY)

Dr. Camille Anne Martina is a research assistant professor at the University of Rochester, in the School of Medicine and Dentistry. She received her PhD in 2005 from the University of Rochester in education, in the Division of Teaching and Curriculum. Her primary appointment is in Community and Preventive Medicine, Division of Social and Behavioral Medicine with a secondary appointment in Environmental Medicine. She serves on the University of Rochester Medical Center's Office of Medical Education Academic Faculty Advisory Board and is an active member of the Master of Science Medical/Health Professionals Education Working Group (a new degree, MSEd, program across three colleges in the university: School of Medicine and Dentistry, School of Nursing and the Warner Graduate School of Education and Human Development).

Dr. Martina is currently a co-investigator on several NIH and CDC grants and in the past has been a co-investigator on AAMC medical education grants. Her research interests in education are looking at the structure and function of social contexts, institutional culture and agency in promoting academic achievement in underrepresented populations, as well as educational and institutional policies that prevent innovative and integrated instruction.

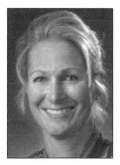

Angela M. McNelis, PhD, RN
Associate Professor & Director of Undergraduate
Special Programs
Indiana University School of Nursing (Indianapolis, IN)

Dr. Angela McNelis is an associate professor and director of undergraduate special programs at Indiana University School of Nursing. She has expertise in study design, curriculum development, use of technology and innovative strategies, data collection and analysis, and evaluation. Her research and scholarship focus is on best practices in teaching and learning, and she has received funding to assess, develop, and evaluate innovative approaches to utilize in clinical, classroom, and online teaching. She has been awarded numerous grants to support her research and has received several awards for teaching and research excellence given by Sigma Theta Tau International, Indiana University, and Indiana University School of Nursing.

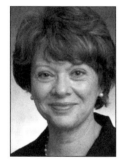

Susan Randles Moscato, EdD, RN
Associate Dean for Graduate Programs & Professor
University of Portland (Portland, OR)

Dr. Susan Randles Moscato is a graduate of the University of Portland and began her nursing career as a Navy nurse at Philadelphia Naval Hospital, the East Coast center for amputees during the Vietnam War. Dr. Moscato has a master's from UCLA with a clinical nurse specialty in rehabilitation. She joined the faculty at UP in 1977 as an adjunct clinical instructor and completed her doctorate in education administration at Portland State University in 1986. She served in various adjunct teaching and administrative roles until 1993, when she served as a nurse consultant to health care organizations concerned with organizational and systems issues.

Dr. Moscato is a qualitative researcher. Her work includes serving as co-principal investigator on a multisite national study for the Kaiser Permanente Health Care System on telephone nursing advice and a study of organizational cultural change at Providence St. Vincent Medical Center for the Robert Wood Johnson Foundation. Since 2002, she has been actively involved in the implementation of the Dedicated Education Unit (DEU) model of clinical teaching and has served as clinical faculty coordinator, DEU coordinator, author and DEU consultant nationally and internationally. Her service activities include Parish Nurse Coordinator and board memberships for both Northwest Parish Nurse Ministry and Macdonald Center and Residence, and leadership in the Omicron Upsilon Chapter, Sigma Theta Tau International.

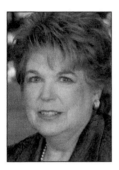

Linda D. Norman, DSN, RN, FAAN
Professor & Senior Associate Dean for Academics
Vanderbilt University School of Nursing (Nashville, TN)

Dr. Linda Norman received a BSN and MSN in adult health from the University of Virginia and a DSN from the University of Alabama at Birmingham. She has been involved in nursing education for over 30 years, serving in administrative positions for the past 20 years.

Dr. Norman focused her career on developing innovative quality improvement curricula that has been tested, published, and presented for a decade through various interdisciplinary and international forums. She was a member of the evaluation team for the Johnson & Johnson Media Campaign and has been the Evaluation Director for the RWJF/NWHF Partners Investing in Nursing's Future project since 2006.

She was recently elected to the NLNAC Board of Commissioners, and has been a program evaluator and a member of the Evaluation Review Panel for several years. She is a member of the NLN Nursing Education Workforce Development Advisory Council (NEWDAC) and a founding member of the NLN/NLNAC Global Task Force: International Nursing Education Service and Accreditation.

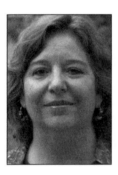

Beth Phillips Cusatis, MSN, RN, CNE
Assistant Clinical Professor
Duke University School of Nursing (Durham, NC)

Ms. Beth Phillips has been in nursing education since 1996. She became a Certified Nurse Educator through the NLN in 2006. Currently, she teaches in the Accelerated Baccalaureate in Nursing Program, where she coordinates the first two clinical courses covering foundational concepts and adult health nursing. She organizes and delivers content and concepts both in the classroom and lab setting as well as oversees the clinical progress of students. She has a passion for creative, interactive classes and labs and has been instrumental in using simulation and unfolding cases to the classroom and lab. She works with new clinical instructors to guide and mentor them and was the lead developer for the 2008 Duke Clinical Instructor Development Intensive for local schools of nursing.

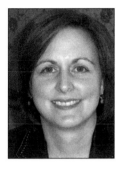

Kristen J. Rogers, MSN, RN, CNE
Service Excellence Director
Washington Hospital (Washington, PA)

Ms. Kristen Rogers has been a part of the nursing profession for 20 years, with 15 years focused on nursing education. In her present position as service excellence director, she collaborates with health care team members to enhance the patient and family experience. In her previous position as assistant director of the school of nursing, she conducted ongoing evaluation of the curriculum and facilitated program evaluation in accordance with NLNAC standards and criteria and State Board of Nursing standards. Her recent professional activities include membership on the NLN Task Group on Clinical Nursing Education, the NLN Education Technology and Information Management Advisory Council and NLN 2009 Summit Planning Workgroup. Her recent publications include contributions to Headlines from the NLN in the July/August 2008 *Nursing Education Perspectives* and co-authoring two chapters in *Simulation in Nursing Education: From Conceptualization to Evaluation*. She has also been a presenter at national conferences on simulation in nursing education.

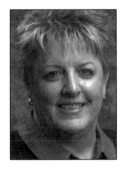

Karen Saewert, PhD, RN, CPHQ, CNE
Clinical Associate Professor & Associate Director for
Evaluation Arizona State University College of Nursing &
Health Innovation (Phoenix, AZ)

Dr. Saewert is a clinical associate professor and associate director for evaluation at Arizona State University College of Nursing & Health Innovation. Her 32-year professional nursing career reflects experience in a variety of direct care, nursing management, program management, hospital management, research, consultation, grants management and nursing education positions. Dr. Saewert received a BSN (1977) and Master of Science (1990; community mental health psychiatric nursing) from Arizona State University and a PhD (2003) in clinical nursing research (major)/public administration and policy (minor) from the University of Arizona. She has numerous certifications in psychiatric and mental health nursing, as a Professional in Healthcare Quality and as a Nurse Educator.

Dr. Saewert has expertise in evaluation and accreditation in the practice and academic sectors. She is an evidence-based practice Advancing Research & Clinical Practice through Close Collaboration (ARCC) Mentor engaged in ongoing Center for the Advancement of Evidence-Based Practice related educational and research initiatives. She holds elected office as chair-elect (2007-2009)/chair (2009-2011) for the NLN Evaluation of Learning Advisory Council (ELAC). Dr. Saewert co-authored two recent articles in *Nursing Education Perspectives* reporting the 2007 NLN ELAC national survey findings.

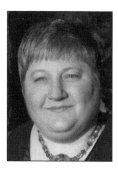

Mary Schoessler, EdD, RN-BC
Director of Nursing Education
Providence Portland Medical Center (Portland, OR)

Dr. Mary Schoessler is director of nursing education at Providence Portland Medical Center in Portland Oregon. She is a Clinical Education Project co-director for the Oregon Consortium for Nursing Education (OCNE) working on the redesign of clinical education. She is the principal developer and educator of the RN Development Program, supporting the transition of newly graduated nurses into practice, and has developed a model that describes key aspects of this transition. She maintains a program of research focusing on strategies to support nurses' development toward expert level practice. Dr. Schoessler has been a member of the NLN since the early 1990s.

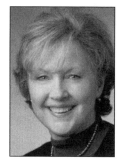

Gwen D. Sherwood, PhD, RN, FAAN
Professor & Associate Dean for Academic Affairs
University of North Carolina at Chapel Hill School of Nursing

Dr. Gwen D. Sherwood is professor and associate dean for Academic Affairs at the University of North Carolina at Chapel Hill School of Nursing. She is co-investigator on Phases I, II, and III of the Quality and Safety Education for Nurses (QSEN) initiative funded by the Robert Wood Johnson Foundation to transform curriculum to prepare nurses in quality and safety for redesigned health care systems. She is nursing leader for the University of North Carolina at Chapel Hill and Duke University Interprofessional Patient Safety Education Collaborative. Through funding from the North Carolina Foundation of GSK, the group designed and implemented a study to measure effectiveness of teaching modalities for interdisciplinary teamwork training involving nursing and medical students. While at the University of Texas-Houston Health Science Center School of Nursing, she was nurse leader with the Medical School's Center for Patient Safety and co-director for the Methodist Hospital's Center for Professional Excellence. She participates in the annual Telluride Science Institute program on interprofessional education with the University of Illinois at Chicago and is a member of the National Patient Safety Foundation Research Committee. She is past president of the International Association for Human Caring and vice president of Sigma Theta Tau International Honor Society of Nursing. She is co-editor of the newly published *International Textbook on Reflective Practice*.

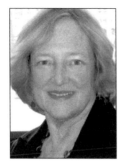

Nancy Spector, PhD, RN
Director of Education
National Council of State Boards of Nursing (Chicago, IL)

Dr. Nancy Spector has been director of education at the National Council of State Boards of Nursing (NCSBN) since August 2002. She has 20 years of experience in nursing education, where she has taught at the undergraduate and graduate levels. While in academia, Dr. Spector studied palliative care nursing, receiving internal and external funding and publishing on symptom control management. More recently, she has been in nursing regulation, where she provides leadership in nursing education issues to the Boards of Nursing and serves as a liaison between nurse educators and NCSBN. Dr. Spector is the editor of *Leader to Leader*, an NCSBN newsletter that is sent to all nurse educators biannually, and she coordinates the publication of NCSBN columns in JONA's Healthcare Law, Ethics, and Regulation, a quarterly journal. She staffs various NCSBN committees, including Transition to Practice, Faculty Qualifications and Innovations in Education Regulation. Dr. Spector presents and publishes on regulatory issues in nursing education.

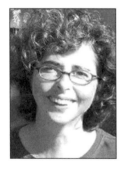

Molly Sutphen, PhD
Assistant Adjunct Professor in Social and Behavioral Sciences
University of California, San Francisco

Dr. Molly Sutphen is a Research Scholar at the Carnegie Foundation for the Advancement of Learning. She is also assistant adjunct professor in the Department of Social and Behavioral Sciences at the University of California, San Francisco, where she teaches in the Global Health Sciences program. She received her master's in anatomy from Duke University and her PhD in the history of medicine from Yale University on the evolution of international health as well as on the history of public health and nursing education. In 2004, she began a study on nursing education for the Carnegie Foundation for the Advancement of Teaching. The study is part of a five-year initiative on the preparation for careers in the law, the clergy, engineering, medicine, and nursing. One purpose of the study is to analyze across disciplines how institutions teach nursing knowledge and science, clinical judgment, and ethical comportment. She co-authored *Educating Nurses: A Radical Call for Transformation*, which will appear in 2009.

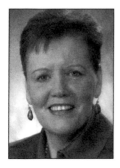

Elaine Tagliareni, EdD, RN
Professor & Independence Foundation Chair
Community College of Philadelphia School of Nursing
(Philadelphia, PA)

Dr. M. Elaine Tagliareni is currently a professor of nursing and the Independence Foundation Chair in Community Health Nursing Education at Community College of Philadelphia. She has been an associate degree nursing educator for over 25 years. She received her BSN from Georgetown University School of Nursing, a master's degree in mental health and community nursing from the University of California, San Francisco and her doctorate from Teachers College, Columbia University with an emphasis on the role of the nurse educator in community colleges.

Currently, Dr. Tagliareni is president of the National League for Nursing (NLN) (2007-2009) and is a member of the NLN Board of Governors. As president, she advocates for excellence in nursing education through pedagogical research and promotes dialogue about successful strategies to prepare a diverse nursing workforce and promote academic progression within nursing.

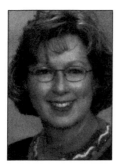

Sharon Tanner, EdD, RN
Executive Director
National League for Nursing Accrediting Commission, Inc.
(Atlanta, GA)

Dr. Sharon Tanner has served as the NLNAC Executive Director since fall 2006. She has been a recognized leader in nursing education and nursing service administration for more than 25 years. She has served as a faculty member, associate dean and academic dean for all nursing program types. In addition, she has been a leader in innovation including various modalities of delivery and integration of new technologies in nursing education. Most recently, Dr. Tanner served as associate vice president for Instruction and Distance Learning for the North Carolina Community College System.

Dr. Tanner holds a doctorate from the University of Tennessee, Knoxville in administration and policy studies in higher education with a concentration in assessment and evaluation. She also holds a master's in nursing with concentrations in primary and secondary care in maternal-child nursing and women's health. Her primary research focus has been on accountability policies and practices in higher education. In addition, she has practiced in a number of nursing service and administration roles, including advanced practice as a clinical nurse specialist. Active professionally, Dr. Tanner has been involved in regional, state, and national organizations.

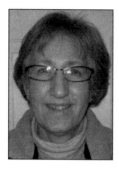

Sharon Vinten, MSN, RNC, WHNP, CNE
Staff Nurse
Carolinas Medical Center (Charlotte, NC)

Ms. Sharon Vinten is an emeritus clinical associate professor at Indiana University School of Nursing and currently teaches online for Indiana University. Her area of expertise is obstetrics and women's health. Ms. Vinten has taught both theory and clinical during her career in LPN to ASN transition programs, ASN, BSN, and MSN programs. She has presented throughout the United States discussing clinical faculty work, development, and has co-authored an online clinical faculty orientation program that she currently teaches.

Ms. Vinten has participated in NLN task groups and has published articles and chapters concerning clinical and faculty development. She also teaches state board reviews on a national basis. Ms. Vinten currently is a staff member in the Carolinas Healthcare System where she is works in uro-gynecology.

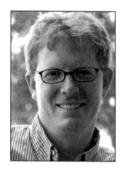

Andrew Wall, PhD
Assistant Professor
Warner School of Education, University of Rochester (Rochester, NY)

Dr. Andrew Wall is an assistant professor in Educational Leadership at the University of Rochester Warner Graduate School of Education and Human Development. He received his PhD in 2005 from University of Illinois at Urbana-Champaign. Dr. Wall has a professional background in student affairs, higher education administration, social policy research and evaluation. He teaches classes in organization and governance of higher education, higher education policy, and evaluation in education. Dr. Wall's research is in three domains: college student health and learning, assessment and evaluation, and organization, governance and policy of higher education. He has been the primary investigator on grant projects that examine alcohol abuse prevention, recent teacher graduates, state education funding formulas, and entrepreneurial leadership in higher education. Dr. Wall's recently published research focuses on college student alcohol use, assessment and evaluation in higher education, and organizational factors related to student success in higher education.

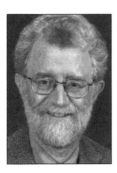

Denham Ward, MD, PhD
Professor & Chair, Department of Anesthesiology
Associate Dean for Faculty Development
University of Rochester (Rochester, NY)

Dr. Denham Ward is professor of biomedical engineering and anesthesiology, and chair of the Department of Anesthesiology. An internationally recognized expert in the field of anesthesiology, as chair, he helped create one of the first international conferences on the use of simulation in anesthesiology education and co-authored a textbook on operating room management. While on sabbatical at the University of Leiden in The Netherlands in 2001, he continued his study on the control of breathing, and also edited a major book, *Pharmacology and Pathophysiology of the Control of Breathing*.

In 2006, Dr. Ward was named associate dean for Faculty Development-Medical Education, charged with developing programs and training sessions to improve the School of Medicine faculty's teaching skills at the University of Rochester School of Medicine and Dentistry. In this role, he has developed an interdisciplinary master's degree in health professions education in conjunction with the schools of Education and Nursing.

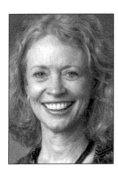

Joanne Rains Warner, DNS, RN
Dean & Professor
University of Portland (Portland, OR)

Dr. Joanne Warner's career as a nurse educator and administrator includes traditional academic and clinical appointments, as well as a range of nontraditional political and policy advocacy roles. Each of her three degrees is in nursing: a baccalaureate from Augustana College in Sioux Falls, SD; a master's in medical-surgical nursing from the University of Iowa; and a doctorate from Indiana University. Her doctoral work combined her clinical specialty — community health nursing — and health policy analysis. Since joining the University of Portland in 2005, she has served as faculty, associate and interim dean, and in January 2008 was appointed dean.

Long-time national leadership with the Friends Committee on National Legislation (1988 to present) has provided significant engagement in legislative policy development and advocacy, and has given expression to her Quaker and community health values of peace and social justice. Electoral campaign management has been another application of her policy interests, including six successful local and state political campaigns, and participating/consulting in other elections. She delights in the scholarship of integration, focusing on political competence and socialization of health professionals into the political role; spirituality related to health and health professionals; and participatory action research within the community.

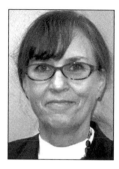

Suzanne Yarbrough, PhD, RN
Associate Dean for Undergraduate Programs
The University of Texas Health Science Center at San Antonio

Dr. Yarbrough received her PhD (nursing science) from Texas Woman's University in Houston, TX in 1994, and her MS (community health, education) from the same institution in 1991. She is currently employed as the associate dean for Undergraduate Programs and associate professor at the University of Texas Health Science Center at San Antonio, and had prior experiences in academia and as a community health nurse.

She has been a member of the Evaluation of Learning Advisory Council committee for the NLN since 2005 and served as co-investigator of a descriptive survey of assessment and evaluation strategies and grading practices in all settings and across domains of learning. That study was conducted in 2007 and resulted in two publications. Dr. Yarbrough has numerous other publications and presentations regarding nursing education, particularly clinical evaluation.

Appendix B

ANNOTATED LITERATURE REVIEW OF
CLINICAL NURSING EDUCATION

Annotated Literature Review of Clinical Nursing Education

Abrahamson, K. L. (1999). Effective clinical teaching behaviors as perceived by associate and baccalaureate degree nursing students (Doctoral dissertation, Grand Valley State University, Michigan, 1999). *ProQuest Dissertations and Theses*, AAT 1396010.

> *Discusses a research study identifying the most effective clinical teaching behaviors. Results indicated that the behaviors were similar between programs but ranked differently.*

Alderman, C. (2001). Best placed…the problem of clinical placements. *Nursing Standard, 15*(29), 14-15.

> *Discusses the enormous gap between theory and clinical and the changes made such as: lectures in hospital setting, increased number of clinical experiences, taking advantage of hospital experiences when presented rather than waiting for "check-offs" first, preclinical preparation, linking students and preceptors, clinicals located in one place for entire training. (Great Britain)*

Allison-Jones, L. L., & Hirt, J. B. (2004). Comparing the teaching effectiveness of part-time and full-time clinical nurse faculty. *Nursing Education Perspectives, 25*, 238-243.

> *Discusses the comparison of students' perception of effectiveness of part-time vs. full-time clinical faculty.*

Amelia, E. J., Brown, L., Resnick, B., & McArthur, D. B. (2001). Partners in NP education: The 1999 AANP preceptor and faculty survey. *Journal of the American Academy of Nurse Practitioners, 13*, 517-523.

> *Discusses and evaluates the preceptor model used in NP education.*

American Association of Colleges of Nursing (AACN). (2007). Nursing shortage. Retrieved February 8, 2008, from www.aacn.nche.edu/Media/FactSheets/NursingShortage.htm

> *Discusses the impact of the nursing shortage on education and practice.*

Andal, E. M. (2006). [Education News]. Technology in nursing education: Clinical evaluation, assessment, and resources at the point of care. *Nursing Education Perspectives, 27*, 66.

> *Discusses a computerized evaluation tool on handheld computers and PDAs in the clinical setting.*

Anderson, B. A. (1999). An orthopaedic workshop and skills laboratory: Providing nursing students with skills to practice effectively in a changing work environment. *Orthopaedic Nursing, 18*(3), 57-61.

> *Discusses how to combine lecture and lab experiences to facilitate student learning.*

Andrus, N. C., & Bennett, N. M. (2006). Developing an interdisciplinary, community-based education program for health professions students: The Rochester experience. *Academic Medicine, 81*, 326-331.

> *Discusses how to blend health disciplines educationally.*

Arcand, L. L., & Neuman, J. (2005). Nursing competency assessment across the continuum of care. *Journal of Continuing Education in Nursing, 36*, 247-254.

> *Discusses how competencies can be measured in the clinical setting to meet the standards of accrediting bodies.*

Aston, L., & Molassiotis, A. (2002). Supervising and supporting student nurses in clinical placements: The peer support initiative. *Nurse Education Today, 23*, 202-210.

> *Discusses a study with senior students (mentors) supervising and supporting junior students in clinical placement. All being supervised by clinical mentor. Peers provided encouragement, and assisted with developing independence. Difficulty is that senior students do not know their role*

or how to implement it, and therefore need to be taught how to mentor peers; may neglect own studies. Great value in formalizing peer support. (Great Britain)

August-Brady, M. M. (2005). Teaching undergraduate research from a process perspective. *Journal of Nursing Education, 44*, 519-521.
Course incorporates clinical practicum as foundation for learning research concepts and process.

Azzarello, J., & Wood, D. E. (2006). Assessing dynamic mental models: Unfolding case studies. *Nurse Educator, 31*, 10-14.
Discusses how to use a general mental model versus a situational mental model in developing case studies for clinical learning.

Baldwin, K. B. (2007). Friday night in the pediatric emergency department: A simulated exercise to promote clinical reasoning in the classroom. *Nurse Educator, 32*, 24-29.
Discusses the use of clinical scenarios presented in the classroom to promote clinical decision making.

Ballard, P., & Trowbridge, C. (2004). Critical care experience for novice students: Reinforcing basic nursing skills. *Nurse Educator, 29*, 103-106.
Discusses how to match students' learning priorities with their practicum experiences.

Baltimore, J. (2004). The hospital clinical preceptor: Essential preparation for success. *Journal of Continuing Education in Nursing, 35*, 133-140.
Discusses the characteristics of preceptors as they orient new nurses. Same characteristics apply to preceptors with nursing students. Teaching strategies also included: name tents, brainstorming, skill instruction exercises, group discussion and sharing.

Bantz, D., Dancer, M. M., Hodson-Carlton, K., & Van Hove, S. (2007). A daylong clinical laboratory: From gaming to high-fidelity simulators. *Nurse Educator, 32*, 274-277.
Discusses how an entire clinical day can occur in a clinical lab setting and provides ideas for multiple stations.

Barn, L. (1996). Preceptorship: A review of the literature. *Journal of Advanced Nursing, 24*, 104-107.
Discusses the concept of preceptorship and findings in the literature.
Barnard, A., Nash, R., & O'Brien, M. (2005). Information literacy: Developing lifelong skills through nursing education. *Journal of Nursing Education, 44*, 505-510.
Discusses the use of information formats, teaching learning approaches, paradigm shift, collaboration with librarians.

Barnsteiner, J. H., Disch, J. M., Hall, L., Mayer, D., & Moore, S. M. (2007). Promoting interprofessional education. *Nursing Outlook, 55*, 144-150.
Discusses how nursing education needs to look at the concept of interprofessional education (IPE) and how to incorporate multiple disciplines in the overall educational process - facilitating the understanding of roles and teamwork.

Barrett, C., & Myrick, F. (1998). Job satisfaction in preceptorship and its effect on the clinical performance of the preceptee. *Journal of Advanced Nursing, 27*, 364-371.
Discusses a research study examining the relationship between the precteptor, preceptee job satisfaction, and clinical performance.

Bartlett, R., Bland, A., Rossen, E., Kautz, D., Benfield, S., & Carnevale, T. (2008). Evaluation of the outcome-present state test model as a way to teach clinical reasoning. *Journal of Nursing Education, 47*, 337-344.

> *Discusses the Outcome-Present State Test Model of Clinical Reasoning, which was designed to assist the student with clinical reasoning. The model was used with 43 students who demonstrated a significant difference in clinical reasoning before teaching the student the model and afterwards.*

Bartz, C., & Dean-Baar, S. (2003). Reshaping clinical nursing education: An academic-service partnership. *Journal of Professional Nursing, 19*, 216-222.

> *Discusses how service and academia partner to provide clinical education.*

Baxter, P. E., & Boblin, S. (2008). Decision making by baccalaureate nursing students in the clinical setting. *Journal of Nursing Education, 47*, 345-350.

> *Discusses the factors that influenced nursing students' decision making throughout a baccalaureate degree program. Nineteen students participated in the qualitative study and described five key types of decisions: assessment, intervention, resource, communication, and action.*

Baxter, P., & Rideout, E. (2006). Second-year baccalaureate nursing students' decision making in the clinical setting. *Journal of Nursing Education, 45*, 121-127.

> *Discusses how students determine need to make a clinical decision whether emotion-based or knowledge-based in response to clinical situations.*

Bearnson, C. S., & Wiker, K. M. (2005, September). Human patient simulators? A new face in baccalaureate nursing education at Brigham Young University. *Journal of Nursing Education, 44*, 421-425.

> *Discusses the benefits and limitations of using an HPS as patient substitute.*

Becker, C. (2004). Workforce Report 2004. Taking initiative on training. providers push expansion of nurse education. *Modern Healthcare, 34*(24), 26, 34.

> *Discusses how a regional hospital took the initiative on developing a partnership with a community college - resulting in simulation lab and clinical placements.*

Becker, K. L., Rose, L. W., Berg, J. B., Park, H., & Shatzer, J. H. (Apr 2006). The teaching effectiveness of standardized patients. *Journal of Nursing Education, 45*, 103-110.

> *Discusses a research study using standardized patients.*

Benner, P. (2004). Using the Dreyfus model of skill acquisition to describe and interpret skill acquisition and clinical judgment in nursing practice and education. *Bulletin of Science, Technology & Society, 24*, 188-199.

> *Examines the use of the Dreyfus model to understand the acquisition of skills.*

Bentley, R., & Ellison, K. J. (2005). Impact of a service-learning project on nursing students. *Nursing Education Perspectives, 26*, 287-290.

> *Discusses service learning in nursing clinicals.*

Berg, C. L., & Lindseth, G. (2004). Students' perspectives of effective and ineffective nursing instructors. *Journal of Nursing Education, 43*, 565-568.

> *Discusses a descriptive study that identified the characteristics of a quality classroom instructor.*

Berry, J. (2005). A student and RN partnered clinical experience. *Nurse Educator, 30*, 240-241.

> *Discusses a preceptor model developed to match student with preceptor, based on learning styles and personality inventories taken by preceptor and student. Results found greater immersion, increased socialization, and positive changes seen by all.*

Bess, J. (2005). Truer to life. *Hospitals & Health Networks, 79*(9), 22, 24.
  Discusses the use of a clinical information system in a simulation lab.

Bjork, I. T., & Kirkevold, M. (1999). Issues in nurses' practical skill development in the clinical setting. *Journal of Nursing Care Quality, 14*(1), 72-84.
  Discusses the development of practical nursing skills and their transfer to the actual clinical setting.

Blum, C. A. (2009). Development of a clinical preceptor model. *Nurse Educator, 34,* 29-33.
  Discusses a study with a purpose of creating a preceptor-guided practice education model.

Bosek, M. S., Li, S., & Hicks, F. D. (2007). Working with standardized patients: A primer. *International Journal of Nursing Education Scholarship, 4,* 1-12, Article 16.
  Discusses the use of standardized patients to teach and evaluate students in the clinical setting.

Botti, M., & Reeve, R. (2002). Role of knowledge and ability in student nurses' clinical decision-making. *Nursing & Health Sciences, 5,* 39-49.
  Discusses the acquisition of decision-making skills and how to measure them in the clinical setting.

Boutain, D. M. (2005). Social justice as a framework for professional nursing. *Journal of Nursing Education, 44,* 404-407.
  Discusses aspects of nursing education to incorporate social concepts into the educational process.

Boutain, D. M. (2008). Social justice as a framework for undergraduate community health clinical experiences in the United States. *International Journal of Nursing Education Scholarship, 5,* 1-23, Article 35.
  Discusses the use of a clinical evaluation tool that enables faculty and students to address the concept of social justice in the community setting.

Bradley, P., Bond, V., & Bradely, P. (2006). A questionnaire survey of students' perceptions of nurse tutor teaching in clinical skills learning program. *Medical Teacher, 28*(1), 49-52.
  Discusses a research study where nurses were used to teach skills to medical students.

Bradshaw, A. (1998). Defining "competency" in nursing (part II): An analytical review. *Journal of Clinical Nursing, 7,* 103-111.
  Discusses how clinical rotations/experiences assist in developing competence.

Bradshaw, M. J., & Woodring, B. (1999). Clinical pathways: A tool to evaluate clinical learning. *Journal of the Society of Pediatric Nurses, 4*(1), 37-40.
  Discusses how clinical pathways could be used to assist a student to objectively progress toward clinical outcomes.

Brancato, V. C. (2006). An innovative clinical practicum to teach evidence-based practice. *Nurse Educator, 31,* 195-199.
  Describes how one nursing program modified clinical rotations to include EBP as required components of the rotation.

Brasler, M. E. (1993). Predictors of clinical performance of new graduate nurses participating in preceptor orientation programs. *Journal of Continuing Education in Nursing, 24,* 158-165.
  Discusses how the current clinical model "prepares" students for clinical practice.

Bremmer, M. N., Aduddell, K., Bennett, D. N., & VanGeest, J. B. (2006). The use of human patient simulators: Best practices with novice nursing students. *Nurse Educator, 31*, 170-174.
Describes a qualitative/quantitative research study addressing the thoughts of students using HPS as a component of clinical experiences.

Brockopp, D., Hardin-Pierce, M., & Welsh, J., (2006). Educational innovation. An agency-financed capstone experience for graduating seniors. *Journal of Nursing Education, 45,* 137-40.
Discusses how agencies have an option in providing a stipend to a student during capstone experience, although this stipend is more often being offered as a scholarship and loan repayment contract if student works for facility.

Broussard, L. (2008). Simulation-based learning: How simulators help nurses improve clinical skills and preserve patient safety. *Nursing for Women's Health Care, 12*, 521-524.
Discusses how simulators are helping nursery nurses to improve their clinical skills and promote safety with their smallest patients.

Brown D., White J., & Leibbrandt, L. (2006). Collaborative partnerships for nursing faculties and health service providers: What can nursing learn from business literature? *Journal of Nursing Management, 14*, 170-179.
Discusses a study using business literature as basis for best practice guidelines. Characteristics of successful partnerships were identified as: definite; clear; valuable reason for collaboration; clear goals; high stakes; best possible participants; leadership; strong, balanced relationships; trust; respect; communication; formalized process.

Brown, G., Alpers, R. R., Jarrell, K., & Wotring, R. (2008). Decisions: Faculty versus students choice: Lessons learned from a community health clinical course. *Teaching and Learning in Nursing, 3*, 108-109.
Discusses a learner-centered approach to clinical education - allowing students to have a choice in community clinical placements. Challenges experienced: establishing and maintaining community partnerships and preceptor preparation; student investment of time, energy, and relationship building; and how to deal with a clinical site(s) not selected by students after negotiating student placement.

Cagle, C. S., Walker, C. A., & Newcomb, P. (2006). Using imaginative literature in clinical courses to improve student outcomes. *Journal of Theory Construction & Testing, 10*(1), 6-10.
Discusses the use of literature (books) to facilitate learning regarding cultural and ethical care in the clinical setting.

Cameron, C., Miller, F., McMillan, C., & Greco, M. (2006) Practice education facilitators-From theory to practice. *Journal of Community Nursing, 20*(4), 18-21.
Discusses the theory-practice gap and support mechanisms. (Scotland)

Campbell, S. E., & Dudley, K. (2005). Clinical partner model: Benefits for education and service. *Nurse Educator, 30*, 271-274.
Discusses the concept of clinical partners between education and service and sharing of resources; provides job descriptions for education and service for all partners involved with nursing education.

Campbell, S. L., Prater, M., Schwartz, C., & Ridenour, N. (2001). Building an empowering academic and practice partnership model. *Nursing Administration Quarterly, 26*(1), 35-44.
Discusses how one nursing program partnered with a hospital to provide an "empowered" clinical learning environment for both staff and students.

Cangelosi, P. R., (2004). A lack of qualified faculty: One school's solution. *Nurse Educator, 29*, 186-188.
 Discusses a faculty mentoring program developed for tenure-track faculty to combat the nursing shortage.

Casey, A. (2000). Nursing competencies for 2010. [Editorial]. *Paediatric Nursing, 12*(5), 3.
 Discusses the definition of professional and clinical competencies.

Castledine, G. (2006). Value of clinical teaching must be recognized. *British Journal of Nursing, 12*, 1355.
 Discusses the discrepancy between universities and clinical sites. (Scotland)

Challis, M. (2001). Building an effective programme for clinical teachers: The role of the staff developer. *Medical Teacher, 23*, 270-275.
 Discusses a variety of methods to enhance strategies for clinical teachers.

Chan, D. S. K. (2002). Association between student learning outcomes from their clinical placement and their perceptions of the social climate of the clinical learning environment. *International Journal of Nursing Studies, 39*, 517-524.
 Study looking at learning outcomes of students based upon site of placement.

Chan, S. W., & Wai-tong, C. (2000). Implementing contract learning in a clinical context: Report on a study. *Journal of Advanced Nursing, 31*, 298-305.
 Discusses the use of learning contracts in the clinical setting and the enhancement of autonomy and motivation of students. (Hong Kong)

Charleston, R., & Happell, B. (2004). Evaluating the impact of a preceptorship course on mental health nursing practice. International *Journal of Mental Health Nursing, 13*, 191-197.
 Discusses how a preceptorship in mental health clinical experiences was utilized to "recruit" new grads into the specialty area.

Charleston, R., & Happell, B. (2005a). Attempting to accomplish connectedness within the preceptorship experience: The perceptions of mental health nurses. *International Journal of Mental Health Nursing, 14*, 54-61.
 Discusses a research study to explore the experience of mental health preceptors and their relationships with students.

Charleston, R., & Happell, B. (2005b). Coping with uncertainty within the preceptorship experience: The perceptions of nursing students. *Journal of Psychiatric and Mental Health Nursing, 12*, 303-309.
 Discusses a research study addressing student perceptions of preceptors in mental health settings.

Charon, R. (2001). Narrative medicine: A model for empathy, reflection, profession, and trust. *Journal of the American Medical Association, 286*, 1897-1902.
 Discusses using literature and reflective writing to allow the examination of four central narrative situations: physician and patient; physician and self; physician and colleagues, and physician and society - all allowing growth regarding respect, empathy, and nourishing medical care.

Charron, S. A., & Parns, M. (2004). Promoting emotional wellness: Undergraduate clinical experiences in elementary schools. *Nurse Educator, 29*, 208-211.
 Discusses use of elementary school as site for mental health clinicals. Included are the program framework, project overview, outcomes and evaluation.

Childs, J. C., & Sepples, S. (2006). Clinical teaching by simulation: Lessons learned from a complex patient care scenario. *Nursing Education Perspectives, 27*, 154-158.
> *Discusses how to incorporate the use of the lab in learning complex patient situations and how to stage the various areas to promote progression.*

Cholowski, K. M., & Whan, L. K. S. (2004). Cognitive factors in student nurses' clinical problem solving. *Journal of Evaluation in Clinical Practice, 10*, 85-95.
> *Discusses a study evaluating students' clinical reasoning based on a model of motivational orientation, prior knowledge, diagnostic reasoning, and diagnostic solutions.*

Clarke, D., Davies, J., & McNee, P. (2002). The case of children's skills laboratory. *Paediatric Nursing, 14*(7), 36-39.
> *Discusses how clinical placement may impact a student's ability to achieve skills and thereby necessitating the need for labs. (Wales)*

Comer, S. K. (2005a). Clinical reasoning: Turning your students into clinical detectives. *Nurse Educator, 30*, 235-237.
> *Discusses a tool developed to assist nursing students in organizing and synthesizing their patients' clinical data.*

Comer, S. K. (2005b). Patient care simulations: Role playing to enhance clinical understanding. *Nursing Education Perspectives, 26*, 357-361.
> *Discusses how to develop an effective patient simulation in the lab using role playing.*

Conger, M. M., & Mezza, I. (1996). Fostering critical thinking in nursing students in the clinical setting. *Nurse Educator, 21*, 11-15.
> *Discusses how critical thinking can be developed in a clinical setting.*

Cox, L. S. (2002). Focused learning: 2 weeks of class - 2 weeks of clinical. *Nurse Educator, 27*, 15.
> *Discusses a new approach used by a nursing program - two weeks in class and then two weeks of clinical. The pilot in 1999 was very positive and became the underlying structure for the nursing program.*

Coyle-Rogers, P., & Putman, C. (2006). Using experiential learning: Facilitating hands-on basic patient skills. *Journal of Nursing Education, 45*, 142-143.
> *Discusses the concept of partnering students with Certified Nurse Assistants.*

Craik, R. L. (2008). Does clinical education need a series of tools to assess success? *Physcial Therapy, 88*, 1106-1108.
> *Discusses how physical therapists do not seem to consider the need to evaluate the outcome of clinical education experiences in the same way they have begun to quantify outcomes of clinical intervention - supports the need to develop a tool to assess clinical education.*

Davies, J., & Clarke, D. (2004). Clinical skills acquisition in children's nursing: An international perspective. *Paediatric Nursing, 16*(2), 23-26.
> *Discusses how clinical skills can be learned in a laboratory setting in adjunct to clinicals.*

DeLashmutt, M. B., & Rankin, E. A. (2005). A different kind of clinical experience: Poverty up close and personal. *Nurse Educator, 30*, 143-9.
> *Discusses students' experience of reality shock while caring for clients in poverty.*

Dieckhaus, K., Vontell, S., Pfeiffer, C., and Williams, A. (2005). The use of standardized patient encounters for evaluation of a clinical education program on the development of HIV/AIDS-related clinical skills. *Journal of HIV/AIDS and Social Services, 4*(2), 9-26.
> *Discusses the development and use of a "novel" evaluation tool to measure the development of HIV-specific clinical skills using Standardized Patient Encounters (SPEs).*

Diefenbeck, C. A., Plowfield, L. A., & Herrman, J. W. (2006). Clinical immersion: A residency model for nursing education. *Nursing Education Perspectives, 27*, 72-79.
> *Discusses how field experience, simulation lab, and work experience were used for clinical hours in a baccalaureate program. Students participated in varying experiences during the first three years with three days/week clinical practice during senior year.*

Dornan, T., Arno, M., Hadfield, J., Scherpbier, A., & Boshuizen, H. (2006). Student evaluation of the clinical curriculum in action. *Medical Education, 40*, 667-674.
> *Discusses a study examining the students' evaluations of the environment, process, and outcome of clinical learning in a medical program.*

Doubt, L., Paterson, M., & O'Riordan, A. (2004). Clinical education in private practice: An interdisciplinary project. *Journal of Allied Health, 33*(1), 47-50.
> *Discusses the use of a private practice arena for clinicals in multiple disciplines.*

Duffin, C. (2004). Simulated "skills labs" to ease pressure on training. *Nursing Standard, 18*(39), 7.
> *Discusses the use of "labs" to provide additional clinical time. (Great Britain)*

Dunn, S., & Burnett, P. (1995). The development of a clinical learning environment scale. *Journal of Advanced Nursing, 22*, 1166-1173.
> *Discusses an instrument used to assess clinical learning environment factors predictive of positive student learning outcomes. (Australia)*

Dunn, S.V., & Hansford, B. (1997). Undergraduate nursing student's perceptions of their clinical learning environment. *Journal of Advanced Nursing, 25*, 1299-1306.
> *Discusses a qualitative research study addressing how students view their clinical experiences; provides recommendations on how to make the experiences "better."*

Durak, H. I., Caliskan, S. A., Bor, S., & Van Der Vleuten, C. (2007). Use of case-based exams as an instructional teaching tool to teach clinical reasoning. *Medical Teacher, 29*, 170-174.
> *Discusses the strategic use of an assessment tool in the clinical setting.*

Edwards, M., Jones, S., & Murphy, F. (2007). Handheld video for clinical skills teaching. *Innovations in Education and Teaching International, 44*, 401-408.
> *Discusses how situations can be videoed in the clinical setting and then used in the classroom setting to teach.*

Ehrenberg, A. C., & Haggblom, M. (2007). Problem-based learning in clinical nursing education: Integrating theory and practice. *Nurse Education in Practice, 7*(2), 67-74.
> *Discusses a study using PBL and preceptors for clinical experiences and how this assisted in bridging the gap between theory and practice.*

Eide, P. J., Hahn, L., Bayne, T., Allen, C. B., & Swain, D. (2006). The population-focused analysis project for teaching community health. *Nursing Education Perspectives, 27*, 22-27.
> *Discusses how a clinical course can encompass community assessment, teaching, and meeting clinical objectives.*

Elisha, S. (2008). An educational curriculum used to improve the knowledge and the perceptions of certified registered nurse anesthetist clinical educators. *AANA Journal, 76,* 287-292.
> *Discusses a study looking at the effects of an 8-hour course had on modifying behavioral perceptions and knowledge of clinical educators.*

Epp, S. (2008). The value of reflective journaling in undergraduate nursing education: A literature review. *International Journal of Nursing Studies, 45,* 1379-1388.
> *Discusses a literature review on reflective journaling and its use in nursing education.*

Eriksen, H. M., Bergdahl, J., & Bergdahl, M. (2008). A patient-centered approach to teaching and learning in dental student clinical practice. *European Journal of Dental Education, 12,* 170-175.
> *Discusses how the treatment plan is based primarily on the patients' perceived needs and how students are trained to retrieve information from the patient in this context, with faculty serving as facilitators versus experts. (Norway)*

Errichetti, A., Gimpel, J., & Boulet, J. (2002). State of the art in standardized patient programs: A survey of osteopathic medical schools. *Journal of the American Osteopathic Association, 102,* 627-631.
> *Discusses how standardized patients are used for learning to: assess skills, develop knowledge base, and for evaluation. The overall goals were to ensure graduates have necessary outcomes, and have capability to "see" that they do.*

Faugier, J. (2005). Be proud of your skills. *Nursing Standard, 19*(25), 18-19.
> *Discusses skills essential for nurses and how these may be obtained.*

Fault, D. R., & Ternus, M. P. (2004). Strategies for teaching public policy in nursing: A creative approach. *Nurse Educator, 29,* 99-102.
> *Nursing education can be delivered through the use of technology and cyberspace. Nursing also needs to develop the voice to communicate their knowledge to others.*

Ferguson, S. (1996). The lived experience of clinical educators. *Journal of Advanced Nursing, 23,* 835-841.
> *Discusses a qualitative study looking at the role of clinical educators in nursing.*

Firth, J. (1986). Levels and sources of stress in medical students. *British Medical Journal, 92,* 1177-1180.
> *Discusses the stresses of clinical education.*

Fitzpatrick, J. J. (2006). [Editorial]. Blinking: The art of clinical judgment? *Nursing Education Perspectives, 27,* 5.
> *Discusses clinical judgment and art of nursing.*

Fletcher, M. (2005). Unique lab broadens education options. *The Canadian Nurse, 101,* 2, 10.
> *Discusses the use of the lab and its use in clinical education. (Canada)*

Fu-in, T., Shieu-ming, C., Hsien-hsien, C. (2005). Students' perceptions of effective and ineffective clinical instructors. *Journal of Nursing Education, 44,* 187-192.
> *Discusses a research study to determine the perceived differences between effective and ineffective clinical faculty. (Taiwan)*

Geller, A. C., Prout, M. N., Sun, T., Krane, R., Schroy, P. C., Demierre, M. F., et al. (2000). Cancer skill laboratories for medical students: A promising approach for cancer education. *Journal of Cancer Education, 15,* 196-199.
> *Discusses how specialized labs can facilitate skill acquisition for medical students.*

Gibbons, S. W., Adamo, G., Padden, D., Ricciardi, R., Graziano, M., Levine, E., et al. (2002). Clinical evaluation in advanced practice nursing education: Using standardized patients in health assessment. *Journal of Nursing Education, 41*, 215-222.
>   *Discusses how standardized patients can make an authentic clinical experience.*

Giddens, J. (2006). Comparing the frequency of physical examination techniques performed by associate and baccalaureate degree prepared nurses in clinical practice: Does education make a difference? *Journal of Nursing Education, 45*, 136-139.
>   *Discusses the impact of the educational level on the frequency of performing a physical assessment in the clinical setting.*

Gillespie, M. (2005). Student-teacher connection: A place of possibility. *Journal of Advanced Nursing, 52*, 211-219.
>   *Discusses the relationship between students and faculty and its potential impact on learning in a variety of settings - including clinical.*

Greiner, A., & Knebel, E. (Eds.). (2003). *Health professions education: A bridge to quality.* Washington, DC: Institute of Medicine, National Academies Press.
>   *Discusses the five characteristics that need to be part of all health care professionals education: interdisciplinary practice, technology, evidence-based practice, patient-centered care, quality improvement. (Chapter 3, p. 45).*

Griffin-Sobel, J. P. (2006). Nursing education in peril. *Clinical Journal of Oncology Nursing, 10*(3), 309.
>   *An editorial on how clinical instruction needs to change.*

Gubrud-Howe, P., & Schoessler, M. (2008). From random access opportunity to a clinical education curriculum. *Journal of Nursing Education, 47*, 3-4.
>   *Discusses a variety of learning models that can be utilized in clinical education.*

Hall-Long, B. (2004). Partners in action: A public health program for baccalaureate nursing students. *Family & Community Health, 27*, 338-345.
>   *Discusses the development of the partnership between the public health department and a nursing program.*

Hall-Long, B. A., Perez, G. B., & Allbright, P. K. (2001). A public health-academic education partnership. *Journal of Public Health Management Practice, 7*(1), 60-66.
>   *Discusses the needs assessment in the development of a formal partnership between service and academia.*

Halse, K., & Hage, A. M. (2006). An acute hospital ward, densely populated with students during a 12-week clinical study period. *Journal of Nursing Education, 45*, 133-136.
>   *Discusses peer learning, situated learning, different ways to organize clinical studies.*

Hansman, C. A., & Wilson, A. L. (1998, May 15-16). *Cognition and practice: Adult learning situated in everyday activity.* Paper presented at the 39th Annual Adult Education Research Conference Proceedings in San Antonio, TX.
>   *Discusses adult learners and the tools, activities and culture necessary for their learning.*

Happell, B. (1999a). Nurse education: Is it responding to the forces of supply and demand? *Nursing Economics, 17*, 252-256.
>   *Discusses a study that looked at the congruence between the areas of nursing that students found appealing and those areas where nurses were needed.*

Happell, B. (1999b). When I grow up I want to be a…? Where undergraduate student nurses want to work after graduation. *Journal of Advanced Nursing, 29*, 499-505.
Discusses a study investigating where students want to work upon graduation and the factors impacting their decision.

Happell, B. (2000). "Love is all you need"? Student nurses' interest in working with children. *Journal of the Society of Pediatric Nurses (JSPN), 5*, 167-173.
Discusses a study that was done to investigate the impact of student clinical experiences and their attitudes toward working with children upon graduation.

Happell, B., & Charleston, R. (2004). Good preceptorship: The way forward. *Australian Nursing Journal, 12*(3), 39.
Discusses the concept of preceptors. (Australia)

Hartigan-Rogers, J. A., Cobbett, S. L., Amirault, M. A., & Muise-Davis, M. E. (2007). Nursing graduates' perceptions of their undergraduate clinical placement. *International Journal of Nursing Education Scholarship, 4*, 1-12, Article 9.
Discusses a study that described third and fourth year nursing students' perception of their clinical placements and recommendations for future placements.

Haskvitz, L. M., & Koop, E. C. (2004). Students struggling in clinical? A new role for the patient simulator. *Journal of Nursing Education, 43*, 181-184.
Discusses how simulators can be used for remediation for clinicals.

Hayes, A. (2005). A mental health nursing clinical experience with hospice patients. *Nurse Educator, 30*, 85-88.
Discusses an eight-week clinical experience for students in mental health and describes how students felt their use of therapeutic communication improved, they were more empathetic and had a better understanding of death and dying.

Hayman-White, K. (2004). Positive experiences key to recruitment. Australian Nursing Journal, 12(3), 35.
Discusses how clinical experiences of students may be the key to recruiting future nurses. (Australia)

Henderson, A., Heel, A., & Twentyman, B. L. (2006). Pre-test and post-test evaluation of students' perceptions of a collaborative clinical education model on the learning environment. Australian *Journal of Advanced Nursing, 23*(4), 8-14.
Discusses a collaborative clinical education model and students' perception of learning environment. (Australia)

Henderson, A., Heel, A., & Twentyman, M. (2007). Enabling student placement through strategic partnerships between a health-care organization and tertiary institutions. *Journal of Nursing Management, 15*, 91-96.
Discusses the partnership that was established to facilitate student learning in clinical rotations.

Henneman, E. A., & Cunningham, H. (2005). Using clinical simulation to teach patient safety in an acute/critical care nursing course. *Nurse Educator, 30*, 172-178.
Discusses the process and method of developing and implementing high-fidelity simulation experiences for senior nursing students.

Hewlett, P. O., & Eichelberger, L. W. (1999). Creating academic/service partnerships through nursing competency models. *Journal of Nursing Education, 38*, 295-298.
Discusses how service and academia worked together to develop a clinical competency model.

Hill, C. M. (2006). Integrating clinical experiences into the concept mapping process. *Nurse Educator, 31*, 36-39.
>   *Discusses how students integrate clinical experiences into a concept map and how the map changes through the work with the client. Evaluation is in postconference with positive student feedback.*

Hill, K. S., & Walker, L. (2004). Partnerships pack recruitment power. *Nursing Management, 35*(12), 14.
>   *Discusses the partnership between academia and service - benefits for both.*

Hoffart, N., Diani, J. A., Connors, M., & Moynihan, P. (2006). Outcomes of cooperative education in a baccalaureate program in nursing. *Nursing Education Perspectives, 27*, 136-143.
>   *Discusses how cooperative education has been used in one school since 1964 and the research behind its success.*

Hofler, L. D. (2008). Nursing education and transition to the work environment: A synthesis of national reports. *Journal of Nursing Education, 47*, 5-12.
>   *Review and synthesis of reports from 1995-2005 responding to need of nursing profession to provide adequate number of nurses and assist students to transition from educational setting to workforce.*

Hoke, M. M. (1999). Community health nursing clinical specialists' views of graduate community health nursing competencies (Doctoral dissertation, New Mexico State University, Las Cruces). *ProQuest Dissertations and Theses*, AAT 9925886.
>   *Discusses a study addressing the clinical competencies needed by graduates of a master's program in community health.*

Hosoda, Y. (2006). Development and testing of a Clinical Learning Environment Diagnostic Inventory for baccalaureate nursing students. *Journal of Advanced Nursing, 56*, 480-490.
>   *Discusses the development of an instrument to assess the clinical learning environment in a clinical setting.*

Howard, E. P., & Steinberg, S. (2002). Evaluations of clinical learning in a managed care environment. *Nursing Forum, 37*(1), 12-20.
>   *A study that obtained evaluative data about the clinical learning experiences for graduate nursing students based on competency domains.*

Howard, V. B., & Tasota, F. J. (2004). How to spell relief for the nursing shortage: S-T-U-D-E-N-T-S. *Nursing, 34*(9), hn14-hn16
>   *Discusses how a positive clinical environment enriches learning and can aid in recruitment efforts.*

Hsu, L. L. (2000). A curriculum module for the improvement of clinical teaching in nursing education (Doctoral dissertation, Columbia University Teachers College, New York, NY). *ProQuest Dissertations and Theses*, AAT 3007538.
>   *Discusses the development and evaluation of a curriculum module for nurse educators to use to enhance the quality of their teaching in the clinical setting.*

Hughes, D. G. (2005). Teaching students in the classroom and clinical skills environment. *Nursing Standard, 19*(35), 41-47.
>   *Discusses how to develop a "lesson plan" for teaching clinical skills.*

Hutchings, A., Williamson, G. R., & Humphreys, A. (2005). Supporting learners in clinical practice: Capacity issues. *Journal of Clinical Nursing, 14*, 945-955.
>   *Discusses a study of the needs of students in the clinical setting to facilitate their learning. (Great Britain)*

Ironside, P. M. (2005). Teaching thinking and reaching the limits of memorization: Enacting new pedagogies. *Journal of Nursing Education, 44*, 441-448.
Discusses how to teach students the thinking that contemporary clinical situations require.

Issenberg, S. B., McGahie, W. C., Gordon, D. L., Symes, S., Petrusa, E. R., Hart, I.R., et al. (2002). Effectiveness of a cardiology review course for internal medicine residents using simulation technology and deliberate practice. *Teaching and Learning in Medicine, 14*, 223-228.
Discusses ways to improve the skills of medical students using simulation.

Jackson, D., & Mannix, J. (2001). Clinical nurses as teachers: Insights from students of nursing in their first semester of study. *Journal of Clinical Education, 10*, 270-277.
Discusses a study addressing insights about clinical nursing staff regarding the planned clinical experiences of students.

Jacobs, L. A. (2001). Interprofessional clinical education and practice. *Theory into Practice, 26*, 116-123.
Discusses how to develop a model of clinical education incorporating various health care professions (interprofessional).

Jacobson, L., & Grindel, C. (2006). [Headlines from the NLN]. What is happening in pre-licensure RN clinical nursing education? *Nursing Education Perspectives, 27*(2), 108-109.
Discusses the reform of basic nursing education that is needed.

James R. (2005). Reducing overcrowding on student practice placements. *Nursing Times, 101*(48), 28-32.
Discusses a framework used between a mental health institution and higher education to schedule increased numbers of nursing students for clinical rotations. (Great Britain).

Jeffries, P. (2001). Computer versus lecture: A comparison of two methods of teaching oral medication administration in a nursing skills laboratory. *Journal of Nursing Education, 40*, 323-329.
Discusses how skills can be taught in a variety of ways.

Jenkins, P., & Turick-Gibson, T. (1999). An exercise in critical thinking using role playing. *Nurse Educator, 24*, 11-14.
Discusses role playing in student learning about persons with diabetes and relays the steps involved in learning process, including positive student response.

Jerlock, M., & Severinsson, E. (2003). Academic nursing education guidelines: Tool for bridging the gap between theory, research, and practice. *Nursing and Health Sciences, 5*, 219-228.
Discusses a study describing the nursing competence expected of students and how to integrate theory and research with practice.

Junger, J., Schafer, S., Roth, C., Ben-David, M. F., & Nikendei, C. (2005). Effects of basic clinical skills training on objective structured clinical examination performance. *Medical Education, 39*, 1015-1020.
Discusses the research done to facilitate medical students' development of communication and clinical skills.

Kafel, K. W. (2008). Implementing quality and safety at the unit level in an innovative clinical education model. *NCSBN Leader to Leader, Fall.*
Discusses dedicated educational units being used in Massachusetts.

Kardong-Edgren, S. E., Starkweather, A. R., & Ward, L. D. (2008). The integration of simulation into a clinical foundations of nursing course: Student and faculty perspectives. *International Journal of Nursing Education Scholarship, 5*, 1-15, Article 26.
> *Discusses how one nursing program went about integrating simulation into a foundational clinical course - linking the scenario with didactic information, importance of debriefing, and the need for repetitive practice.*

Keels, C. L. (2004). Doctoring up the nursing profession: Several factors are contributing to the national nursing shortage, but initiatives, perceptions and college programs can nurture industry's growth. *Black Issues in Higher Education, 21*(20), 26-31.
> *Discusses the efforts to encourage African Americans to pursue nursing careers.*

Kelly, C. (2007). Students' perceptions of effective clinical teaching revisited. *Nurse Education Today, 27*, 885-892.
> *Discusses two studies addressing what teacher characteristics and contextual influences impact on students in clinical settings.*

Kelly, R. E. (2006). Engaging baccalaureate clinical faculty. *International Journal of Nursing Education Scholarship, 3*(1), 1-16, Article 14.
> *Discusses an instrument utilized to assess the roles of clinical educators.*

Kemsley, M., & Riegle, E. (2004). A community-campus partnership: Influenza prevention campaign. *Nurse Educator, 29*, 126-129.
> *Discusses how a school of nursing and community partnership fostered service learning and assisted graduate and undergraduate student learning.*

Kenny, A. (2002). Online learning: Enhancing nurse education? *Journal of Advanced Nursing, 38*, 127-135.
> *Discusses online learning and themes associated with use of this technology.*

Kinchin, I. M., Baysan, A., & Cabot, L. B. (2008). Towards a pedagogy for clinical education: Beyond individual learning differences. *Journal of Further and Higher Education, 32*, 373-387.
> *Discusses how teaching in higher education has moved toward a learner-oriented model, which has contributed to "tensions" within the overall system. The article supports moving towards an expertise model, which allows variation between complementary chains of practice and networks of understanding.*

Kirkham, S. R., Harwood, C. H., & Van Hofwegen, L. (2005). Capturing a vision for nursing: Undergraduate nursing students in alternative clinical settings. *Nurse Educator, 30*, 263-270.
> *Discusses several alternative clinical sites and the research conducted on the quality of clinical education for nursing students. (Canada)*

Kirkpatrick, H., Byrne, C., Martin, M. L., & Roth, M. L. (1991). A collaborative model for the clinical education of baccalaureate nursing students. *Journal of Advanced Nursing, 16*, 101-107.
> *Discusses how collaboration between practice and education in nursing provides a schematic of the student learning environment, and the benefits as well as problems with collaboration.*

Kline, K. S., & Hodges, J. (2006). A rational approach to solving the problem of competition for undergraduate clinical sites. *Nursing Education Perspectives, 27*, 80-83.
> *Discusses clinical placement consortium and partnership in site selection.*

Kosir, M. A., Fuller, L., Tyburski, J., Berant, L., & Yu, M. (2008). The Kolb learning cycle in American Board of Surgery In-Training Exam remediation: The Accelerated Clinical Education in Surgery course. *American Journal of Surgery, 196*(5), 657-662.
Discusses how using the Kolb cycle facilitated learning in surgical students who had previously failed.

Krautscheid, L., Kaakinen, J., & Warner, J. R. (2008). Clinical faculty development: Using simulation to demonstrate and practice clinical teaching. *Journal of Nursing Education, 47*, 431-433.
Discusses how simulation can be utilized in the orientation of new clinical faculty to prepare and support them for their teaching roles in the clinical setting.

Kuiper, R. A. (2005). Self-regulated learning during clinical preceptorship. *Nursing Education Perspectives, 26*, 351-356.
Discusses the self-regulated learning model, a research study, and how it could be used in clinical nursing education.

Kyrkjebo, J. M. (2006). Teaching quality improvement in the classroom and clinic: Getting it wrong and getting it right. *Journal of Nursing Education, 45*, 109-116.
Discusses how to improve quality of care while learning care

Ladyshewsky, R. K. (2000). Peer-assisted learning in clinical education: A review of terms and learning principles. *Journal of Physical Therapy Education, 14*(2), 15-22.
Discusses how cooperative learning was used in clinical with PT students.

Laitinen-Väänänen, S., Talvitie, U., & Luukka, M.-R. (2007). Clinical supervision as an interaction between the clinical educator and the student. *Physiotherapy Theory and Practice, 23*(2), 95-103.
Discusses a study reviewing the interaction between clinical educators and students during supervised learning treatment sessions. (Finland)

Lambert, V., & Glacken, M. (2005). Clinical education facilitators: A literature review. *Journal of Clinical Nursing, 14*, 664-73.
Discusses the conflicting demands for those educating students and the gap as to who has prime responsibility for clinical teaching. Suggestions are made on how to correct this situation. (Ireland)

Larew, C., Lessans, S., Spunt, D., Foster, D., & Covington, B. G. (2006). Innovations in clinical simulation: Application of Benner's theory in an interactive patient care simulation. *Nursing Education Perspectives, 27*, 16-21.
Discusses the development of a clinical scenario used in the clinical lab to engage students in the learning process incorporating "clinical" components.

Lasater, K., Luce, L., Yolpin, M., Terwilliger, A., & Wold, J. (2007). When it works: Learning community health nursing concepts from clinical experience. *Nursing Education Perspectives, 28*, 88-92.
Discusses how one nursing program combined mental health and community clinicals to meet competencies.

Laschinger, S., Medves, J., Pulling, C., McGraw, R., Waytuck, B., Harrison, M.B., et al. (2008). Effectiveness of simulation on health profession students' knowledge, skills, confidence and satisfaction. *International Journal of Evidence-Based Healthcare, 6*, 278-302.
Discusses a review (1995-2006) to identify the best available evidence on the effectiveness of using simulated learning experiences in pre-licensure health professions education.

Lashley, M. (2005). Teaching health assessment in the virtual classroom. *Journal of Nursing Education, 44*, 348-350.
> *Discusses how health assessment skills can be taught outside a traditional clinical/lab setting.*

Lauder, W., Reynolds, W., & Angus, N. (1999). Transfer of knowledge and skills: Some implications for nursing and nurse education. *Nurse Education Today, 19*, 480-487.
> *Discusses the challenges students have in transferring skills from the lab to the clinical setting.*

Lee, D. T. F. (1996). The clinical role of the nurse teacher: A review of the dispute. *Journal of Advanced Nursing, 23*, 1127-1134.
> *Discusses the controversies regarding the role of nurse educators, especially in the clinical setting.*

Lee-Hsieh, J., Kuo, C. L., & Tseng, H. F. (2005). Application and evaluation of a caring code in clinical nursing education. *Journal of Nursing Education, 44*, 177-184.
> *Discusses how to teach caring in the clinical environment and the research regarding the use of a caring code.*

Lehmann, S. & Brighton, V. (2005). The clinical orientation manual: A student/preceptor educational resource. *Nurse Educator, 30*, 47-49.
> *Discusses how to orient students and preceptors to their roles.*

Leners, D., Sitzman, K., & Hessler, K. L. (2006). Perceptions of nursing student clinical placement experiences. *International Journal of Nursing Education Scholarship, 3*(1), 1-17, Article 24.
> *Discusses a qualitative study investigating the clinical placement of students and the participants involved.*

Leung, G. M., Johnston, M., Tin, K. Y. K., & Wong, O. L. (2003). Randomized controlled trial of clinical decision support tools to improve learning of evidence-based medicine in medical students. British *Medical Journal, 327*, 1090-1093.
> *Discusses the use of a handheld computer support tool and pocket card during clinical experiences. (Great Britain)*

Levett-Jones, T. (2004). Clinical assessment increases confidence. *Australian Nursing Journal, 12*(5), 31.
> *Discusses the development of a one-day assessment, observed by "specially trained assessors," of how nursing students do in the clinical setting. (Australia)*

Leyshon, S. (2005). Making the most of teams in the mentorship of students. *British Journal of Community Nursing, 10* (1), 21-23.
> *Discusses the use of a mentorship model, using mentoring teams to provide clinical education. (Great Britain)*

Ligeikis-Clayton, C., & Denman, J. (2005). Service learning across the curriculum. *Nurse Educator, 30*, 191-192 .
> *Discusses a model for service learning beginning with first semester in community college program that had positive outcomes: enhancement of personal and civic responsibilities, critical reflective practice, health promotion, teaching, and one-on-one client care.*

Lindh, I. B., Severinsson, E., & Berg, A. (2008). Exploring student nurses' reflections on moral responsibility in practice. *Reflective Practice, 9*, 437-448.
> *Discusses a small qualitative study to gain an understanding of students' perception of moral responsibility in the clinical setting. (Norway & Sweden)*

Lingard, L., Reznick, R., DeVito, I., & Espin, S. (2002). Forming professional identities on the health care team: Discursive constructions on the "other" in the operating room. *Medical Education, 36*, 728-734.
> *Discusses the concept of interprofessional groups and how clinicals provide opportunities to develop professional identities.*

Little, M. A., & Milliken, P. J. (2007). Practicing what we preach: Balancing teaching and clinical practice competencies. *International Journal of Nursing Education Scholarship, 4*(1), 1-14, Article 6.
> *Discusses the challenge that nursing faculty have of maintaining both clinical and teaching competencies.*

Lofmark, A., & Thorell-Ekstrand, I. (2000). Evaluation by nurses and students of a new assessment form for clinical nursing education. *Scandinavian Journal of Caring Science, 14*, 89-96.
> *Discusses the development of a clinical evaluation tool based on higher education regulation and international guidelines regardless of the level of the program or clinical specialty. (Sweden)*

Lopez, V. (2002). Clinical teachers as caring mothers from the perspectives of Jordanian nursing students. *International Journal of Nursing Studies, 40*, 51-60.
> *Discusses a qualitative study looking at the attributes of nursing clinical faculty. (Jordan)*

Lundberg, K. M. (2008). Promoting self-confidence in clinical nursing students. *Nurse Educator, 33*, 86-89.
> *Discusses how clinical faculty can instill confidence in students - strategies and teaching behaviors.*

Lundy, K. (1999). Developing clinical learning sites for undergraduate nursing students. *AORN Journal, 70*(1), 64-71.
> *Discusses how students can have input into their clinical sites.*

Lusk, J., Winne, M., & DeLeskey, K. (2007). Nurses' perceptions of working with students in the clinical setting. *Nurse Educator, 32*, 102-103.
> *Discusses a study looking at the impact of an increased number of nursing students in the clinical setting and the use of preceptors.*

Mallette, S., Loury, S., Engelke, M., & Andrews, A. (2005). The integrative clinical preceptor model: A new method for teaching undergraduate community health nursing. *Nurse Educator, 30*, 21-26.
> *Discusses a cooperative model with clinical faculty, preceptor and students in the clinical setting that had several positive outcomes: community project, interactive clinical seminar, and reflective clinical journal; found increased interactivity among members of group and better rapport, and the faculty became a resource to preceptor.*

Mamchur, C., & Myrick, F. (2003). Preceptorship and interpersonal conflict: A multidisciplinary study. *Journal of Advanced Nursing, 43*, 188-196.
> *Discusses pros and cons of a preceptorship model in clinical education.*

Martin, T., & Happell, B. (2001). Undergraduate nursing students' views of mental health nursing in the forensic environment. *Australian and New Zealand Journal of Mental Health Nursing, 10*, 116-125.
> *Discusses the evaluation of clinical placements. (Australia/New Zealand)*

Mason, S. R., & Ellershaw, J. E. (2008). Preparing for palliative medicine; evaluation of an education programme for fourth year medical undergraduates. *Palliative Medicine, 22*, 687-692.
> *Discusses a study to determine how prepared medical students were to practice palliative care and their overall attitudes toward care. (Great Britain)*

Matsumura, G., Callister, L. C., Palmer, S., Cox, A. H., & Larsen, L. (2004). Staff nurse perceptions of the contributions of students to clinical agencies. *Nursing Education Perspectives, 25,* 297-303.
> *Discusses the perceived benefits of having students on clinical units and the perceptions of the students themselves.*

Mayne, W., Jootun, D., Young, B., Marland, G., Harris, M., & Lyttle, P. (2004). Enabling students to develop confidence in basic clinical skills. *Nursing Times, 100*(24), 36-39.
> *Discusses how one nursing program used a skills lab to guarantee development of "common foundational" skills to assist when there was an increased number of students in clinical setting.*

McAllister, L., Higgs, J., & Smith, D. (2008). Facing and managing dilemmas as a clinical educator. *Higher Education Research & Development, 27*(1), 1-13.
> *Discusses a qualitative study that sought to increase the understanding and appreciation of the roles and responsibilities of being a clinical educator in speech pathology. The results have potential implications for the preparation and professional development of clinical educators, especially concerning the complexity, challenges, and dilemmas inherent in the role.*

McAllister, M., Tower, M., & Walker, R. (2007). Gentle interruptions: Transformative approaches to clinical teaching. *Journal of Nursing Education, 46,* 304-312.
> *Discusses the concept of transformative learning and how it can be utilized in the clinical setting.*

McCallum, C. (2004). Clinical education in a nursing home setting: A structured framework for student learning. *International Journal of Therapy and Rehabilitation, 11,* 374-380.
> *Discusses how nursing homes can serve the needs of PT students in three areas: clinical experiences, administrative experiences, and research experiences.*

McCartney, P., & Morin, K., (2005). Where is the evidence for teaching methods used in nursing education? *American Journal of Maternal Child Nursing, 30,* 406-412.
> *There does not appear to be well documented research on traditional clinical nursing education methods.*

McDonough, J. P., & Osterbrink, J. (2005). Learning styles: An issue in clinical education? *AANA Journal, 73*(2), 89-93.
> *Discusses whether the learning style of anesthesia students plays a role in their success clinically.*

McLean, M. (2006). Clinical role models are important in the early years of a problem-based learning curriculum. *Medical Teacher, 28,* 64-69.
> *Discusses a study addressing role models identified by students in a traditional medical program.*

McManus, E. S., & Sieler, P. A. (1998). Freedom to enjoy learning in the 21st century: Developing an active learning culture in nursing. *Nurse Education Today, 18,* 322-328.
> *Discusses an active learning approach and its application to nursing education. (Great Britain)*

McNamara, S. A. (2006). Perioperative nursing in nursing school curricula. *Association of Operating Room Nurses (AORN) Journal, 83,* 301-304.
> *Discusses clinical experience in perioperative areas.*

Medley, C. F., & Horne, C. (2005). Using simulation technology for undergraduate nursing education. *Journal of Nursing Education, 44,* 31-34.
> *Discusses how simulation can be used as clinical time.*

Memshick, M. T., & Shepard, K. F. (1996). Physical therapy clinical education in a 2:1 student-instructor education model. *Physical Therapy, 76*, 968-981.
Discusses 2:1 model and provides a conceptual framework of clinical educational experiences.

Miller, J., Shaw-Kokot, J. R., Arnold, M. S., Boggin, T., Crowell, K. E., Allegri, F., et al. (2005). A study of personal digital assistants to enhance undergraduate clinical nursing education. *Journal of Nursing Education, 44*, 19-26.
Information-seeking behaviors; incorporation of PDAs into practice.

Mogensen, E., Elinder, G., Widstrom, A. M., & Winbladh, B. (2002). Centres for clinical education (CCE): Developing the health care education of tomorrow - A preliminary report. *Education for Health, 15*(1), 10-18.
Discusses the development of centers designed to address both community health needs and educational opportunities for health care profession students.

Moran, R. (2005). Enriching clinical learning experiences in community health nursing through the use of discussion boards. *International Journal of Nursing Education Scholarship, 2*(1), 1-13, Article 23.
Discusses a constructivist approach to learning, namely, that an Internet-based discussion board can be used to support the reflection and dialogue of registered nurse students in a community health course.

Morgan, P. J., Cleave-Hogg, D., Desousa, S., & Lam-McCulloch, J. (2006). Applying theory to practice in undergraduate education using high fidelity simulation. *Medical Teacher, 28*, 10-15.
Discusses the use of a high fidelity simulation lab for anesthesia students.

Morris, J. (2006). Audit of use of a common undergraduate physiotherapy clinical assessment form. *International Journal of Therapy and Rehabilitation, 13*, 407-413.
Discusses a means of assessing students' performance in the clinical setting.

Morton, N. (2005). Medication evaluation teaching strategy. *Journal of Nursing Education, 44*, 575-576.
Discusses how to evaluate teaching strategies used for administering medications; effects of large classes, and prerequisite courses.

Moscato, S. R., Miller, J., Logsdon, K., & Weinburg, S. (2007). Dedicated education unit: An innovative clinical partner education model. *Nursing Outlook, 55*, 31-37.
Discusses the concept of a clinical unit dedicated to clinical education and the partnership between the facility and academia. (Great Britain)

Mossop, M., & Wilkinson, T. (2006). Nursing education in gerontological clinical settings. *Journal of Gerontological Nursing, 32*(6), 49-56.
Discusses the concepts of ethics, pace, and undervaluing special knowledge and skills found in a gerontological clinical setting.

Mullen, A., & Murray, L. (2002). Clinical placements in mental health: Are clinicians doing enough for undergraduate nursing students? *International Journal of Mental Health Nursing, 11*, 61-68.
Discusses an innovative student program designed and implemented by clinicians who were committed to providing a quality clinical placement for students.

Murphy, F. A. (2000). Collaborating with practitioners in teaching and research: A model for developing the role of the nurse lecturer in practice areas. *Journal of Advanced Nursing, 31*, 704-714.
Discusses a model to develop the clinical role of a lecturer.

Murray, T. A. (2007). Expanding educational capacity through an innovative practice education partnership. *Journal of Nursing Education, 46*, 330-334.

Discusses how additional students were educated based upon a practice/academia partnership.

Myrick, F., & Tamlyn, D. (2007). Teaching can never be innocent: Fostering an enlightening educational experience. *Journal of Nursing Education, 46*, 299-303.

Discusses the complexities and subtle incongruities in teachers' intentions and practice in teaching students critical thinking.

Myrick, F., & Yonge, O. (2004). Enhancing critical thinking in the preceptorship experience in nursing education. *Journal of Advanced Nursing 45*, 371-380.

Discusses a study to examine the preceptor experience and its role in the enhancement of critical thinking in graduate education.

Napthine, R. (1996). Clinical education: A system under a pressure. *Australian Nursing Journal, 3*(9), 20-25.

Discusses how clinical education "completes the education begun in the classrooms and laboratories," provides examples of what "A good clinical educator must...", and notes the principles of good quality clinical education. (Australia)

Niedringhaus, L. K. (2001). Using student writing assignments to assess critical thinking skills: A holistic approach. *Holistic Nursing Practice, 15*(3), 9-17.

Discusses how one program developed a variety of assessment tools for critical thinking that included appropriateness of clinical interventions.

Novak, R. E. (2006). Challenges to our professions over the next 10 years: New models for professional education (Part II). *American Speech-Language-Hearing Association Leader, 11*(2), 6-11.

Discusses models used in speech-language pathology and the need for change.

Nugent, L. L. B. (1992). Factors influencing implementation of innovations in clinical nursing education (Doctoral dissertation, University of Arizona, Tucson). *ProQuest Dissertations and Theses,* AAT 9225183.

Discusses a study that assessed whether ADN programs were using innovations in the clinical curricula; most had implemented changes that are currently being used in today's clinical education - 15 years later.

Oermann, M. (2008). Ideas for postclinical conferences. *Teaching and Learning in Nursing, 3*, 90-93.

Discusses guidelines for nursing faculty in planning postclinical conferences, with various types described.

Ogilvie, L. D., Paul, P., & Burgess-Pinto, E. (2007). International dimensions of higher education in nursing in Canada: Tapping the wisdom of the 20th century while embracing possibilities for the 21st century. *International Journal of Nursing Education Scholarship, 4*(1), 1-32, Article 7.

Discusses how knowledge from the 20th century can be used to generate current international initiatives regarding nursing education. (Canada)

Olesinski, R. L. (1998). From student laboratory to clinical environment. *Clinical Laboratory Science, 11*(3), 167-173.

Discusses how a 6-hour "shift" could be simulated for Clinical Laboratory Sciences program outside the hospital setting.

Palmer, S. P., Cox, A. H., Callister, L. C., Johnsen, V., & Matsumura, G. (2005). Nursing education and service collaboration: Making a difference in the clinical learning environment. *Journal of Continuing Education in Nursing, 36,* 271-276.

> *Discusses the relationship between academia and service, and provides practical suggestions and steps to improve relationship between academia and service.*

Parkes, R. (1995). Educating for the future. *Australian Nursing Journal, 2*(7), 22-27.

> *Discusses the 12 principles of good quality clinical education. (Australia)*

Parish, C. (2000). Brighton flock...a one-year common foundation programme and longer continuous placements. *Nursing Standard, 15*(9), 14-15.

> *Discusses the benefits of students who stay in same hospital setting and share common early portion of nursing education. (Great Britain)*

Paterson, B. L. (2003). Learning from each other: Critics have suggested hospital-based nursing education relies too much on skill acquisition without theory. *Canadian Nurse, 99*(2), 23-26.

> *Discusses how changes in theory and clinical will involve all stakeholders. (Canada)*

Pharez, M. E., Walls, N. D., Roussel, L. A., & Broome, B. A. (2008). Combining creativity and community partnership in mental health clinical experiences. *Nursing Education Perspectives, 29,* 100-104.

> *Discusses practical and creative ways to approach mental health clinicals from a nontraditional approach.*

Pollard, H. P. (2004). Supporting clinical skills developments. *Nursing Standard, 18*(35), 31-36.

> *Discusses the development of centers (labs) to teach clinical skills to nurses and physicians. (Great Britain)*

Ponzer, S., Hylin, U., Kusoffsky, A., Lauffs, M., Lonka, K., Mattisson, A. C., et al. (2004). Interprofessional training in the context of clinical practice: Goals and students' perceptions on clinical education wards. *Medical Education, 38,* 727-736.

> *Discusses the model of training two or more professions associated with health or social care together - interdisciplinary courses with a clinical component.*

Porter, J., & Baker, E. L. (2005). The management moment: Partnering essentials. *Journal of Public Health Management Practice, 11,* 174-177.

> *Discusses the essential elements needed in an effective partnership between sites - hospitals, community, academia.*

Preheim, G., Casey, K., & Krugman, M. (2006). Clinical scholar model: Providing excellence in clinical supervision of nursing students. *Journal for Nurses in Staff Development, 22*(1), 15-20.

> *Discusses clinical scholars partnership with school of nursing educators.*

Prince K., Boshuizen, H., van der Vleuten, C., & Scherpbier, A. (2005). Students' opinions about their preparation for clinical practice. *Medical Education, 39,* 704-712.

> *Discusses how students feel they are prepared for clinical experiences. (Netherlands)*

Purcell, C. (2006). Commentary on clinical education facilitators: A literature review. *Journal of Clinical Nursing, 15,* 647-648.

> *Provides comments on the need for the development of clinical nursing skills - see article by Lambert & Glacken, which this article makes comments about. (Great Britain)*

Radcliffe, C., & Lester, H. (2003). Perceived stress during undergraduate medical training: A qualitative study. *Medical Education, 37*, 32-8.
   Discusses the stressful nature of transition in the clinical setting. (Great Britain)

Radhakrishnan, K., Roche, J. P., & Cunningham, H. (2007). Measuring clinical practice parameters with human patient simulation: A pilot study. *International Journal of Nursing Education Scholarship, 4*(1), 1-11, Article 8.
   Discusses a quasi-experimental pilot study designed to evaluate the effects of simulation on clinical performance.

Ranse, K., & Grealish, L. (2007). Nursing students perceptions of learning in the clinical setting of the dedicated education unit. *Journal of Advanced Nursing, 58*, 171-179.
   Research study to explore the nursing students' experiences on a dedicated educational unit for clinical practice.

Redding, S. R., & Graham, P. (2006). Promoting an active clinical learning environment for associate degree nursing students. *Nurse Educator, 31*, 175-177.
   Discusses how one nursing program developed a positive learning environment in the clinical settings.

Reising, D. L., Shea, R. A., Allen, P. N., Laux, M. M., Hensel, D., & Watts, P. A. (2008). Using service-learning to develop health promotion and research skills in nursing students. *International Journal of Nursing Education Scholarship, 5*, 1-15, Article 29.
   Discusses how service learning can be used in a community clinical course and meet the health promotion needs of the community.

Rice, R. (2003). Collaboration as a tool for resolving the nursing shortage. *Journal of Nursing Education, 42*, 147-148.
   Discusses the Colleagues in Caring (CIC) project promoting articulation from educational setting to work environment and how it has improved the competencies at all levels of nursing education.

Richardson, L., Resnick, L., Leonardo, M., & Pearsall, C. (2009). Undergraduate students as standardized patients to assess advanced practice nursing student competencies. *Nurse Educator, 34*, 12-16.
   Discusses the use of undergraduate nursing students as standardized patients for graduate advanced practice nursing students - primarily for a distance education program.

Ridely, R. T. (2004). Creative collaborative clinical quickies. *Nurse Educator, 29*, 135-136.
   Discusses several short learning activities to use in a maternal child clinical setting during those "slow periods" of clinical.

Roberts, D. (2008). Commentary on Secomb, J.: A systematic review of peer teaching and learning in clinical education. *Journal of Clinical Nursing, 17*(20), 2793-2794.
   Discusses the author's views on the article by Secomb and the fact the article only discussed "formal" peer teaching while there are "informal" elements that are also important.

Rose, S. R. (2008). The utilization and role of the preceptor in undergraduate nursing programs. *Teaching and Learning in Nursing, 3*, 105-107.
   Discusses the concept of preceptors: their role and necessary guidance for a successful preceptor experience.

Rowe, M. M., & Sherlock, H. (2005). Stress and verbal abuse in nursing: Do burned out nurses eat their young? *Journal of Nursing Management, 13*, 242-248.
Discusses how negative clinical staff can be toward nursing students in their clinical rotations.

Ryan-Nicholls, K. D. (2004). Preceptor recruitment and retention. *Canadian Nurse, 100*(6), 18-22.
Discusses the clinical teaching associate model and the use of preceptors. (Canada)

Saarikoski, M., Isoaho, H., Leino-Kilpi, H., & Warne, T. (2005). Validation of the clinical learning environment and supervision scale. *International Journal of Nursing Education Scholarship, 2*(1), 1-16, Article 9.
Discusses a study to validate a research instrument to evaluate the quality of the clinical learning environment and the supervision given to nursing students by qualified staff nurses.

Salyers, V. L. (2007). Teaching psychomotor skills to beginning nursing students using a web-enhanced approach: A quasi-experimental study. *International Journal of Nursing Education Scholarship, 4*(1), 1-12, Article 11.
Discusses a study that looked at the mode for teaching psychomotor skills.

Schaffer, M. A., Nelson, P., & Litt, E. (2005). Using portfolios to evaluate achievement of population-based public health nursing competencies in baccalaureate nursing students. *Nursing Education Perspectives, 26*, 104-112.
Discusses how clinical competencies can be measured using portfolios in the community setting.

Scherer, Y. K., Bruce, S. A., & Runkawatt, V. (2007). A comparison of clinical simulation and case study presentation on nurse practitioner students' knowledge and confidence in managing a cardiac event. *International Journal of Nursing Education Scholarship, 4*(1), 1-14, Article 22.
Discusses a study that compared case studies versus simulation in students' knowledge and confidence in managing a cardiac event.

Schlenker, E. C., & Kerber, C. H. S. (2006). The CARE case study method for teaching community health nursing. *Journal of Nursing Education, 45*, 144.
Discusses methods to stimulate critical thinking and apply theory to practice.

Schmidt, L. (2007). Camp nursing: Innovative opportunities for nursing students to work with children. *Nurse Educator, 32*, 246-250.
Discusses alternative clinical site for pediatrics.

Schoenfelder, D. P., & Valde, J. G. (2009). Creative practicum leadership experiences in rural settings. *Nurse Educator, 34*, 38-42.
Discusses the development, implementation, and evaluation of a rural clinical leadership practicum in a prelicensure course.

Schuster, P. M. (2000). Reducing clinical care plan paperwork and increasing learning. *Nurse Educator, 25*, 76-81.
Discusses ways to maximize clinical learning.

Scott, S. D. (2008). "New professionalism" - Shifting relationships between nursing education and nursing practice. *Nurse Education Today, 28*, 240-245.
Discusses the challenges currently experienced in nursing education and the potential impact of service-education partnerships.

Secomb, J. (2008). A systematic review of peer teaching and learning in clinical education. *Journal of Clinical Nursing, 17*, 703-716.

Discusses a review of the literature and the effectiveness of using peers to teach in the clinical setting.

Seibert, D. C., Guthrie, J. T., & Adamo, G. (2004). Improving learning outcomes: Integration of standardized patients and telemedicine technology. *Nursing Education Perspectives, 25*, 232-237.

Discusses a study examining the relationship between technology-based strategies and the improvement of knowledge outcomes and competencies.

Sevean, P. A., Poole, K., & Strickland, D. S. (2005). Actualizing scholarship in senior baccalaureate nursing students. *Journal of Nursing Education, 44*, 473-476.

Discusses the concept of clinical scholarship and means to operationalize this in the clinical setting.

Shawler, C. (2008). Standardized patients: A creative teaching strategy for psychiatric-mental health nurse practitioner students. *Journal of Nursing Education, 47*, 528-531.

Discusses a learning strategy to use in psychiatric-mental health clinical settings and the students' experiences with standardized patients.

Shayne, P., Hellpern, K., Andoer, D., & Palmer-Smith, V. (2002). Protected clinical teaching time and a bedside clinical evaluation instrument in an emergency medicine training program. *Academic Emergency Medicine, 9*, 1342-1349.

Discusses graduate medical education, clinical skills, teaching, clinical competency, emergency medicine, and residents.

Singleton, J., & Levin, R. (2008). Strategies for learning evidence-based pratice: Critically appraising clinical practice guidelines. *Journal of Nursing Education, 47*, 380-383.

Discusses a teaching-learning strategy to help students learn how to critically appraise clinical practice guidelines using a specific instrument.

Siuk H. M., Laschinger, H. K. S., & Vingilis, E. (2005). The effect of problem-based learning on nursing students' perceptions of empowerment. *Journal of Nursing Education, 44*, 459-469.

Discusses Kanter's structural empowerment theory, structural and psychological empowerment, and their impact on learning.

Sizer, S. (2001). Reality check…student placements. *Nursing Standard, 15*(50), 14-15.

Discusses an exchange experience comparing the U.S. and British clinical systems. U.S. nurses felt a need for faculty to be present so they could concentrate on patient care. (Great Britain)

Skhal, K. J. (2008). A full revolution: Offering 360 degree library services to clinical clerkship students. *Medical Reference Services Quarterly, 27*, 249-259.

Discusses the positive effects of having a librarian on the clinical team to assist medical students/ residents find answers quickly.

Smee, S. (2003). Skill based assessment. *British Medical Journal, 326*, 703-706.

Describes the use of an oral examination and "long case" to assess clinical competence. Interaction with the patient is not directly observed. (Great Britain)

Snyder, M. D., Fitzloff, B. M., Fiedler, R., & Lambke, M. R. (2000). Preparing nursing students for contemporary practice: Restructuring the psychomotor skills laboratory. *Journal of Nursing Education, 39*, 229-230.

Discusses how educators need to "prepare the learner with knowledge and technical skills mitigated with flexibility, creativity, and active involvement."

Sorenson, D., & Dieter, C. (2005). From beginning to end: Video-based introductory, instructional, and evaluation applications. *Nurse Educator, 30*, 40-43.
   Discusses how videos are incorporated into distance education courses to identify students who need remediation.

Sowan, N. A., Moffatt, S. G., & Canales, M. K. (2004). Creating a mentoring partnership model: A university-department of health experience. *Family & Community Health, 27*, 326-337.
   Discusses the model developed between a university and the State Health Department to increase the number of students rotating to their sites for clinical experiences.

Sowers, J., & Smith, M. R. (2004). Evaluation of the effects of an inservice training program on nursing faculty members' perceptions, knowledge, and concerns about students with disabilities. *Journal of Nursing Education, 43*, 248-252.
   Discusses students with disabilities, patient safety concerns, and clinical/academic standards.

Speziale, H. J. S., & Jacobson, L. (2005). Trends in registered nurse education programs 1998-2008. *Nursing Education Perspectives, 26*, 230-235.
   Discusses the last ten years in nursing education - classroom and clinical.

Stevens, R. H., & Roper, W. L. (2004). The North Carolina experiment: Academia-practice partnerships. *Journal of Public Health Management Practice, 10*, 316-326.
   Discusses the partnership developed between academia and service.

Strohschein, J., Hagler, P., & May, L. (2002). Assessing the need for change in clinical education practices. *Physical Therapy, 82*, 160-172.
   Discusses 10 models used in PT clinical education, and the pros and cons of each. (Canada)

Sweet, J., Wilson, J., & Pugsley, L. (2008). Chairside teaching and the perceptions of dental teachers in the UK. *British Dental Journal, 205,* 565-569.
   Discusses a study describing how dental tutors at the chairside viewed their teaching and describes what are considered important current issues, requirements and recommendations for good chairside teaching. (Great Britain)

Sweet, J., Wilson, J., Pugsley, L., & Schofield, M. (2008). Tools to share good chairside teaching practice: A clinical scenario and appreciative questionnaire. *British Dental Journal, 205*, 603-606.
   Discusses a scenario to analyze good chairside teaching practice. (Great Britain)

Tadd, W., Clarke, A., Lloyd, L., Leino-Kilpi, H., Strandell, C., Lemonidou, C., et al. (2006). The value of nurses' codes: European nurses' views. *Nursing Ethics, 13*, 376-393.
   Discusses nursing codes - their content and function in clinical practice.

Tang, F., Chou, S., & Chiang, H. (2005). Students' perceptions of effective and ineffective clinical instructors. *Journal of Nursing Education, 44*, 187-192.
   Discusses students' perceptions of the qualities of clinical nursing faculty.

Tanner, C. A. (2002). Clinical education, circa 2010. *Journal of Nursing Education, 41*, 51-52.
   Discusses how clinical education will potentially look in the future.

Tanner, C. A. (2005). [Editorial]. The art and science of clinical teaching. *Journal of Nursing Education, 44*, 151.
   Suggests clinical focus needs to be on learning outcomes; involve a variety of learning activities; integrate simulation; vary student/faculty ratio depending on clinical situation, student level, and clients; incorporate research, and incorporate literature on types of learning experiences.

Tanner, C. A. (2006). [Editorial]. The next transformation: Clinical education. *Journal of Nursing Education, 45*, 99-100.
> *Suggests clinical nursing education is in need of revision, as education is the same as it has been for many years.*

Tanner, C. A., Gubrud-Howe, P., & Shores, L. (2008). The Oregon consortium for nursing education: A response to the nursing shortage. *Policy, Politics, & Nursing Practice, 9*, 203-209.
> *Discusses the development of the coalition, its infrastructure development, creaton of the shared curriculum, redesign of clinical education, faculty development and plans for evaluation.*

Teeley, K. H., Lowe, J. M., Beal, J., & Knapp, M. L. (2002). Incorporating quality improvement concepts and practice into a community health nursing course. *Journal of Nursing Education, 45*, 86-90.
> *Discusses the use of faculty guides, continuous quality improvement (CQI), student satisfaction.*

Thompson, M. D., & Carson, R. L. (2008). Four steps for discovering the beliefs behind your clinical education practices. *Athletic Therapy Today, 13*(5), 6-9.
> *Discusses how personal beliefs affect actions by clinical educators.*

Tobar, K., Wall, D., & Parsh, B. (2007). Use of 12 hour clinical shifts in nursing education: Faculty, staff and student response. *Nurse Educator, 32*, 190-191.
> *Discusses the pros and cons of 12-hour clinical from the perspective of all players.*

Urquhart, G., & Comeau, A. (2002). Maintaining specialized clinical competencies: Continous learning to renew clinical competencies can be difficult to achieve for nurses in acute care and frustrating for the educator. *Canadian Nurse, 98*(8), 25-28.
> *Discusses an approach to assess ongoing competence in the clinical setting. (Canada)*

Usher, K., Nolan, C., Reser, P., Owens, J., & Tellefson, J. (1999). An exploration of the preceptor role: Preceptors' perceptions of benefits, rewards, supports, and commitment to the preceptor role. *Journal of Advanced Nursing, 29*, 506-514.
> *Discusses a study that explored the relationship between preceptors' perceptions of benefits, rewards and support, and their commitment to their role. (Australia)*

Utley-Smith, Q. (2004). Five competencies needed by new baccalaureate graduates. *Nursing Education Perspectives, 25*, 166-170.
> *Discusses what clinical competencies are needed by new graduates.*

Veloski, J., Boex, J. R., Grasberger, M. J., Evans, A., & Wolfson, D. B. (2006). Systematic review of the literature on assessment, feedback and physicians' clinical performance. *Medical Teacher, 28*, 117-128.
> *Discusses a research study that reviewed the impact of assessment and feedback on the clinical performance of physicians.*

Walsch, C. M., & Seldomridge, L. A. (2005). Clinical grades: Upward bound. *Journal of Nursing Education, 44*, 162-168.
> *Discusses how grade inflation exists in clinical evaluation.*

Weber, S. (2005). Measuring quality in clinical education. *Journal of the American Academy of Nurse Practitioners, 17*, 243-244.
> *Discusses how effective clinical education will prepare competent entry-level practitioners in structured and varied experiences; safe, effective practice; and essential skills and behaviors, all under the supervision of competent clinical educators. Each section has a list of qualities that will be present for "high quality."*

Wellard, S. J., Woolf, R., & Gleeson, L. (2007). Exploring the use of clinical laboratories in undergraduate nursing programs in regional Australia. *International Journal of Nursing Education Scholarship, 4*(1), 1-11, Article 4.
> *Discusses a qualitative study looking at how labs are being used in meeting clinical time. Its results indicated a need for rigorous investigation of pedagogies that can support nursing students' preparation for clinical practice. (Australia)*

Welle-Graf, H. M., & Hansman, C. A. (1999). Assessing the perceived importance of preparing health educators to teach adult learners. *International Electronic Journal of Health Education, 2*(4), 170-177.
> *Discusses a study on the need to incorporate adult learning principles in health education professional preparation programs and to delineate current efforts in health education programs to train future health educators in adult education.*

Wheeler, B. K., Powelson, S., & Kim, J. (2007). Interdisciplinary clinical education: Implementing a gerontological home visiting program. *Nurse Educator, 32*, 136-140.
> *Discusses how a medical school and university sent students from a variety of health-related disciplines on home visits together.*

Wheeler, E. C., & Plowfield, L. (2004). Clinical education initiative in the community: Caring for patients with congestive heart failure. *Nursing Education Perspectives, 25*, 16-21.
> *Discusses how to use a community setting to achieve experience with chronic conditions in nursing education.*

White, L. L. (2006). Preparing for clinical: Just-in-time. *Nurse Educator, 31*(2), 57-60.
> *Discusses the use of the Japanese model of Just-in-Time for students to use to prepare for clinical experiences.*

White, A., Allen, P., Goodwin, L., Breckinridge, D., Dowell, J., & Garvy, R. (2005). Infusing PDA technology into nursing education. *Nurse Educator, 30*, 150-154.
> *Discusses how students can no longer retain in their heads all the information needed to practice clinically and how PDAs are a technological alternative that can assist students.*

Wieland, D. M., Altmiller, G. M., Dorr, M. T., & Wolf, Z. R. (2007). Clinical transition of baccalaureate nursing students during preceptored, pregraduation practicums. *Nursing Education Perspectives, 28*, 315-321.
> *Discusses a study that described the experience of pregraduation students during a clinical transition experience.*

Williams, R., Hall, S., & Papenhausen, J. (2005). The collaborative track option for BSN education: The best of both worlds. *Nurse Educator, 30*, 57-61.
> *Moving from the community college to university environment to obtain a BSN. Discussion of barriers and facilitation for students.*

Wilson, M., Sheperd, I., Kelly, C., & Pitzner, J. (2005). Assessment of a low-fidelity human patient simulator for the acquisition of nursing skills. *Nurse Education Today, 25*(1), 56-67.
> *Discusses how user friendly simulators can be and how they can facilitate clinical success.*

Winslow, S., Dunn, P., & Rowlands, A. (2005). Establishment of a hospital-based simulation skills laboratory. *Journal of Nurses in Staff Development, 21*(2), 62-65.
> *Discusses how the laboratory can be used to facilitate the development of skills necessary in today's health care environment.*

Wong, F. K. Y., Cheung, S., Chung, L., Chan, K., Chan, A., To, T., et al. (2008). Framework for adopting a problem-based learning approach in a simulated clinical setting. *Journal of Nursing Education, 47*, 508-514.

> *Discusses how problem-based learning can be utilized in a simulated clinical setting. Reveals six key manifestations of this learning environment: collection of information, data analysis, formulation of hypotheses, validation, discussion and reflection, and learning synthesis. (Hong Kong)*

Wong, F. K. Y., & Lee, W. M. (2000). A phenomenological study of early nursing experiences in Hong Kong. *Journal of Advanced Nursing, 31*(6), 1509-1517.

> *Discusses the impact that effective clinical education has on the initial experiences and thereby the retention of nurses. (Hong Kong)*

Suggested Reading

Billings, D. M., & Halstead, J. A. (Eds.). (2005). *Teaching in nursing: A guide for faculty* (2*nd* ed.). St. Louis, MO: Elsevier.

Emerson, R. J. (2007). *Nursing education in the clinical setting*. St. Louis, MO: Mosby.

Flynn, J. P., & Stack, M .C. (2006). *The role of the preceptor: A guide for nurse educators, clinicians, and managers* (2nd ed.). New York: Springer Publishing.

National Council of State Boards of Nursing Practice, Regulation and Education Committee. (2005). [Position paper]. Clinical instruction in prelicensure nursing programs. Retrieved from https://www.ncsbn.org/Final_Clinical_Instr_Pre_Nsg_programs.pdf
Nursing education experiences should be across the lifespan; clinical education should be with actual patients, supervised by qualified faculty who provide feedback and facilitate reflection. Faculty are responsible to demonstrate that clinical experiences with actual patients meet program outcomes. Research is needed in prelicensure nursing education and clinical competency development.

O'Connor, A. B. (2006). *Clinical instruction and evaluation: A teaching resource. Sudbury*, MA: Jones and Bartlett.

Rose, M., & Best, D. (Eds.). (2006). *Transforming practice through clinical education, professional supervision, and mentoring*. London: Elsevier.

Sigma Theta Tau International Clinical Scholarship Task Force. (1999). *Clinical Scholarship White Paper.* Indianapolis, IN: Author. Retrieved June 9, 2009 from http://www.nursingsociety.org/aboutus/PositionPapers/Documents/clinical_scholarship_paper.pdf

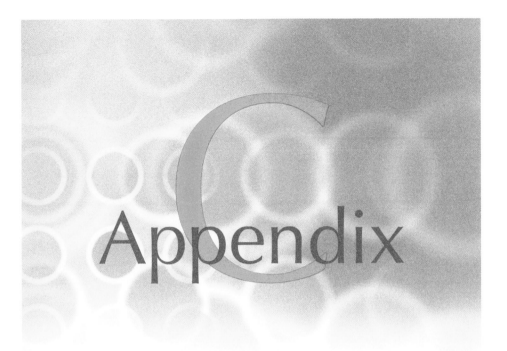

FINAL REPORT OF THE NLN TASK GROUP ON CLINICAL NURSING EDUCATION DECEMBER 2008

IDEAS FOR POSITION STATEMENT OVERVIEW OF THE LITERATURE

Final Report of the NLN Task Group on Clinical Nursing Education

FINAL REPORT — DECEMBER 2008

Introduction

This report is being submitted to the Nursing Education Advisory Council (NEAC) for the purpose of summarizing the activities and accomplishments of the Task Group on Clinical Nursing Education. The group was initially constituted in 2006, with membership consisting of seven (7) individuals representing a broad distribution of education programs/regions and one (1) NEAC liaison member. The group had two members withdraw during its existence (one occurring within the first few months). The Chair of the Task Group (Nell Ard) remained consistent for the duration of the Task Group.

Charge

The charge of the Task Group was: to encourage and promote excellence and innovation in nursing education's approaches to clinical and laboratory teaching and the evaluation of learning in the clinical and laboratory settings. With this overall purpose, the group was charged with completing a number of specific tasks, which served as the framework that guided the activities of the Clinical Nursing Education Task Group over the three-year period of its existence. The specific tasks were as follows:

- Revise, renew and/or write a Position Statement on Clinical Nursing Education that encourages and promotes (a) the development and implementation of innovative teaching/learning models and (b) research about clinical learning.

- Compile a comprehensive synthesis of the literature from nursing and other health profession fields that focuses on clinical/laboratory/simulation teaching and evaluation.

- Disseminate information about factors that promote or inhibit the development and implementation of innovative clinical/laboratory teaching and evaluation strategies.

- Add information about clinical and laboratory teaching and evaluation to the literature database in order to expand the repository of evidence on this topic.

- Develop and monitor an electronic "community" on the topic of clinical/laboratory teaching and evaluation.

Framework for Activities and Accomplishments

The Clinical Nursing Education Task Group (hereafter referred to as TG) began an extensive review of the literature regarding clinical education in nursing and other higher education disciplines with clinical or experiential requirements after their very first conference call. This literature review continued throughout the TG's existence and has resulted in an extensive annotated bibliography on clinical education.

At the first face-to-face meeting in June 2006, after a discussion regarding numerous issues related to clinical education in nursing, the TG thought that it would be helpful to reflect on five significant questions about clinical education: What is it? Why do it? When does it occur? Where is it done? Who is involved? The results of this reflection soon became the driving force behind the TG's future activities and presentations.

The TG believes clinical education:

- is a holistic experience that attends to the intellectual (knowledge, critical thinking, decision-making, priority setting, transfer of knowledge and understanding from one situation to another, etc.), physical (presence), and passion (values, psychosocial elements, professional involvement, etc.) components of learning what it means to be a nurse and developing one's identity as a nurse. It requires the involvement of four (4) "players" if it is to be called "clinical": the student, the teacher, the patient (family unit/community), and the clinical staff (health care team).

- is the most effective way to help prepare students to meet the health care needs of society. Clinical education also assists the student in "pulling it all together" so abstract didactic concepts become real. Students learn to think on the spot, with limited or conflicting information and in ambiguous, uncertain, unpredictable situations. In clinical education, the student has the opportunity to operationalize the three (3) components (i.e., intellectual, physical, and passion) in the context of the four (4) players (i.e., student, teacher, patient/family, and clinical staff).

- can occur in any setting that provides for integration of the intellectual, physical, and passion components of what it means to be a nurse and involves all four players. Where the student actually does their clinical learning should be determined by (1) the learning outcomes/goals that have been developed mutually by students and faculty, and (2) the ability to integrate the three components and four players. Clinical "placements" should not be determined by required rotations through medical specialty areas or by a specified number of hours that have to be "put in."

- should occur throughout the nursing program. The group also believes that some type of immersion experience should occur at some point during the program, preferably toward the end of the program.

- includes four players. The student must be fully engaged in the learning process. He/She should collaborate with the faculty member to identify learning outcomes and seek out and take responsibility for obtaining experiences that will facilitate achievement of those learning outcomes. The role of the teacher is to work with the student to develop learning outcomes, help arrange experiences, and work with the clinical agency to provide a positive environment where learning objectives can be realized. The teacher does not necessarily need to be physically present, but neither should he/she abandon the student. There are two very important roles of the teacher: (1) to help students survey their learning as they engage in reflective exercises, and (2) to facilitate/guide/critique/evaluate the student's performance. The patient/family/ community does not need to be a physiological entity — in other words, it can be a simulator or geographic community or group including standardized patients and patients being seen via telehealth. The final player is the clinical staff/team, who are expected to facilitate student learning in order to help meet the outcomes. They do not need to be physically present at all times, but like faculty should never abandon the student.

- When staff are used a preceptors, they should be carefully selected, properly prepared for the role, and expected to supervise student performance, oversee and help plan the student's day-to-day experiences, and contribute input to the student's evaluation.

Activities And Accomplishments

The TG initially had the opportunity to present at Summit 2006. The session entitled, Providing Optimal Clinical Experiences for Student Nurses: A Dialogue, addressed many of the issues and challenges that either contribute to or detract from a student's clinical experience. In the course of the session, the TG presented suggested principles of quality clinical education:

- Quality clinical education is an activity of shared interest between higher education and health care providers.
- Clinical and theoretical components of nursing should be as closely integrated as possible.
- Clinical placements should have clear learning objectives.
- Planning for clinical education should be a joint endeavor of both faculty and student.
- Student evaluation and feedback on clinical placements should occur routinely.
- Clinical experience should represent the curriculum with a broad span of clinical areas.
- The main emphasis should be on experiential learning, not on observation.
- Placement should be aimed at depth — especially when placements are of short duration.
- Clinical placements should be structured to match the organization of work and promote continuity of care.
- Quality clinical education maximizes the student's time spent in nursing activities — those contributing to clinical skills and understanding.
- Assessment of student performance should be conducted by university faculty in cooperation with staff with whom the student has regular contact. (Parkes, 1995).

The TG encouraged faculty to focus on the positives, focus on learning, and focus on communication to assist in providing optimal learning environments for students in clinical settings.

In March 2007, based upon beliefs regarding clinical education, the TG developed a survey that was disseminated to all NLN members. Using a 4-point Likert scale, the participants responded to 51 statements using Strongly Agree to Strongly Disagree. The survey had 2218 nursing educators respond as well as 28 individuals associated with Boards of Nursing across the United States. Overall, the majority of the participants agreed with the statements. (Ard, Rogers, & Vinten, 2008).

The TG had opportunity to present at the 2007 Education Summit with a session entitled, An Emerging Framework for Clinical Education in the 21st Century. This session provided participants with an overview of the results of the clinical education survey.

In April 2008, the TG chair participated in a Think Tank on Clinical Education. The annotated bibliography developed by the TG was distributed to the group as a component of preparing for the dialogue. The think tank validated many of the ideas and thoughts of the TG. The think tank had a variety of participants representing faculty, nursing education leaders, the NLN Blue Ribbon Panel, nursing accreditation, and nursing regulation. The work of the TG as well as the national think tank validated the need for additional research specific to clinical education and a national research project on the topic was launched by NLN in fall 2008.

The TG continued to review the literature and utilized some of the information gathered in a final educational symposium entitled, 21st Century Models of Clinical Education, at the 2008 Education Summit. This symposium provided the participants with the "current" educational models used in nursing education versus "future" models of clinical education to consider.

Work To Be Completed In The Future/Remaining Work

The TG is writing a review of the literature to be included in a book about clinical education that is scheduled for publication in 2009. This book will also include the complete annotated bibliography developed by the group.

The TG did not initiate an e-community on clinical education. This was primarily due to technical issues with e-communities, rather than the group's unwillingness to set such a thing up. The TG believes an e-community could provide an avenue for opening the dialogue about clinical education, its challenges and successes, for interested educators.

The TG also did not complete a position statement regarding clinical education. The TG believes it is vital that a position statement be developed. This task was not completed for two primary reasons: (1) lack of time to develop a position statement, and (2) the fact that additional data regarding clinical education is being obtained with the fall data collection by the NLN on clinical education. To draft a potential position statement prior to this important collection of information would be premature. Ideas for the position statement can be found in Appendix A to this Report. Appendix B to this Report includes a brief overview of the literature regarding the what, why, where, when, and who of clinical education that could also be included in the preface of a position statement.

Recommendations

The TG has made the following recommendations to the NEAC:

- The focus of Summit 2009, or some future Education Summit, should be on clinical education.

- A position statement on clinical education should be developed with NLNAC and NCSBN co-authoring. This position statement should be developed after the research study in fall 2008 is completed and be combined with the Think Tank on Clinical Education results.

- Another TG on Clinical Education should be formed to focus on a position statement and research.

- Clinical Evaluation could also be a focus of a future Task Group.

- The literature database on clinical education should be continued. Additional emphasis may be spent specifically on an international element.

- Research questions to be addressed: What percentage of clinical can be simulation and still accomplish the "why" of clinical? Do clinicals need to occur on specialty units? When relationships between students and staff change, what impact does this have on student learning? What alternative methods/models of clinical have positive outcomes? What benefits are there to having an immersion experience?

Conclusion

It is our hope that the leadership and the membership of the National League for Nursing continue to champion efforts directed at clinical education. The report of this TG hopefully represents only the beginning, and not the end, of this very important aspect of nursing education.

The membership of this TG is to be commended for its tireless work and accomplishments. The TG has been highly productive and made important and lasting contributions to the scholarship of clinical education. I would like to close by formally naming and thanking each individual who participated in this effort during these past three years.

Sheila Cox Sullivan, PhD, RN, CNE
Nancy Mosbaek, PhD, RN
Kristen J. Rogers, MSN, RN, CNE
Ana Stoehr, MSN, RN
Sharon Vinten, MSN, RNC, WHNP
Cindy Krueger, MSN, RN (NEAC Liason)
Terry Valiga, EdD, RN, FAAN (NLN Staff)

Respectfully submitted,

Nell Ard, PhD, CNS, RNC, CNE
Chair, Task Group on Clinical Nursing Education

References

Ard, N., Rogers, K., & Vinten, S. (2008). [Headlines from the NLN]: Summary of the survey on clinical education in nursing. *Nursing Education Perspectives, 29*, 238-245.

Parkes, R. (1995). Educating for the future. *Australian Nursing Journal, 2*(7), 22-27.

Task Group on Clinical Nursing Education
Ideas for Position Statement

This TG has been charged to do the following: *Revise, renew and/or write a Position Statement on Clinical Nursing Education that encourages and promotes (a) the development and implementation of innovative teaching/learning models and (b) research about clinical learning.* In order to facilitate the preparation of such a position statement, all TG members are asked to share their thinking about what this position statement should address.

What are the most significant issues related to clinical nursing education that should be addressed in a position statement issued by the NLN?

- Clinical is not "X" number of hours. It is the quality of the experience. Is the term "clinical" too broad/general? Clinical encompasses many activities — conferences, simulation, observational experiences, direct care experiences…What percentage of clinical can involve these various experiences?

- Encourage the exploration of other ways to stimulate student thinking, apply concepts/processes, develop ability to analyze situation and take action, evaluate action outcomes with the student to determine potential benefits, explore other options not take (why?), and what the student would do differently the next time

- Must have a very strong statement about simulation and how it should be used in programs.

- Number of clinical faculty and nurse educators will not change quickly enough to decrease the need for educators and clinical faculty at any time in the foreseeable future.

- To increase number of clinical faculty
    - the profession has to be attractive from a financial perspective
    - faculty have to be respected
    - they need to be prepared for educational role and responsibilities by the university
    - they need to be able to maintain clinical expertise
    - clinical and education roles of nursing cannot be mutually exclusive. Need to develop a single role that allows faculty to physically, financially, and emotionally maintain a balance between university, practice environment and life; i.e., faculty cannot meet requirements of two plus settings. How is medicine faculty doing this?

- Clinical nursing education must keep up with pace of health care reforms.

- Nursing has worked in isolation for many years, but with the nature of clinical education, it has to become much more collaborative with other disciplines

- A specific model will not meet the needs of both LPN and varying levels of RN students, nor will one model meet the needs of all types of schools. Variety is positive as long as appropriate student outcomes are achieved, state board scores are within passing range, and new nurses can care for patients well.

- Models need to be developed, piloted and, based on the evidence, shared with not only the nursing community, but with other health care disciplines.

Should this statement address all kinds of programs (practical nurse, prelicensure RN, graduate)? Why or why not?

- Currently, prelicensure programs and graduate programs vary as to what is "clinical." Graduate programs are focused on a specific area — education, curriculum, administration. Prelicensure programs are focused on a variety of areas.

- A position on student-faculty ratio that addresses patient safety should be seriously considered

- The position statement should address all levels of pre-licensure, including LVN/LPN and RN. If NLN supports LPN through PhD programs, then some concepts will be general and apply to all types of nursing programs; others will be for undergraduate and graduate programs. If the current emphasis is on the RN programs, to suddenly begin including LPNs in NLN work may not be kindly accepted, and may require negotiation and discussion with those who currently provide guidance to the LPN group.

- In a position statement, suggest addressing prelicensure RN only. Rationale: The goals of nursing and progression through programs can best be applied if the programs remain of the same type. Graduate nursing education must certainly be addressed after the foundation and clinical evidence has been established.

What would you like to see as the impact of a position statement on clinical education that is issued by the NLN? What difference could it make?

- Stimulates thinking of educators and licensing boards about "what is clinical" for a prelicensure program. The current picture of "what is clinical" has been around for a while. What are the core outcomes of clinical experiences?

- A position supporting the use of an immersion experience at the end of the program.

- Voice heard in health care settings:
  - Congress and legislators listen to a larger, representative body (NLN) as the educational influence of the profession. Nursing education has to provide ideas, leadership, keep itself in the public eye, offer suggestions for change based on evidence available, and begin change.

- Increased funding for nursing education on federal, local and state levels.

- Nursing education and the service setting partner work cooperatively to develop, implement and evaluate a new clinical education model

What kinds of recommendations from the NLN (for faculty, deans/directors, boards of nursing, clinical facilities, the NLN itself, other organizations, etc.) would be beneficial to stimulate action and enhance the clinical learning experience for students?

Clinical is not a set number of hours. It is experiences that offer students the time to apply concepts/processes, opportunities to grow their "thinking," learn through application, enhance their skills (not just psychomotor).

For all groups listed below:

The nursing shortage is a nationwide issue as part of our US health care crisis. Problems cannot be resolved by or dependent upon one group of individuals (nurse educators). Clinical education is only one section of the larger problem.

A system of cooperation and a sense of responsibility among universities, colleges, educational settings and the health care systems need to be developed and implemented. Think of nursing education without the hospital. Take the university setting and the best of the service aspects of nursing education and combine them. We have the history and clinical competence associated with service and the evidence being developed and sought after by education.

- **Recommendations for Faculty**

  Study, trial, implement a system of shared employment between practice and the university. (done now but only to a small degree)

  There can be different levels of educators as we have different types of nurses. Maintain the MSN with an education core of courses as a basis for an educator in a university setting.

  Other models may include: 1) MSN and education credentials as lead faculty with faculty who are working on both of these as responsible for clinical education and working under lead faculty. 2) LPNs, if they are a separate group from the NLN, can have other educators with BSN plus education credits as faculty.

- **For Deans/Directors/Chairpersons**

  Support faculty in a role that incorporates service and education. Faculty have a right to a family and their own life and the demands of both the service and university setting are tremendous. Meld those roles, pay them well for their skills without burning faculty out.

  Support faculty and graduate students in furthering their education but, as above, faculty have a right to a family and a life.

  Support collaboration between colleges and universities in a geographic area. Create new faculty development models that facilitate clinical and educational expertise. Support, foster, build clinical relationships so that all parties involved in clinical education feel as they are working toward a common goal.

- **Clinical Facilities**
  - Education cannot be accomplished without you!
  - In our society, health care reform will only work when the society is desperate. We aren't there yet, but….Financial rewards seem to hold the highest value in our society.
    - Federal and state dollars added to hospital revenue for utilizing a cooperative model with the collegiate system.
    - Financial rewards for working with the education of students, and graduating a certain number of nurses each year. (Not the system we use today, but one of shared responsibility.)

Overview of the Literature on Clinical Education

"What" Clinical Nursing Education

What does the nursing literature say about clinical education and what is needed both now and in the future? As a basis, Jacobson and Speziale (2005) discussed trends projected for nursing education, with informatics and diversity seen to have greater emphasis, along with active learning promoting critical thinking, and self-directed, interdisciplinary teaching and learning. These trends support core competencies of the Institute of Medicine, especially as delineated in Health Professions Education: A Bridge to Quality (Greiner & Knebel, 2003).

The intellectual components of nursing encompass knowledge acquisition, critical thinking, decision making, priority setting, and transfer of knowledge, in addition to many other concepts. New ways of doing things, advancing clinical judgment, decision making, management of care, and application of technology in the clinical setting are all integral to the advancement of health care as we move into the 21st century (Sigma Theta Tau, 1999). Nursing is paying more attention to developing strategies incorporating thinking into clinical (Conger & Mezza, 1996; O'Connor, 2001; Rowles & Brigham, 2005; Schuster, 2000) as well as didactic settings (Ironside, 2004; Ironside, 2005).

The physical components of nursing are observable by clients, nurses, families and members of the community as all interact on multiple levels with nursing. Physical components of nursing are also impacted by the physical environment where patient care and learning takes place. The importance/emphasis of this active involvement is underscored by state boards of nursing requiring a particular number of hours to be spent in the learning lab or on the clinical unit to meet course completion requirements.

The passion of nursing is often equated with values, psychosocial aspects of caring for self or clients, and involvement with the professional. Subjective values are difficult to define and measure (Beck, 2001). Caring has been the most widely studied value as faculty work to define, teach and evaluate student caring (Beck, 1999; Lee-Hsieh, Kuo, & Tseng, 2005). Green-Hernandez (1991) divided caring into "nature caring and professional caring" and describes the first as presence, social support, giving, physical touch, and reciprocity while professional caring is communication, personal involvement, listening, and professional experience. Given these two different views, caring encompasses not only the care given to clients, but the caring utilized in maintaining and advancing one's career. Professional development, in continuing education units, to maintain and enhance clinical expertise is inherent in the role of the nurse and is monitored by state boards of nursing as a requirement in many states for licensure renewal.

The role of clinical educator is multifaceted and complex. Educators now have more information available concerning learning styles and needs of students (Skiba, 2007) as lecturing is becoming a least preferred method of transfer of knowledge. Since the 1970s, the education profession has been incorporating active learning into the educational environment and nursing is following suit. Web-based nursing courses (Buckley, Beyna, & Dudley-Brown, 2005; Dodge, 2008) as well as didactic and clinical student experiences are now incorporating active learning in multiple ways. (Brancato, 2006; Fay, Johnson, & Selz, 2006; Herrman, 2006).

Service and education are beginning to seriously collaborate to further the care and safety of patients and to improve the learning of students (Berry, 2005). Many ideas have been developed, trialed, and published, but no broad definitive changes have occurred. The subject is continually being discussed from both the education and service setting perspective (Kline & Hodges, 2006; Palmer, Cox, Callister, Johnsen, & Matsumura, 2006; Preheim, Casey, & Krugman, 2006).

"Why" Clinical Nursing Education

Clinical nursing education is the environment for transformation from novice learner to novice nurse. Within the environment, the novice learner is immersed in experiences that foster self-discovery. During this journey of self-discovery, the learner encounters anticipated and unanticipated phenomena. These phenomena challenge the learner to integrate assessment skills, communication skills, technical skills, and critical thinking skills to determine a plan of care within a specific context. The learner is guided on this journey by an educator. The educator utilizes various pedagogies (the art and science of teaching) to create opportunities that facilitate the transformation to novice nurse.

"Where" Clinical Nursing Education

Attempts to form collaborative relationships between education and practice continue (Brown, White, & Leibbrandt, 2006). Challenges exist and will need to be addressed. Many variables exist in these interactions, indicating that there is not a "one size fits all" solution. Joint appointments, a culture of valuing and fostering, student participation in unit activities and a staff position as education liaison are but a few suggestions to facilitate a climate of learning (Matsumura, Callister, Palmer, Cox, & Larsen, 2004).

Where do these students obtain their clinical experiences? This calls forth creativity and reviewing course outcomes, and faculty have done that to develop nontraditional clinical experiences (Andrus & Bennett, 2006). Kirkham, Harwood and Hofwegen (2005) discuss non-hospital-based settings as shifting students' perceptions about themselves, self-initiated learning, and integrating students and nursing into the community. Articles discuss teaming the service setting with academia (Bartz & Dean-Baar, 2003). Yet others explore developing clinical settings where education is a major focus (Moscato, Miller, Logsdon, & Weinberg, 2007; Schmidt, 2007).

"When" Clinical Nursing Education

When clinical occurs during a nursing curriculum has always been a point of consideration. Should clinical specialty areas be in conjunction with didactic content? Should students have split clinical days or back-to-back clinical days? When should certain types of clinicals be scheduled within a curriculum? Should there be clinical experiences across the curriculum? Should students have an immersion experience at some point during the curriculum? If so, where should this immersion occur? What are the merits of day-shift clinicals versus evening shift versus weekend?

The literature has a limited number of articles dealing specifically with the "When" of clinical education. Cox (2002) discusses how two weeks of class and then two weeks of clinical works throughout a nursing curriculum. The overall pilot was very positive. Another article discusses how three days per week in the final year (clinical immersion) benefited the students in the program (Diefenbeck, Plowfield, & Herrman, 2006). The article also discusses "alternative" clinical experiences utilized throughout the program.

Additional research needs to be conducted on "when" clinical education should/could occur and have the best impact on the learners' outcomes and overall retention both in a nursing program and in the nursing profession. Since clinicals are where the student is "able to put all the pieces together" and is the ultimate nursing role, it is imperative that nurse educators address the "when" of clinical education.

"Who" of Clinical Education

Who is responsible for the education of the nursing students? The obvious answer is that of the student and the nursing faculty. This is true; however, the responsibility also lies with many others.

There is no research on who is responsible for education of the nursing student. If the topic is reviewed, it will become clear that there are many individuals that impact student learning.

As previously stated, the faculty plays a big role in the clinical educational process, because without the faculty there would no knowledge shared with the students.

The students are also responsible for their clinical learning experiences. They need to do further reading on their patients. At the same time, they need to seek out learning opportunities within the clinical setting. They need to challenge themselves each and every clinical day

The clinical staff is also responsible for educating our students. It is their experiences that will give students information about what to do if they encounter a similar situation. It is the staff that will be able to guide the student to a learning opportunity within that clinical site.

The physicians have a responsibility to teach the nursing students about their patients. At the same time, they need to ask questions of the nursing student that require the student to critically think through the situation. Also, if the physician knows that there is an opportunity for the student to observe or participate in a procedure, then the physician must seek out the student.

In addition, clinical education includes any member of the health care team. This may be social work, physical/occupational therapy, case management, dietary, environmental engineering and members of the administrative team (CEO, CNE, COO, etc.).

The patient has a role in the clinical education of the nursing student, although it is not as direct as other members of the health care team. The patients provide, each and every time a nursing student cares for them, an opportunity to learn something new or to expand what they already know.

References

Andrus, N. C., & Bennett, N. M. (2006). Developing an interdisciplinary, community-based education program for health professions students: The Rochester experience. *Academic Medicine, 81*, 326-331.

Bartz, C., & Dean-Baar, S. (2003). Reshaping clinical nursing education: An academic-service partnership. *Journal of Professional Nursing, 19*, 216-222.

Beck, C.T. (1999). Quantitative measurement of caring. *Journal of Advanced Nursing, 30*(1), 24-32.

Beck, C.T. (2001). Caring within nursing education: A metasynthesis. *Journal of Nursing Education, 40*, 101-109.

Berry, J. (2005). A student and RN partnered clinical experience. *Nurse Educator,30*, 240-241.

Brancato, V.C. (2006). Innovative clinical practicum to teach evidence-based practice. *Nurse Educator, 31*, 195-199.

Brown, D., White, J., & Leibbrandt, L. (2006). Collaborative partnerships for nursing faculties and health service providers: What can nursing learn from business literature? *Journal of Nursing Management, 14*, 170-179.

Buckley, K. M., Beyna, B., & Dudley-Brown, S. (2005). Promoting active learning through on-line discussion boards. *Nurse Educator, 30*, 32-36.

Conger, M. M., & Mezza, I., (1996). Fostering critical thinking in nursing students in the clinical setting. *Nurse Educator, 21*, 11-15.

Cox, L. S. (2002). Focused learning: 2 weeks of class — 2 weeks of clinical. *Nurse Educator, 27*, 15.

Diefenbeck, C. A., Plowfield, L. A., & Herrman, J. W. (2006). Clinical immersion: A residency model for nursing education. *Nursing Education Perspectives, 27*, 72-79.

Dodge, B. (2008). Active learning on the Web. Retrieved January 30, 2008, from http://edweb. sdsu.edu/people/bdodge/Active/ActiveLearning.html

Fay, V. P., Johnson, J., & Selz, N. (2006). Active learning in nursing education. *Nurse Educator, 31*, 65-68.

Green-Hernandez, C. (1991). Professional nurse caring: A conceptual model for nursing. In R.M. Neil & R. Watts (Eds.), *Caring and nursing: Explorations in feminist perspectives* (pp. 85-96). New York: NLN Center of Human Caring.

Greiner, A., & Knebel, E. (Eds.). (2003) *Health professions education: A bridge to quality.* Washington, DC: Institute of Medicine, National Academies Press.

Herrman, J. W. (2006). Using film clips to enhance nursing education. *Nurse Educator, 31*, 264-269.

Ironside, P. (2004). Covering content and teaching thinking: Deconstructing the additive curriculum. *Journal of Nursing Education, 43*, 5-12.

Ironside, P. (2005). Teaching thinking and reaching the limits of memorization: Enacting new pedagogies. Journal of *Nursing Education, 44*, 441-449.

Kirkham, S. R., Harwood, C. H., & Hofwegen, L.V. (2005). Capturing a vision for nursing: Undergraduate nursing students in alternative clinical settings. *Nurse Educator, 30*, 263-270.

Kline, K. S., & Hodges, J. (2006). A rational approach to solving the problem of competition for undergraduate clinical sites. *Nursing Education Perspectives, 27*, 80-83.

Lee-Hsieh, J., Kuo, C., & Tseng, H. (2005). Application and evaluation of a caring code in clinical nursing education. *Journal of Nursing Education, 44*, 177-184.

Matsumura, G., Callister, L.C., Palmer, S., Cox, A. H., & Larsen, L. (2004). Staff nurse perceptions of the contributions of students to clinical agencies. *Nursing Education Perspectives, 25*, 297-303.

Moscato, S. R., Miller, J., Logsdon, K., & Weinberg, S. (2007). Dedicated education unit: An innovative clinical partner education model. *Nursing Outlook, 55*, 31-37.

O'Connor, A. B. (2001). *Clinical instruction and evaluation: A teaching resource.* New York: National League for Nursing.

Palmer, S., Cox, A. H., Callister, L. C, Johnsen, V., & Matsumura, G. (2005). Nursing education and service collaboration: Making a difference in the clinical learning environment. *Journal of Continuing Education in Nursing, 36*, 271-276.

Preheim, G., Casey, K., & Krugman, M. (2006). Clinical scholar model: Providing excellence in clinical supervision of nursing students. *Journal for Nurses in Staff Development, 22*(1), 15-20.

Rowles, C. J., & Brigham, C. (2005). Strategies to promote critical thinking and active learning. In D. M. Billings & J. A. Halstead (Eds.), *Teaching in nursing: A guide for faculty* (2nd ed.) (pp. 283-315). St. Louis, MO: Elsevier.

Schmidt, L. (2007). Camp nursing: Innovative opportunities for nursing students to work with children. *Nurse Educator, 32*, 246-250.

Schuster, P. M. (2000). Reducing clinical care plan paperwork and increasing learning. *Nurse Educator, 25*, 76-81.

Sigma Theta Tau International Clinical Scholarship Task Force. (1999). *Clinical Scholarship White Paper.* Indianapolis, IN: Author. Retrieved June 9, 2009 from http://www.nursingsociety.org/aboutus/PositionPapers/Documents/clinical_scholarship_paper.pdf

Skiba, D. J. (2007). *The Net Generation: Implications for Nursing Education and Practice.* National League for Nursing Living Book. Retrieved February 4, 2008, from http://www.electronicvision.com/nln/chapter01/index.htm

Speziale, H. J. S., & Jacobson, L. (2005) Trends in registered nurse education programs 1998-2008. *Nursing Education Perspectives, 26*, 230-235.

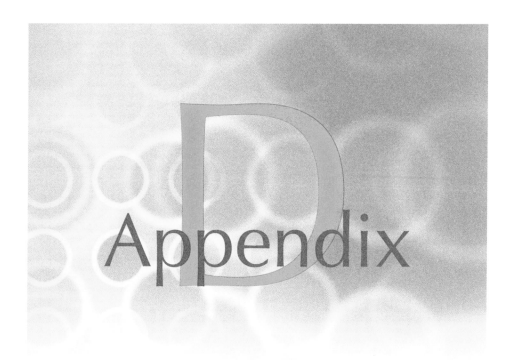

ABBREVIATED FINAL REPORT OF THE NLN THINK TANK ON TRANSFORMING CLINICAL NURSING EDUCATION

APRIL 14 – 15, 2008
INDIANAPOLIS, INDIANA

Abbreviated Final Report of the NLN Think Tank on Clinical Nursing Education

April 14 – 15, 2008
Indianapolis, Indiana

The idea of sponsoring the Think Tank on Transforming Clinical Nursing Education arose from the NLN's Blue Ribbon Panel discussion of the priorities for research in nursing education. Extended dialogue about the most pressing issues in nursing education brought the Blue Ribbon Panel back, again and again, to the topic of clinical education; the recommendation of these leaders and scholars in nursing education was that the NLN sponsor a national, interdisciplinary think tank on the topic.

The invitational think tank met on April 14 – 15, 2008 to lay a foundation that would help the National League for Nursing and its members answer the following questions:

- What does it mean to teach a practice?
- What are the most effective ways to help students learn the practice of nursing?
- What are the most effective ways to assess the clinical performance of nursing students in prelicensure RN programs?
- What meaning do these questions have for teaching diverse student populations to care for diverse patient populations?

Twenty-one individuals were invited to participate in this important dialogue; these individuals included the NLN's Blue Ribbon Panel, the chair of the NLN's Nursing Education Research Advisory Council, the chair of the NLN's Task Group on Clinical Nursing Education, faculty teaching in various types of nursing education programs, leaders from the practice setting, representatives from nursing regulatory and accrediting bodies, educational scholars from outside nursing, and a colleague from medicine.

In addition, several individuals were invited to observe the dialogue and contribute ideas at designated times during the session. The "observers" included the 11 individuals participating in the NLN/Johnson & Johnson Mentor/Protégé program, the executive director of the NLN Foundation, a Laerdal partner, and a nurse working with the Robert Wood Johnson Foundation.

The think tank was co-facilitated by Dr. Pamela Ironside and Dr. Christine Tanner, both of whom serve on the Blue Ribbon Panel. The NLN president and CEO were actively engaged in the discussion. Finally, the work of the think tank was supported by the NLN's chief program officer and a student enrolled in the nursing PhD program at Villanova University, who was completing course requirements through an internship at the National League for Nursing. The complete list of participants, including a brief biography for each, is included as Appendix A.

In planning the think tank, the Blue Ribbon Panel and NLN staff outlined several expected outcomes:

- Achieve consensus on the need to transform clinical nursing education, particularly in prelicensure RN programs.
- Achieve consensus on the structures that support or interfere with such transformation.
- Explore approaches that have the potential to effectively facilitate the integration of clinical teaching and classroom teaching.

- Consider promising integrative clinical education models, pedagogies, and methods for clinical performance assessment.
- Identify research priorities for clinical education and assessment of clinical performance in prelicensure RN programs.
- Make explicit the professional's scholarly thinking about clinical education.

The meeting commenced with welcomes given by Dr. Ironside and Dr. Tanner. NLN president Dr. Elaine Tagliareni also welcomed the group and provided a context for their work by reviewing the NLN's strategic plan and core values. She noted that clinical nursing education is the most critical component of transforming nursing education and the NLN's support of this kind of dialogue makes explicit the organization's goal of "doing the right thing" for the nursing education community.

Later in the meeting, NLN CEO Dr. Beverly Malone also addressed the importance of this group's work in helping the NLN fulfill its mission of excellence in nursing education. She noted that educators need to keep in mind that their connection to patients and collaboration with practice is essential, and she reminded participants that our students and clinicians "live in both worlds" (education and practice). Finally, Dr. Malone clarified that this think tank is a step in the journey toward excellence, and the NLN is committed to leading that journey.

All participants, observers, and staff were introduced and each shared thoughts about the significance of the discussions about to be undertaken. In addition, the role of the observers in the group was clarified: listening critically, helping the group fill in "gaps" as ideas are discussed, and helping the group clarify the assumptions they may be making.

The first topic of discussion was the most important or "pressing" issues related to clinical nursing education. The following were identified:

Faculty Issues

- Finding qualified faculty who understand the "big picture" of the school's curriculum
- Orienting/Preparing/Mentoring clinical (and other new) faculty
- Finding ways to help faculty stay "connected" to clinical practice and remain current
- Preparing faculty as teachers/educators

Student/Learning Issues

- Managing the differences in learning styles between faculty and learners
- Rethinking what students actually do during their clinical experiences and how the time spent in clinical settings can be most effective in helping them learn the practice
- Providing opportunities through which students can examine skills related to multi-tasking (including its value and its danger) and the ability to manage systems
- Lack of student (and teacher) recognition of the need to be a lifelong learner
- Preparing students for developing and sustaining relationships with patients, team members, and others
- Helping students learn how to continually pursue development of "self"
- Creating environments where "thinking outside the box" is encouraged and expected

- Meeting the challenges of preparing students for the role of clinician
- Integrating learning across the classroom, clinical setting, and laboratory

Clinical Setting Issues

- Finding appropriate clinical venues for quality student learning experiences
- Finding ways to effectively support clinical staff who are overburdened with patient care responsibilities and then are asked to participate in educational responsibilities as well
- Clarifying strategies to access and use resources in the clinical area (e.g., technology, other team members, etc.)

General Issues

- Resolving the seeming disconnect between assertions that schools are preparing generalists, yet clinical experiences often are in specialized areas
- Thinking of new ways to conceptualize the clinical component of nursing education and create an evidence base for current and new educational practices, particularly in light of the lack of significant funding for research on education
- Creating opportunities for effective, positive interprofessional teamwork, particularly those that focus on communication and systemwide concerns
- Developing more visionary and organized approaches to nursing education, particularly in light of the clinical staff and faculty shortages
- Reducing the emphasis on task completion and increasing the focus on critical thinking, clinical judgment, "thinking on one's feet," contributing to the continuity of care, and the development of thoughtful nurses who can practice independently and interdependently and who "think like a nurse"
- Strengthening the value placed on clinical learning and not allowing it to be lost in the name of innovation or a desire to do something unique and different

As part of providing a context for the group's discussion, Dr. Ironside reviewed the model developed by the Blue Ribbon Panel (see Figure 15-1). This model is intended to convey the idea that when one looks at and thinks about clinical education, one should not do it in just in terms of looking at and thinking about what happens in the classroom (i.e., patient-centered teaching) and in the overall context (i.e., system re-design). In some instances, new clinical education models may receive more attention, but the other component must always be in the background. Likewise, emphasis at other times may be on system re-design, but that must be addressed with new clinical education models and patient-centered teaching in the background.

With this background and context, think tank participants broke into small groups to discuss: *what does it mean to teach a practice?* The following ideas were offered:

- Teaching in a context
- Thinking through a situation
- Teaching pattern recognition
- Exploring ways to seek out answers
- Accessing and using resources effectively

- Fostering inquiry and lifelong learning
- Bringing clinical and classroom together…blurring the distinctions between the two and "keeping the patient with us at all times"
- Providing transformative experiences
- Being focused on learning, not hours or task completion
- Teaching mindfulness…the practical mind, the idea mind, and the synthesis mind
- Helping students develop habits of mind for practice; helping them develop wisdom and discernment
- Possessing and drawing upon a body of knowledge and evidence related to practices
- Enacting skills that are tied to knowledge
- Integrating elements of complex and ever-changing situations
- Being and doing informed by research
- Role modeling with students and among colleagues
- Implementing reflective practice
- Engaging in interdisciplinary experiences
- Synthesizing theoretical and experiential learning
- Evaluating outcomes
- Clearly defining endpoints
- Listening and responding to what might show up in practice
- Helping students learn what to pay attention to so they develop a sense of salience

The small groups also discussed the *opportunities and challenges inherent in teaching a practice* and identified the following:

Opportunities

- Have thoughtful conversations about effective use of "clinical time"

  Challenge the assumptions on which our clinical models are built…hours, objective evaluations, predictability, rigidity, etc.
- Develop new and relevant pedagogies
- Learn from other disciplines
- Grade students on the quality of their questions rather than on the accuracy of their answers
- Serve as role models for what we want students to do (e.g., reflective thinking)
- Focus on skills and high-level thinking (e.g., through use of simulation)
- Make visible to students how faculty "puzzle through" problems
- Focus assessment on things other than skill performance

Challenges

- Lack of incentives for clinical teaching

- Being comfortable with subjective evaluations
- Meeting external mandates (e.g., regulators, legislators, accrediting bodies)
- Lack of clarity regarding the real objectives of clinical learning
- Lack of skill in teaching thinking
- The overwhelming number of nurses who need to be educated to meet patient/ family/ community needs
- Role models of teacher/scholars for faculty
- Keeping current with clinical advances when in the faculty role
- Helping students integrate the three apprenticeships

Other Thoughts

- There are skills that cannot be learned any other way than clinical and those skills need to be identified
- The NLN's Task Group on Clinical Education identified that passion and ethical components of nursing are lacking in our current approaches
- Psychomotor skills can be taught outside clinical, but relational aspects cannot be taught without a clinical setting; learning psychomotor skills in a laboratory allows the student to focus on relational aspects of clinical
- There is a need to focus on the hidden curriculum, as well as the intended one
- We need to capitalize on the uniqueness of caring offered by nurses

Think tank participants were then asked to reflect on *what we want students to learn, particularly as a result of clinical experiences.* The following learning goals were identified:

- Knowing what to pay attention to
- Integrating all three apprenticeships (i.e., intellectual, practical, and ethical)
- Thinking critically
- Reasoning soundly
- Being self-aware
  Knowing one's legal and ethical responsibilities
- Working effectively on teams
- Being with patients and families through building relationships
- Understanding the meaning of integrity and accountability in a patient care context
- Knowing how to recognize significant changes and how to respond appropriately
- Surviving and coping with the reality of today's clinical context (i.e., rapid changes, numerous interruptions, etc.)
- Appreciating/understanding systemwide concerns
- Being aware of the outcomes of one's decisions and actions

- Knowing how to talk with colleagues about practice concerns
- Assessing individuals and situations
- Reading the ecology of the practice environment
- Helping people manage chronic illness

These learning goals led the group to address the question: *how do we teach students to cope with the realities of today's clinical environment?* (e.g., dealing with distractions, delegating, and managing one's time). Among the ideas offered were the following:

- There must be conscious attention given to the development of self-awareness and coping skills. We cannot assume individuals will develop such skills simply by being in a clinical setting.
- We must find a way to balance caring for individual patients and attending to the larger context of the clinical environment; we must help students look at the entire system, not only their individual patient(s).
- Students need opportunities to see the results/outcomes of their decisions and actions.
- Practice partnerships need to be advanced.
- Communication and transactional failures must be addressed and resolved.
- Understanding the ecology of an environment is needed, with the allocation of safe and reflective space.

In recognition of the fact that today's clinical environment is complex and presents challenges to both teachers and learners, think tank members brainstormed about what an *ideal clinical education model* would look like. Among the attributes defining the "ideal" were the following:

Integrative Experience

- Clinical education is not fragmented but, instead, integrates all three apprenticeships and focuses on the complexity of the nursing role.
- Students are immersed in the nursing role in a given setting (e.g., a particular acute care unit, a specific community), rather than being exposed to the role only in three- or four-hour blocks of time on one or two days of the week.
- Clinical experiences are flexibly designed as the rigidity of "X" before "Y" is challenged.
- Learning experiences are designed to help students understand and gain an appreciation for the continuum of care and changes in patient status.
- Cross-disciplinary learning experiences are integral.

New Relationships

- Faculty members work closely with clinical nurse managers to focus on patient outcomes rather than on completion of tasks.
- Learning communities are created through immersion experiences and partnerships.
- Paid internships or other mechanisms are in place to help students transition to the RN role.
- The experience is designed to respond to the learner's needs, interests, and concerns.

- Feedback from students is valued and used to drive future planning.

Learning Experiences

- Students do not need to have "total patient care" assignments all the time.
- The teacher-to-student ratio varies depending on the nature of the setting, the learning outcomes to be achieved, etc.
- The experience is an inductive one where students participate in clinical activities, then focus on what they needed to know to care for patients, where to find that information, how to use resources appropriately, and so on.
- Measurement of student success and learning incorporates a 360-degree perspective, including the extent to which patients are satisfied with their care, the extent to which student contributions helped the unit/agency address specific issues of concern to them (e.g., patient falls), the ways in which students and staff collaborated, etc.
- Learners, teachers, and staff address core concepts that are transferable from one setting to another.
- The time spent in the clinical area is determined by the learning goals and the achievement of those goals, rather than the number of hours students put in.
- Not all students necessarily have to have clinical experiences in all areas (i.e., the concept of "completing rotations" does not drive student experiences and placements). Experiences are planned around common health problems and populations rather than around clinical rotations.

Environmental Considerations

- Space and time for discourse and reflection are incorporated.
- Faculty create "safe" space for students to question, make mistakes, propose ideas, etc.

In addition to these ideas, participants expressed support for post-graduation internships/residencies that facilitate integration of all that has been learned. They also noted that faculty need to package these and other concepts in various ways, so as not to expect or try to find a single model that would serve as "the new truth." Thus, various models need to be developed and tested through demonstration projects; then the findings of those tests need to be disseminated so that guiding principles can be articulated, and the notion of what clinical education needs to be is held open for continued discussion and exploration. Finally, we would need to study how nursing practice changes when students are educated through different clinical education models. Such a process would keep the issue of quality and patient safety in the forefront and encourage engagement and integration of education and practice. It was suggested that perhaps the NLN could issue a position statement on this topic.

Some of the new models we are currently seeing include the following:

- Front loading the theory component of a course and concentrating clinical experiences toward the end
- Front loading skills learning and then moving on to learning content while in clinical practice settings as students are confronted with real patient care situations
- Implementing a post-graduation residency
- Investing more extensively in educating preceptors for their role

- Faculty coaching clinical staff to be good clinical teachers

- Growth in the number of DEUs (Dedicated Education Units) in clinical facilities

- Using preceptors throughout the program (not only in the final semester) in ways that are appropriate to the students' learning objectives

We need to be asking what students are really doing while they are in the clinical setting and how they are spending their time. Is their time always focused on learning? How much time do they spend finding information, waiting for the instructor, or other activities that take them away from patients? Do we keep students too safe? Are activities always focused on patient-centered care? What can be done to uncover the hidden curriculum, to appreciate the unintended outcomes of our programs, and to understand what students really learn as a result of their experiences?

In essence, we need to focus on what students need to learn instead of how we deliver education, the number of hours required, the "rotations" students complete, etc.

In light of the QSEN (Quality and Safety Education for Nurses) project and overarching concerns about patient safety, the question was raised: *How do we know if our student can provide safe, effective care?* Responses to this question included the following:

- Patients would express satisfaction with the care they received and the relationships that were built.

- The kinds of questions students ask would be of a higher order.

- Nurse-sensitive indicators would be positive.

- Student and staff narratives would be insightful and reflect deep learning in all three apprenticeships.

- Peers would critically evaluate one another without those evaluations necessarily becoming part of one's formal evaluation.

Think tank participants then worked in small groups to discuss *what stands out as having huge potential for transforming clinical nursing education?* and how could we craft a study to look at its effectiveness? The following elements were identified:

- Advancement of relationship-centered and patient-centered approaches: Students would look at the system as a collective, focus on nurse and patient indicators, write thoughtful narratives about their experiences, and examine their relationships with patients/families, team members, and the overall system. They would come to understand the role of the nurse in all types of relationships.

- Integrating immersion experiences throughout the program, not only at the end: Faculty would rethink the concepts that are introduced (e.g., leadership, systems thinking, quality indicators) and when they are addressed, since some concepts are quite complex and need time to mature in the students' minds. Clinical time would be used differently, and all time would be spent in productive activities. Education/practice partnerships would be strengthened. The concept of rotations would no longer exist. The ways in which part-time/adjunct/clinical faculty are oriented, mentored, used, and guided by role models would be reexamined. Students would be engaged in projects that focus on different patient populations, are completed in different settings, and are implemented in different time frames, rather than all students doing the same thing at the same time.

- Faculty and clinical staff would share accountability for the preparation of students: The practices of "ask me, don't ask the staff" or "ask your instructor, not me" would disappear; the IOM (2003) recommendations would be implemented; a wider array of evaluations would be used; and feedback would be used to guide clinical practices in the setting and to guide students' continued learning.

- Education would be connected to quality indicators from the beginning: A spirit of inquiry would pervade the academic and clinical environments; varied and appropriate teaching strategies would be used; students would engage in higher order thinking; interdisciplinary learning and practice would be evident; and everyone would be engaged in helping students be successful.

With any of these models, we need to ask if the clinical practice of the graduates is different from graduates of programs using more traditional clinical models. We also would be challenged to reflect on what can be learned in a simulated setting and what can be learned only in a clinical setting.

In order to engage in such creative thinking, faculty would need safe spaces where they can seriously explore new ideas, make mistakes, and make their thinking explicit to students, so learners can see how professionals manage ambiguity and uncertainty, make decisions, evaluate available information, and deal with change. If faculty do not make their thinking explicit, how can we expect students to learn such skills?

Finally, the Think Tank on Clinical Nursing Education participants were asked to make recommendations for NLN activities to facilitate the transformation of clinical nursing education. The following suggestions were offered and will be further discussed by the NLN Board of Governors and staff:

- Publish information pieces for faculty about new developments in clinical practice and clinical education (e.g., the work of QSEN, the evolution of DEUs).

- Facilitate links among NLN constituent leagues, local AONE chapters, and nursing workforce centers to engage in dialogue about ideas offered here.

- Conduct a national study on how educational practices (e.g., new clinical education models) affect patient care quality and the practice of nursing.

- Conduct research and provide grants to NLN members to support the study of new models of clinical education.

- Convene a national conference that brings together faculty, clinical partners, regulators, accreditors, students, and maybe even patients to discuss new models for clinical education in nursing.

- Convene a national conference where faculty, local AONE representatives, and workforce center teams would come together to create new models for clinical education.

- Offer a web-based program on new models.

- Publish a Reflection & Dialogue piece on the need for new clinical education models.

- Be purposeful about collecting national data needed to facilitate progress in this area.

- Develop a clear dissemination plan.

- Create global links that may help crystallize thinking about new clinical education models.

- Develop an online repository of innovations being implemented regarding clinical education.

- Schedule sessions at the NLN Education Summit to discuss this topic.
- Submit a manuscript to the Journal of Nursing Administration and the Journal of Staff Development about the need for transformation of clinical nursing education and the significance of education/practice partnerships in such new models.

In closing, Dr. Tagliareni noted that NLN members provide direction for the work of the organization and that there is a renewed energy within the organization to continue to provide leadership in the transformation of nursing education. She also urged the group to keep the diversity issue in mind as it pursues this clinical education initiative.

Dr. Malone then assured the group that the NLN can provide a framework to facilitate work at the local level through our constituent leagues, schools of nursing, NLN members, individual faculty, and so on. She also noted that the shortage of nurses in practice and the shortage of nurse faculty provide a wonderful opportunity to journey together in transforming clinical nursing education.

IOM (Institute of Medicine). (2003). *Health professions education: A bridge to quality.* Washington, DC: National Academies Press.

This report was prepared by Dr. Terry Valiga, NLN chief program officer (through June 2008) and Ms. Tammie Kear, Villanova University College of Nursing PhD student completing a spring 2008 internship at the NLN.

Used with the permission of the National League for Nursing.